J. Gershon-Cohen

Atlas of Mammography

With 300 Figures

Springer-Verlag
Berlin · Heidelberg · New York 1970

Jacob Gershon-Cohen, M.D., D.Sc. (Med.), Professor of Radiologic Research, Temple University School of Medicine; Director Emeritus, Division of Radiology, Albert Einstein Medical Center, Philadelphia, PA/USA

ISBN-13:978-3-642-85680-8 e-ISBN-13: 978-3-642-85678-5
DOI: 10.1007/978-3-642-85678-5

Universitätsdruckerei H. Stürtz AG, Würzburg. Title No. 1661

To my esteemed colleague, Helen Ingleby, M.D., M.R.C.P.; to J.W. Birsner, M.D., President, and Mr. E.C. Reid, Founder, The Lucile Reid Cancer Institute, for preservation of thousands of original mammographic records and for dedicating the initial efforts of this facility to mammography and thermography; and to the loyal medical and surgical staffs of the Albert Einstein Medical Center, without whose devoted collaboration this Atlas would not have been made possible.

J. Gershon-Cohen

Contents

Acknowledgments

It affords me much pleasure to acknowledge with sincerity the able and enthusiastic work and support of my associates and technical assistants.

Dr. Helen Ingleby gave up some ten years of her retired life to devote herself full-time to studies of the pathologic-roentgenographic relationships of breast diseases. She was the senior author of our text, *Comparative Anatomy, Pathology and Roentgenology of the Breast*, published by The University of Pennsylvania Press in 1960. This work summarized our collaborative efforts from which we both derived much new insight into the subject of mammography.

To my colleagues, Drs. Mortimer B. Hermel, Simon M. Berger, Myron Forman, A. G. B. Borden, Ernest J. Pick, Victor Kremens, Herbert S. Klickstein, Robert M. Byrne and Louis S. Bringhurst, I am deeply grateful for their encouragement and sympathetic support while persevering with the many problems which arose during the successful development of this discipline.

To Dr. Henry A. Rothrock, pathologist at the Chester County Hospital, West Chester, and to Drs. Henry Brody and Irving Young, pathologists at the Albert Einstein Medical Center, I am indebted for the many intrusions on their valuable time and experience to resolve the numerous pathologic questions incident to our endeavors. Among the many able technicians who are responsible for enthusiastic application to the technical and administrative problems entailed with our work, I should like to mention particularly Mrs Lolita Moore, Miss Barbara M. Curcio and my dear sister, Miss Sara Cohen. It was my extreme good fortune to enjoy their loyal dedication to the numerous administrative and technical problems which they so successfully tackled.

Without the devoted and able assistance of Mrs. Lillian Cohen and Mrs. Rae B. Smith, the preparation and organization of this contribution could not have occurred. My gratitude for their unremitting editorial assistance is a pleasure to acknowledge.

Finally, I am deeply indebted to all the members of the staff of the Albert Einstein Medical Center and the Chester County Hospital for their mounting interest and encouragement in the prosecution of our work.

I Introduction

The recognition of normal and abnormal patterns in the breast by mammography is a skill that must be acquired through training and experience in the same way the radiologist learns to recognize the normal or abnormal skull, gastrointestinal tract, chest, spine, and other anatomy.

To disseminate information on the breasts to radiologists on a large scale, the most effective method — person-to-person teaching — is obviously impractical. Even postgraduate courses in mammography can reach but a few fellow radiologists. Therefore we have felt for some time that a teaching *Atlas of Mammography* would serve a useful purpose, within the limitations of the method, by bringing to the attention of radiologists and physicians in general the salient features of the X-ray appearance of the normal and the abnormal breast.

In mammography as in no other area of roentgenologic study, technique is of crucial importance. Accurate diagnosis is absolutely dependent upon demonstration of very fine detail, sometimes as delicate as a linear strand or two, or minute specks of calcium. To some extent the pictorial representation embraced by an atlas defeats the teaching objective, for much fine detail is often lost in reproducing radiographs. Every effort has been made to obtain the best possible reproductions of mammograms in this *Atlas,* but some illustrations must of necessity remain unconvincing to the reader. Some of the details described will be appreciated only when viewing a good quality original radiograph. We believe, however, that as mammographic experience accumulates, most of the questions or doubts that arise from unclear illustrations in this *Atlas* will be resolved. There is, after all, no substitute for the actual examination of patients and inspection of original mammograms.

One of the greatest values of mammography is the opportunity it affords to detect a disease process before it is manifested clinically. An outstanding example is the unsuspected or so-called "occult" cancer. An occult cancer in the strict sense is one in which the discovery of a remote symptom or sign, such as localized pain over the spine or an enlarged node in the axilla, arouses suspicion of breast cancer although no mass can be palpated. Many of these cancers can be located only by mammography.

There are three principal ways by which a cancer can continue to escape detection: 1. The malignant tumor is felt but wrongly diagnosed as benign; 2. It is masked by other lesions; 3. It is still too small to be palpable.

In erroneous diagnosis, the mass is felt but is so circumscribed and movable that its malignant nature is not suspected. For example, a duct carcinoma, even when it has reached extensive proportions, is frequently mistaken for a benign tumor and biopsy is likely to be postponed. An X-ray examination in these cases may give an unequivocal answer, convince a reluctant patient to submit to operation, save valuable time and possibly life.

Another reason for mandatory X-ray examination of all lesions is that while the palpable mass may indeed be benign, a small preclinical "silent" carcinoma may be found in another part of the breast. Too often the patient is lulled into a false sense of security by the removal of a cyst or other benign lesion when the real culprit lies latent, to appear perhaps years later when it is no longer curable.

X-ray examination is also indicated in all patients with nodularity or "lumpiness" in one or both breasts, whether or not a dominant mass is present. Finding a cancer in such breasts is very common. In most of them, adenosis is the underlying or masking lesion. In some patients the adenosis has progressed to hyperplastic fibrosis. In a few others, mazoplasia cystica has developed on the basis of adenosis. Rarely, the nodularity is due to multiple fibroadenomas. In the great majority of cases, lumpy breasts are benign and remain so, but should a carcinoma develop it is not likely to be discovered for a very long time. Often the malignant growth is actually remote from the area of the palpable lump, and it is not uncommon for multiple operations to be performed on these breasts without discovering the cancer. Hence the wisdom of roentgenography as a preliminary to biopsy.

All women who present vague, unusual, or unaccountable symptoms referable to the breast should be examined roentgenographically. Pain is sometimes the presenting symptom of a non-palpable carcinoma. Indefinite thickening noted in any part of the breast should likewise come under suspicion. Finally, a negative X-ray examination can reassure the healthy patient with cancerophobia and a positive family history of breast cancer.

Carcinomas may remain asymptomatic for a very long time. X-ray examination leads to their detection long before they can be recognized clinically. We learned this from retrospective studies of the growth rate of cancers whose presence on the original films was missed. Some of these tumors were not discovered until months or years later, when subsequent films and comparison with originals disclosed their slow, insidious development.

The preclinical diagnosis of mammary carcinoma before metastasis has occurred offers much greater hope for surgical removal. For this reason, roentgenography of the breasts should be an integral part of any program for periodic health examination of women. In the case of obvious cancer, X-ray studies, while not mandatory, have proved their worth in a number of ways. They help to rule out an unsuspected cancer in the opposite breast and to determine the type of therapy advisable if operation is not contemplated. Considerable increase in knowledge of breast pathology has resulted from careful study of these cases. Data on precancerous lesions recognized by mammography afford reason to hope that in the future many lesions will be treated in the precancerous stage, probably the most effective approach to the control of this disease.

Many of the comments and explanations in the pages that follow will be quoted or paraphrased from the Ingleby and Gershon-Cohen textbook, *Comparative Anatomy, Pathology and Roentgenology of the Breast,* published by University of Pennsylvania Press, Philadelphia, Pa., 1960.

II Some Pertinent Remarks on Histology of the Breast

Dr. Helen Ingleby, a long-time colleague and a superb pathologist, often remarked that "a thorough knowledge of breast pathology is a sine qua non for interpretation of breast films." Forty-odd years of experience with mammography-pathology correlation attest to the wisdom of her observation.

Unfortunately, pathologic classification of the condition found depends chiefly upon the individual pathologist or surgeon, so that terminology is extremely variable and inexact. Many writers content themselves with imprecise expressions, such as fibrocystic disease, cystic mastitis, mastopathy, and even the long outdated chronic mastitis. They seldom define what they mean and rarely distinguish one form of dysplasia from another. The unfortunate radiologist is apt to be caught in this inchoate welter of terminology to his consternation.

Adding to the confusion it the fact that few pathologists have studied entire breasts. Histologic examination of minute breast sections is of course essential to exact diagnosis, but it does not help the radiologist who must view the organ as a whole and compare it with its fellow, drawing his conclusions from overall observations.

The author realized that progress in X-ray diagnosis could only be made by careful comparison of the film with the actual breast specimen. The method followed was to have the pathologist make whole serial sections of the frozen breast, stain the series, and examine the tissue under the microscope. The sections were then set up alongside the X-ray film and each was compared with the other. The counterpart of opacities seen on the film was studied in the section. Structures seen in the section were studied on the roentgenogram. Furthermore, the films and the sections were matched to the clinical groups as they were revealed by the records. Classification practically made itself (Figs. 1, 2).

Minute histologic study of breast tissue with paraffin sections has been beset by confusion due to variability in the amount of parenchyma; the number, size, and distribution of lobules; and the rate of cyclic growth and regression not only in different women but in different parts of the same breast.

The first stage of development is proliferation of cells at some point in the wall of a duct, probably a prelobular duct, although growth from larger ducts has been noted. The multiplication of cells occurs by amitosis. Mitosis is rare, being seen only in hyperplastic conditions. Soon a lumen appears, the duct grows, and ductules arise from it. Growth and branching continue until a lobule is formed. The epithelial cells are relatively small, with deeply staining nuclei and scanty cytoplasm. The nuclei are basal and lie close together.

After the proliferative phase, the epithelial cells swell. The nuclei are larger and rounder and the particles of chromatin are, as it were, pushed apart by a clear substance. The cytoplasm is also increased and the nuclei no longer contact each other. Granules and at times larger protein masses appear in the cytoplasm.

The protein secretion is seen first as acidophil caps on the surface of the cells. Later, the material forms elongated, then rounded, bodies which become detached and collect in the lumen, where they fuse. Occasionally fatty secretion is also seen, but it is not to be looked for in all cases. During menstruation the basal cells break up and the epithelium is shed into the lumen. In the pre-menstruum the prelobular and intralobular ducts dilate. The individual's fluid intake and output will contribute to the dilatation. The intraductal tissue is loose and edematous, and contains scattered mononuclear cells. After menstruation, it becomes dense and fibrous and fills the gaps left by the degenerated ductules.

The Myoepithelium, Myothelium, or Myoid. The normal mammary duct is lined by two layers of cells. Those impinging on the lumen are cuboid to columnar in shape, and are typically epithelial. The cells of the deeper layers are more irregular in shape but are contiguous. A certain confusion in nomenclature has arisen concerning this layer. It is termed "basal" by some, "myoid" or "myoepithelial" by others. We believe that no element should be considered myoepithelial unless the cytoplasm presents one or more processes.

The shape of the basal cell is determined by its surroundings. When it is free to expand, the cell is rounded or ovoid. Myoid cells are sparse in the larger ducts if no cause for hyperplasia is present. They lie along the basement membrane and are often found between the epithelial cells. The nuclei are elongated or ovoid, sometimes triangular in cross-section, and the fully developed cell stains relatively deeply. Long fibrils are present in the cytoplasm and course lengthwise along the duct.

The myoepithelium is most easily observed in the lobules, especially in the prelobular ducts. Myothelial cells in the prelobular and smaller ducts evolve as follows. At first they are plump with pale vesicular nuclei. They resemble basal cells, except that in good slide preparations one or more cytoplasmic processes may be discerned. The processes are initially blunt and irregular; then striae appear in them. Soon the cell resembles a smooth muscle fiber, which functionally it is, its epithelial origin notwithstanding.

In the smaller prelobular ducts the myoid forms a definite layer, and at times the pointed cytoplasmic processes may be seen streaming into the surrounding fibrillary tissue. In lobules when postmenstrual degeneration is complete, the myoid cells are the last to disappear. Swollen degenerated elements cluster around the disappearing ductules. Their appearance suggests the possibility of a phagocytic function. The nucleus gradually becomes more attenuated and finally disappears. These observations lead to the inescapable conclusion that the connective tissue of the mammary gland proper is of epithelial origin and is derived from the myoid.

Many earlier authors laid great stress on the basement membrane which separates the epithelial cells from the surrounding intraductal fibrillary tissue and on which the myothelial cells rest. This has been a stumbling block to the true conception of what the mammary gland is and how it functions. The basement membrane is very conspicuous, especially when impregnated with silver. To many of the older generation it was an immutable barrier separating mesoblastic from epithelial tissue. Of course myoepithelial cells could not cross it! We have, however, sections showing fibrils from the myoid actually entering into the formation of this membrane.

Years ago, Masson in his textbook illustrated myoid hyperplasia, later called sclerosing adenosis by Urban and Adair (1949), and asserted that the fibers become lost in the connective tissue. The transition of myoid into connective tissue in pathologic conditions is generally conceded. There is, therefore, no *a priori* reason why the normal intraductal tissue of the mammary gland should not also be of myoid origin.

Mammary Vessels. The main arteries supplying the breast arise from the internal and external mammary and from the intercostals. Their number and distribution are very variable, and the same is true of veins. There is no conspicuous, convenient milk vein as is found in dairy animals. The most constant vessel seen on mammograms is a vein which crosses the subareolar region at right angles to the lactiferous ducts and which enlarges considerably during pregnancy. In the breasts of older women calcification of arteries is frequently observed on X-ray films, just as it is in arteries elsewhere in the body.

The vascular supply to lobules and smaller ducts is an example of the correlation between structure and function which prevails in the body generally. Precapillary arterioles anastomose to form a circular mesh at the outer edge of the lobule or duct. They give off enormous numbers of capillaries which traverse the parenchyma as far as the basement membrane. The amount of blood reaching the duct or ductules is controlled by sympathetic fibers to the arterioles. The removal of epithelial debris after menstrual shedding, the presence of congestion and edema in the intraductal connective tissue, the accessibility or inaccessibility of hormones to the mammary parenchyma may be accounted for by the state of relaxation or contraction of these arterioles. This factor may also explain the variability of hormone response encountered in the same breast.

Fig. 1 A
Mammogram of infiltrating duct cell cancer with scirrhus. The irregular, undulating, notched margins of the scirrhus differentiate the lesion from a benign cyst or a fibroadenoma

B
A slicer section which illustrates the gross appearance of the lesion. Roentgenologists can acquire diagnostic skill by such comparisons

Fig. 2 A
Infiltrating duct cell and scirrhous carcinomas with metastasis to mammary and axillary lymph nodes

B
Slicer section of whole breast for comparison

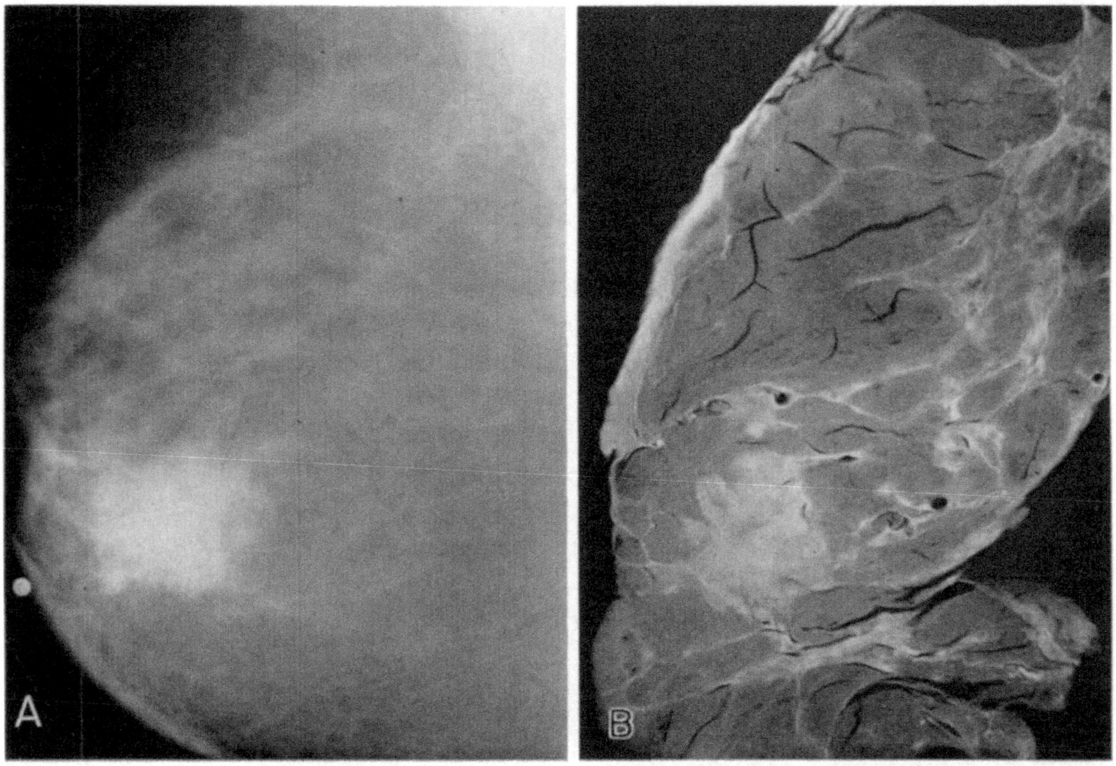

1

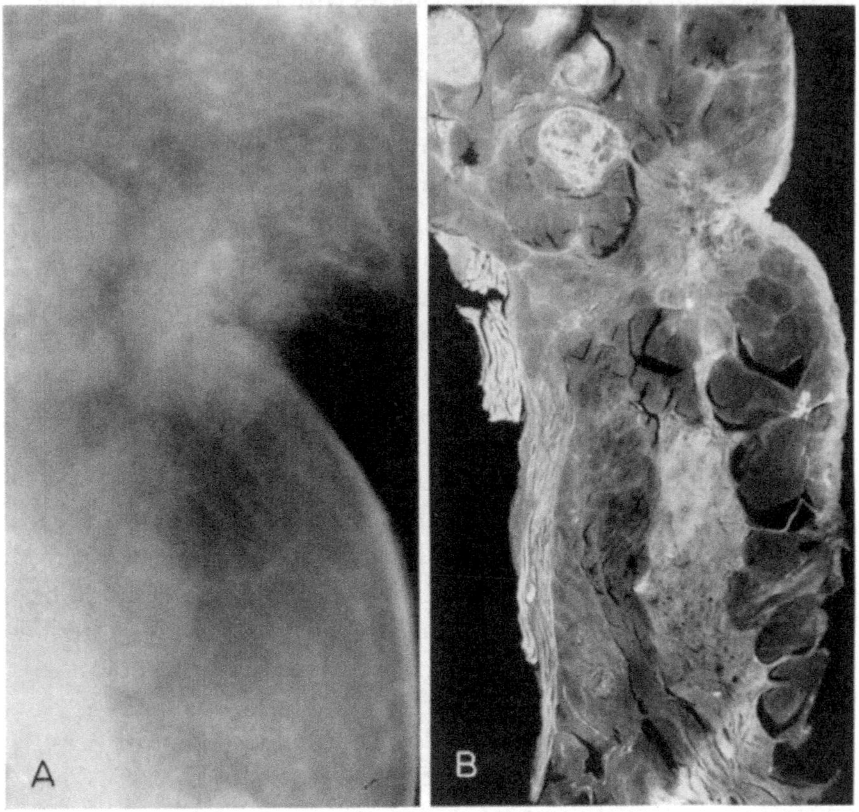

2

III Technique

The principles that make mammography a successful discipline are basic to roentgenology of any other part of the body. Diagnostic accuracy depends chiefly on obtaining excellent films with optimal detail and contrast.

Mammography poses some special problems. These concern

1. the variable size and shape of a soft-tissue organ such as the breast;
2. the progressive changes that occur in the structural components with aging;
3. the impossibility of always projecting the entire organ with a single exposure;
4. the necessity of working with the lowest possible kilovoltage for utmost contrast, which often requires special service adaptation of commercial X-ray apparatus;
5. the selection of proper compromises with regard to focal spot, collimators, filters, type of film, and exposure times so as to obtain good films with the shortest possible exposure;
6. the selection of the most appealing processing techniques;
7. deciding whether it is desirable to use skin markers to indicate an area of special interest, such as the site of symptoms, a palpable mass, or a previous operation.

To achieve optimal contrast in a soft structure like the breast, where differences in density are so slight, we find it best to confine the energy of conventional equipment to between 25 and 33 KV, and if nonscreen film is used (which we prefer), the range is best confined to 25 KV $\pm$ 2 KV. To obtain this range, we found it necessary many years ago to alter the transformer taps of our mobile X-ray apparatus. Good collimation is achieved with flat-sided, lead-lined cones of various sizes. If a focal spot of 0.8 mm is used, without filtration, at a distance of 40 cm, exposures of from 150 to 300 MaS will afford fine detail. The radiation dose provided is minimal — 1 to 2 rads per exposure — and little stress is placed upon the X-ray tube or the apparatus.

Recently, radiographic apparatus specifically designed for mammography became available in the Senograph (Figs. 3—5). This apparatus evolved through the dedication and zeal of Doctor

Charles M. Gros of Strasbourg, long a champion of breast roentgenography and the foremost proponent of mammography on the Continent. He persuaded a French company to make the original prototype, and after appropriate field-testing, Senographs were made generally available, including the United States[1].

All features of the Senograph have been designed to make breast radiography more exact for the radiologist, more easily accomplished by the technician, and more comfortable for the patient. The target is of molybdenum rather than tungsten and is located at the end of the tube instead of in the middle. The "K" radiation wave-edge length of molybdenum is ideally suited for soft-tissue roentgenography, being 0.7 Å versus 0.2 Å for tungsten. The X-rays are sharply collimated by a series of cones of all sizes, varying from one with a diameter of 6 cm for taking spot films to one whose exit diameter is 25 cm. All cones are flat-sided and have rounded edges so that breast compression is accomplished with thoroughness and minimal discomfort to the patient. The apparatus is compact, requiring but 9 square feet of floor space, and operates on a 220 volt line. The tube is water-cooled, requiring one gallon per minute. It can be rotated through 360 degrees, so that the entire examination can be made while the patient remains comfortably seated upon a stool which is raised and lowered hydraulically.

Mammograms made with the Senograph are far superior in contrast and detail to those made with previously available equipment (Fig. 6). We have not been using this equipment for very long, so most of the illustrations that comprise this *Atlas* will have been made with the older, standard equipment. Visualization of microcalcifications, a critical point in locating nonpalpable infiltrating duct cancers, is especially enhanced using the Senograph. However, the radiologist whose eye has been trained to search for these incriminating calcareous particles will also be able to detect them on properly processed mammograms made with standard equipment.

The radiologist recognizes tissues not only by their outlines but by differences in their density. In the breast, such variations in density are relatively slight. The coefficients of absorption of the component structures are close to that of water. On a mammogram, air and fat are almost translucent. Water is less so, having a coefficient of linear absorption of 1.0 compared to 0.92 for fat. The figure for transudates is 1.008, and for blood and pus, 1.06. Thus, cysts containing clear albuminous fluid are

1 Distributed in the United States by Keleket/CGR Co., Waltham, Mass.

discerned rather easily, especially if they are large, because the thickness of the fluid layer and the displacement of other tissues in the area enhance their visibility. Cysts which contain blood or pus, as in chronic abscess, are also easy to see provided their outlines are not masked by inflammatory reaction around them.

Fibrous tissue has a coefficient of 1.2. In practice, this will vary with the amount of water it contains and with its physical and chemical make-up. On a film, the thickness of an area of fibrosis often decides whether other structures such as cysts will be masked by it. The cellular component of the breast has about the same density as the fibrous tissue and is not distinguishable from the fibrous parenchyma.

An absolute increase in density is found in many scirrhous carcinomas. Other tumors show a relatively increased density because in most cases their structure is more compact than that of the breast in which they lie. Very small growths can be discerned in postmenopausal atrophic breasts because they lie in a bed of fat. The glandular breasts of younger women contain a smaller proportion of adipose tissue, and tumors in them are correspondingly more difficult to define. In immature breasts which contain almost no fat, the tumor may have exactly the same density as the surrounding parenchyma, and unless the margin of the tumor is visible, diagnosis may be impossible.

Using our conventional radiographic equipment, suitably serviced for mammography, we experimented with different films. We long ago came to favor nonscreen film as the best compromise, because good contrast can be obtained without sacrificing diagnostic detail and the films can be processed automatically. Many roentgenologists prefer to use industrial film, which requires energy in the range of 33 KV $\pm$ 2 KV in order to take full advantage of this type of film.

The technician is apt to feel that a higher kilovoltage is needed for a large breast than for a small compact one, but invariably the reverse is true. The large breast is usually composed mostly of fat. It requires less kilovoltage than the small, compact, virginal breast, whose density can only be portrayed properly by using higher kilovoltages. It is the amount of glandular tissue as opposed to fat that governs the selection of the optimal kilovoltage, as well as the conventional measurement of the thickness of the tissue to be traversed by the central beam. It is also important to compress the breast properly, without causing discomfort to the patient or buckling the breast tissue (Fig. 7).

It is seldom possible to project the entire breast with a single exposure because the surface of the chest wall curves. Two basic projections are usually routine, the lateral and the cephalocaudad. In addition, it is often necessary to make projections in more anterolateral planes to permit visualization of the *entire* breast (Figs. 8—10). Rarely, additional views of the axillary tail of the breast may be necessary. A skilled technician who has palpated the breast properly will know when to employ these exceptional technical measures.

If the patient has localized symptoms or a palpable mass in which the clinician is interested, we routinely affix a millimeter-sized lead shot over the area with Scotch tape. It must be affixed lightly to avoid factitious thickening of the skin due to the too-tight tape (Fig. 11). If the breasts have been subjected to surgery, we also fasten with Scotch tape a line of these lead shots over the scar or scars. The radiologist, when viewing the films, can readily locate the specific area in which the clinician is interested, and the lines of lead shot over surgical scars identify structural distortions due to previous operations he might otherwise have found diagnostically misleading (Fig. 12).

The processing of mammographic films requires the utmost care and precision. Only relentless surveillance by the technician and the radiologist can assure maintenance of the high standards the discipline demands. Industrial films require hand processing. The automatic film processors are much more rapid and less subject to human error. With these, the skilled technician can examine the film in minutes for technical quality and make any needed corrections before the patient is dismissed. The dedicated roentgenologist will take pains to train technicians to appreciate the difference between "passable" and high-quality mammograms.

It goes without saying that the results of a good history and careful physical examination should always be available on all patients as an integral part of the discipline of mammography.

Localization of Areas of Microcalcifications and Suspected Tumors. Pathologists have always been aware of calcareous deposits in malignant tissue which has undergone necrosis, but it took Leborgne (1951) to recognize their importance in cancer of the breast. Probably 85 per cent of all breast cancers are associated with some microscopic granular calcifications, but only about 35 per cent of them will be found on roentgenograms. Fortunately, they are visible while the cancers are still very small and before signs or symptoms supervene, making their detection and localization very important to diagnosis.

A prerequisite for accurate preoperative localization of a site containing microcalcifications in the absence of a palpable tumor are mammograms which demonstrate the site in two projections at right angles to each other. This is accomplished by means of the routine lateral and cephalocaudad projections, with the breast supported to the degree necessary to profile the nipple and all of the mammary tissue from chest wall to nipple. One cannot overemphasize the necessity of identifying with film markers the various quadrants of the breast. We routinely place these alongside the upper aspect of the breast in the lateral projection and alongside the outer aspect of the breast in the cephalocaudad projection.

A base line is then drawn on the roentgenograms from nipple to chest wall in both projections and the suspect area is suitably marked. We encircle it with crayon, including at least an additional perimeter of 0.5 cm of breast tissue to allow for minute variations in projection. This procedure localizes the lesion to a specific quadrant of the breast, since the lateral projection establishes whether the lesion is above or below the nipple, and the cephalocaudad projection shows whether it is medial or lateral to it (Fig. 13).

Localization of Proper Area for Histologic Section. In addition to localizing the suspicious area for the surgeon, we act also to assure that the proper area has been removed and to aid the pathologist in deciding which area should be studied microscopically. When both the surgeon and the pathologist cooperate, maximum speed of handling the specimen is assured.

The specimen is sent directly from the operating room to the radiology department. There it is placed flat upon a piece of waxed paper with suitable markers affixed to it. A roentgenogram is taken immediately, using factors of 10 to 50 MaS and 25 KV, depending upon the thickness of the tissue. The position of the specimen itself remains unchanged. The original roentgenogram is checked at once and the surgeon informed whether or not removal of the suspected area has been accomplished.

The specimen is then moved via the waxed paper on to a cardboard and covered with damp gauze. Both specimen and the roentgenograms of it are taken with speed to the pathologist's laboratory. Since the specimen has been maintained in the exact position in which it was roentgenographed, accurate localization of supect areas can be made for microscopic study (Fig. 14).

Injection of Contrast Medium for Duct Visualization. The presence of a papilloma can be suspected when there is a history of bloody discharge from the nipple, but very often these tiny lesions cannot be confirmed on mammograms. We have found it wise to try to locate them by using contrast medium injected into the secretory ducts using the technique of Buttenberg. This is done using Renografin, 1 ml, and a 30-gauge needle; no anesthesia is necessary. Patients tolerate the procedure with surprising lack of discomfort, and the additional diagnostic data it affords help to establish the diagnosis of papilloma, to localize the lesion, or to differentiate it from carcinoma in situ (Fig. 15).

Doctor Gros habitually resorts to the introduction of air into evacuated cysts in order to demonstrate any intracystic growths. If radiologists in the United States would subscribe as wholeheartedly to this practice as mammographers abroad do, a wealth of information would be gained by this simple maneuver.

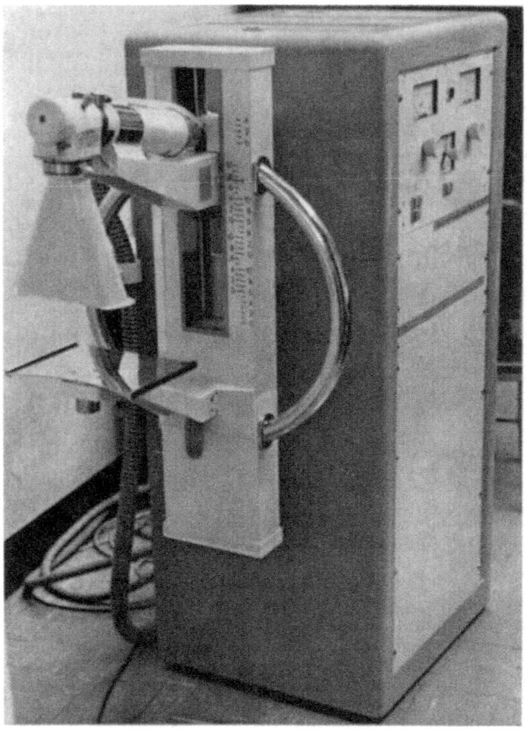

Fig. 3. The Senograph

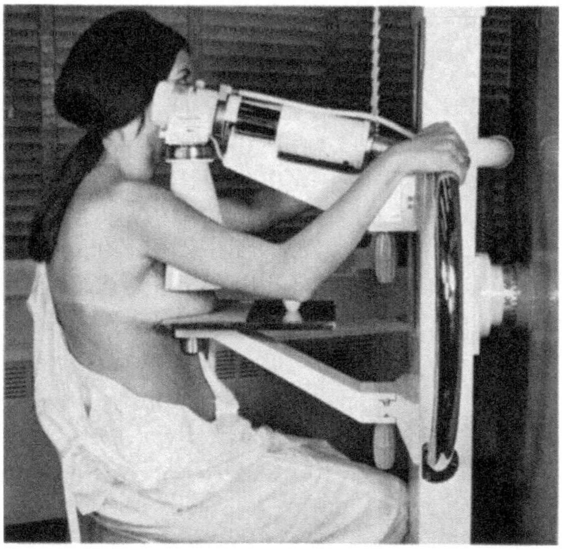

Fig. 4. Senograph in use during cephalocaudad projection with compression of breast

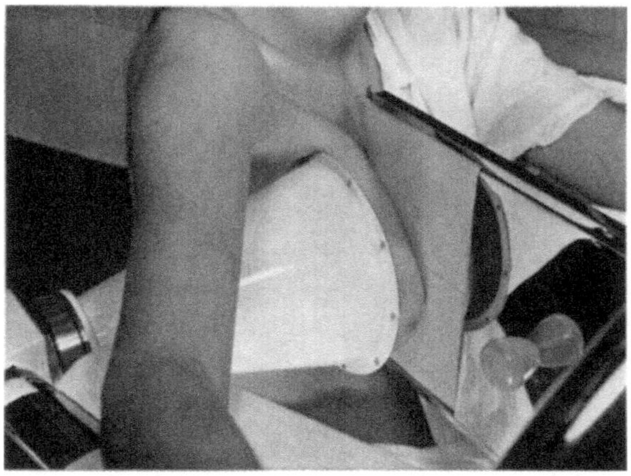

Fig. 5. Lateromedial projection with patient in sitting position

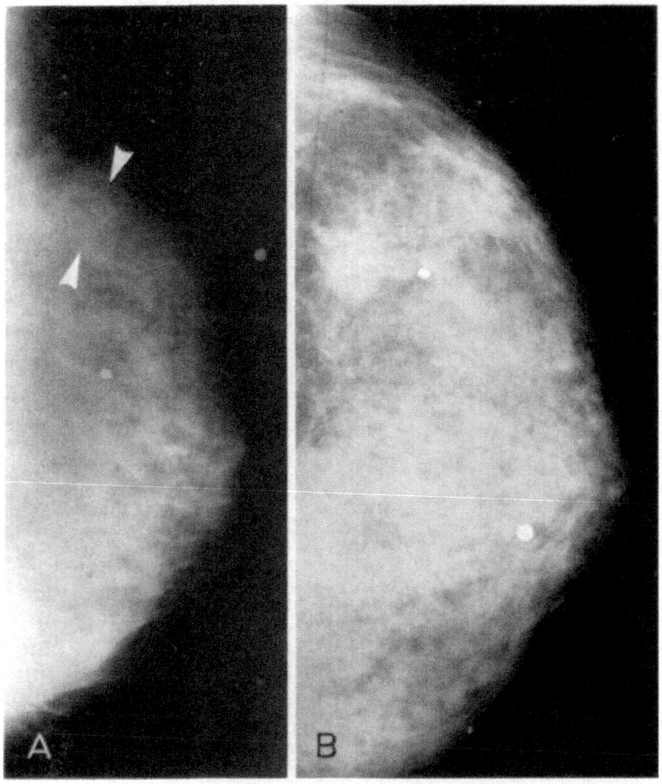

Fig. 6 A
Mammogram made with conventional X-ray apparatus modified for mammography. The tube had a beryllium window and a 0.5 mm Al filter. The factors were 28 KV, 50 Ma, 3 seconds, 18 inches distance, and a 3 mm focal spot on a tungsten target. Nonscreen film was used and was automatically processed

B
Mammogram of the same breast made with the Senograph. The beryllium window was shielded by a molybdenum filter, 30 microns thick. The factors were 30 KV, 40 Ma, 4 seconds, 18 inches distance, a 0.7 mm focal spot on a molybdenum target, and nonscreen film which was processed automatically

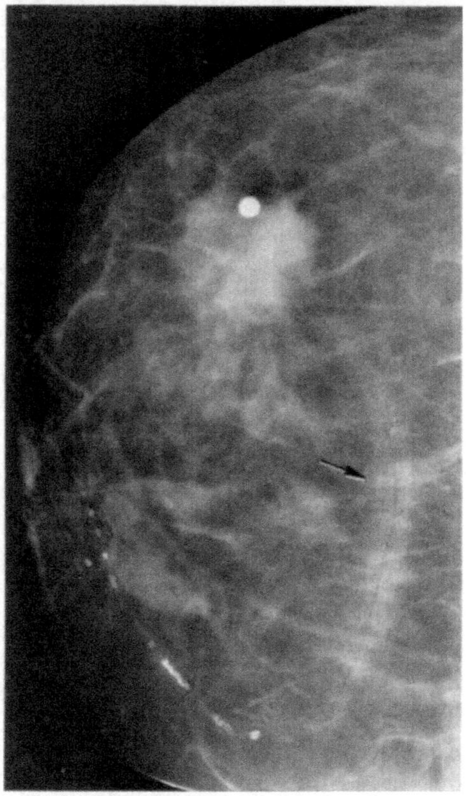

Fig. 7. In positioning the breast, skin buckling must be avoided. The long curving density with its radiolucent midline is due to buckling of the skin of an improperly-positioned breast (arrow). An infiltrating papillary duct cell carcinoma is present, with short strands issuing from the angular margins at site of skin marker

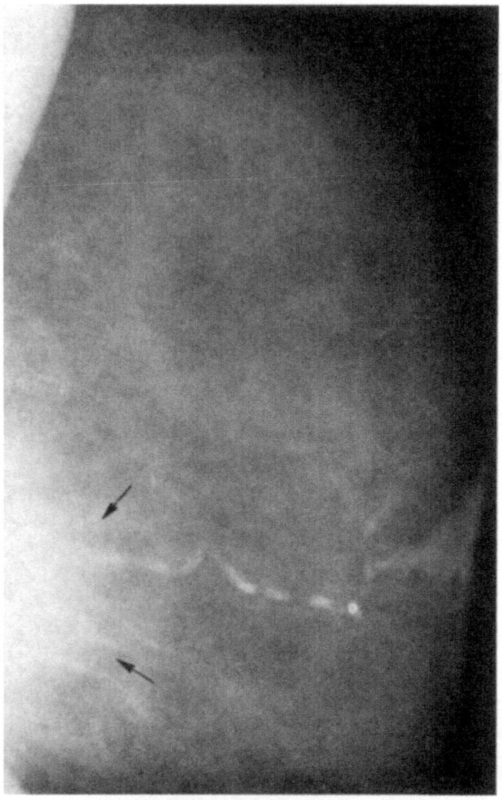

Fig. 8. Improper profiling of the breast in the lateral position may fail ro reveal the prepectoral fat layer. Lesions deep in the breast, such as this infiltrating duct cell carcinoma, may be only partially revealed or completely missed. Selecting the proper kilovoltage for the type of breast and type of film so that optimal contrast is obtained requires training and experience. In this case, contrast is poor and only part of the large cancer can be visualized

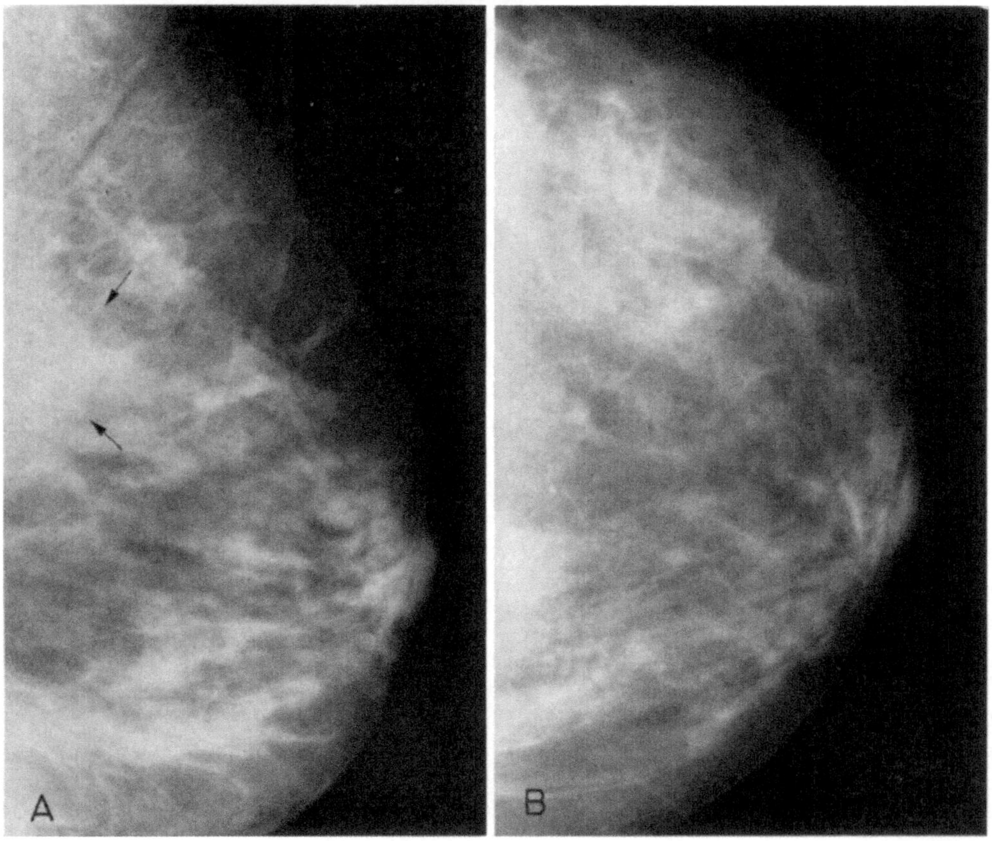

9

Fig. 9 A
Lateral view reveals only a partial aspect of a cancer because of improper profiling of the entire breast

B
No portion of the deep-seated cancer is revealed in the cephalocaudad view

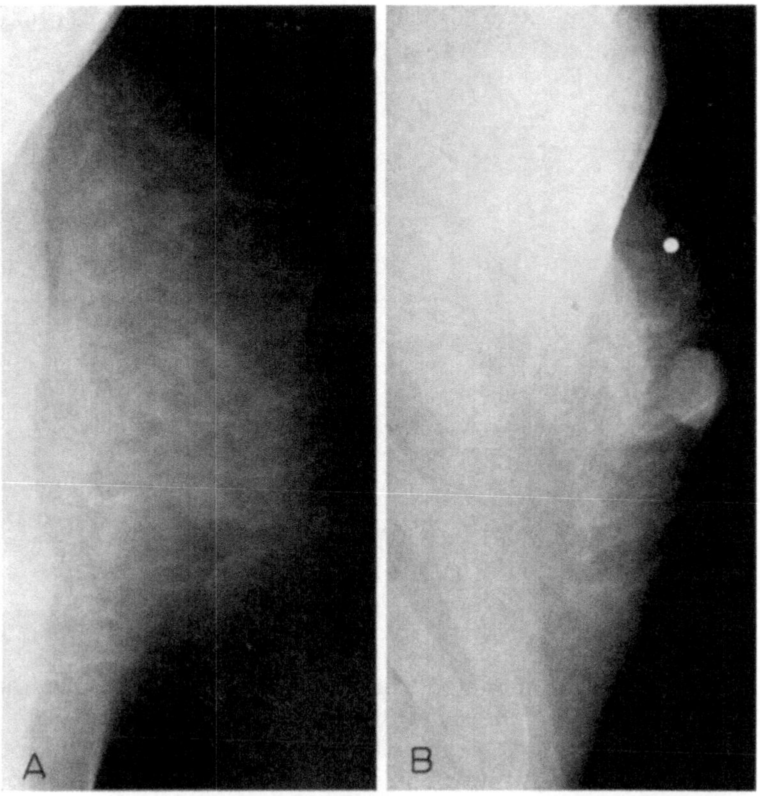

Fig. 10
A. A mass about 2.5 cm in diameter was palpable in the right breast. No skin marker was placed for orientation because the radiologist expected its presence to be clearly discerned on the roentgenogram. To his surprise, this was not the case in either the lateral or cephalocaudad views

B. After placing a skin marker, a special compression film was obtained and a mass was seen. The undulating edges and the fine striae streaming into the perifocal tissues led to a presumptive diagnosis of cancer. The histologist found a lymphosarcoma

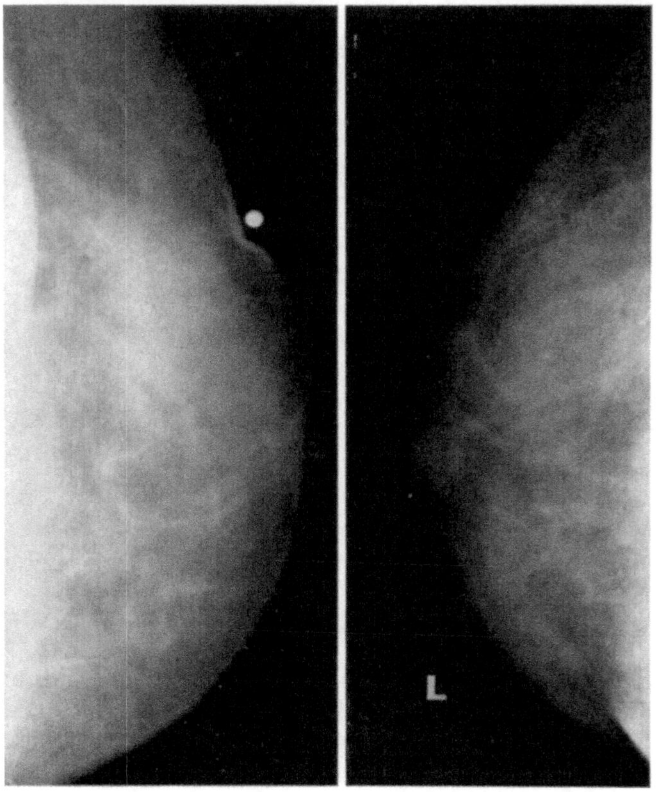

Fig. 11. The skin marker must not be too tightly attached. Infiltrating duct cell cancer may be very difficult to discern in a field of adenosis. In this case, a palpable mass in the right breast was thought to be a cancer by the surgeon, but the mammogram reveals only an area of increased density resembling adenosis. Local edema blurs the structural distortions due to the cancer. Comparison with the opposite (left) breast helps to appreciate the changes in the right, adding credence to the clinical impression. The skin marker was too tightly bound to the skin with Scotch tape, so that the retraction of the underlying skin is an artifact

Fig. 12. Lead shot markers are useful for identifying the location of palpable masses and operative scars. The line of markers on the skin of the right breast has been placed along a scar resulting from an old operation for a benign lesion. In the left breast a nodular scirrhous carcinoma (arrow) was very-difficult to recognize because it is present in an area of mastopathy containing much ductal and lobular fibrous hyperplasia. Immediately apparent is the generalized edema of this breast as compared with the opposite side

Fig. 13. Method of obtaining a localization diagram. Lateral and cephalocaudad mammograms on which the suspected lesion is suitably identified are projected onto a diagram. The depth of the lesion from the skin surface is easily measured directly from the roentgenograms

12
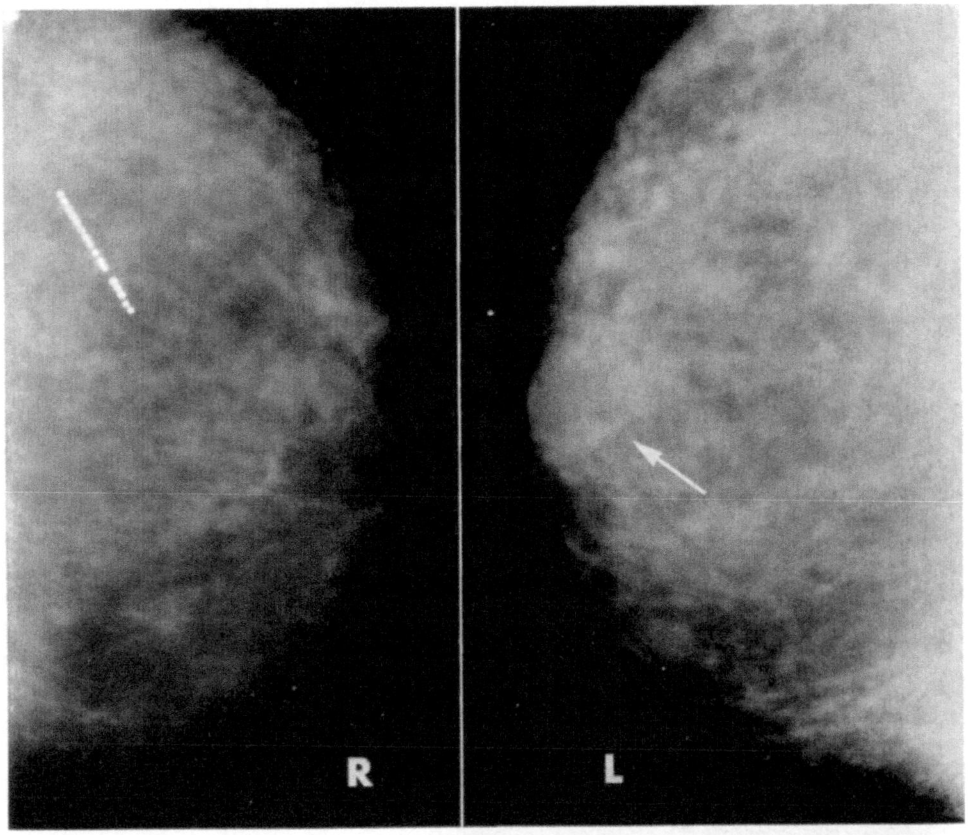
R
L

13
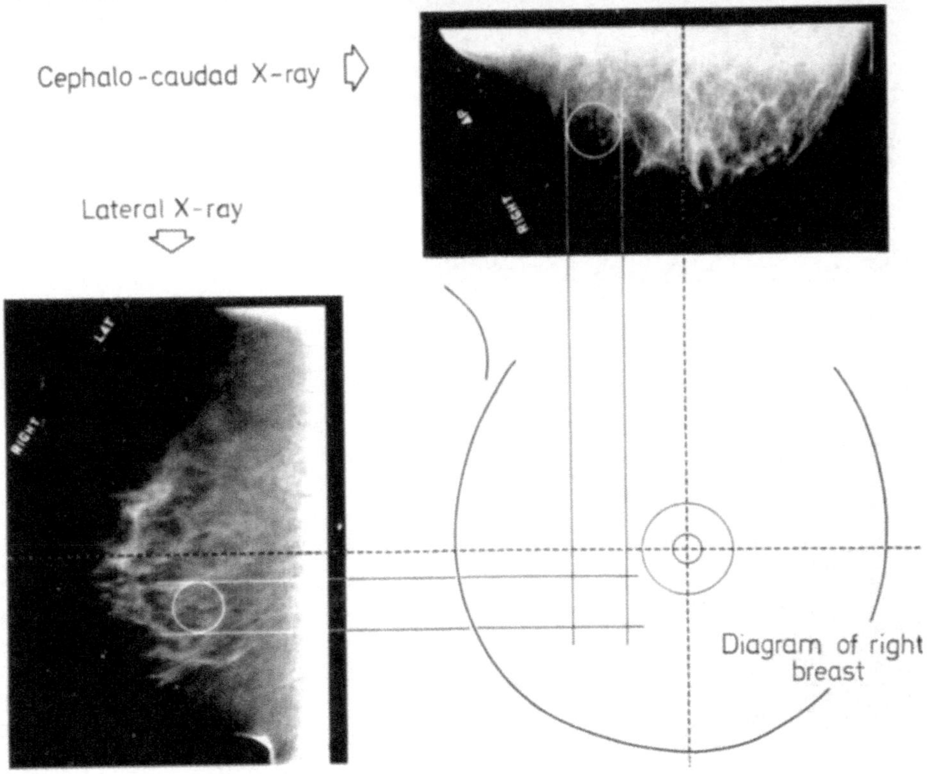
Cephalo-caudad X-ray
Lateral X-ray
Diagram of right breast

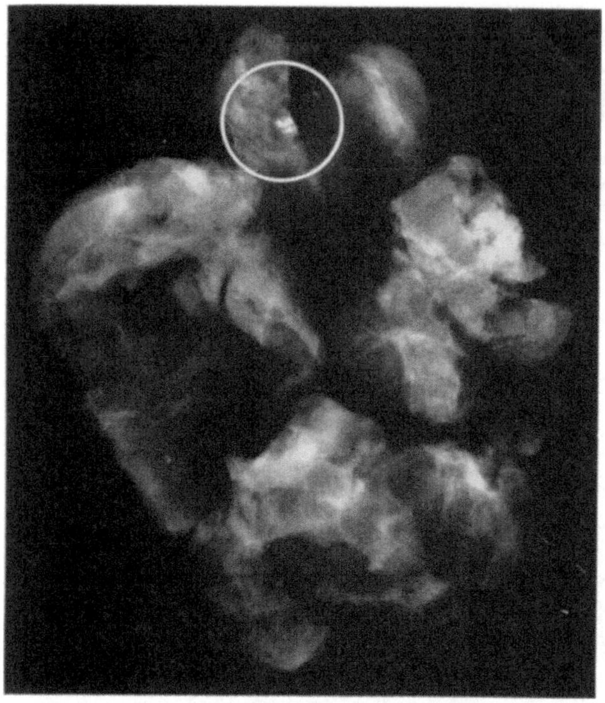

Fig. 14. Roentgenogram of biopsy specimen shows that removal of the area containing suspicious calcific particles has been accomplished. Sections of the area containing these particles revealed the presence of an infiltrating intraductal carcinoma

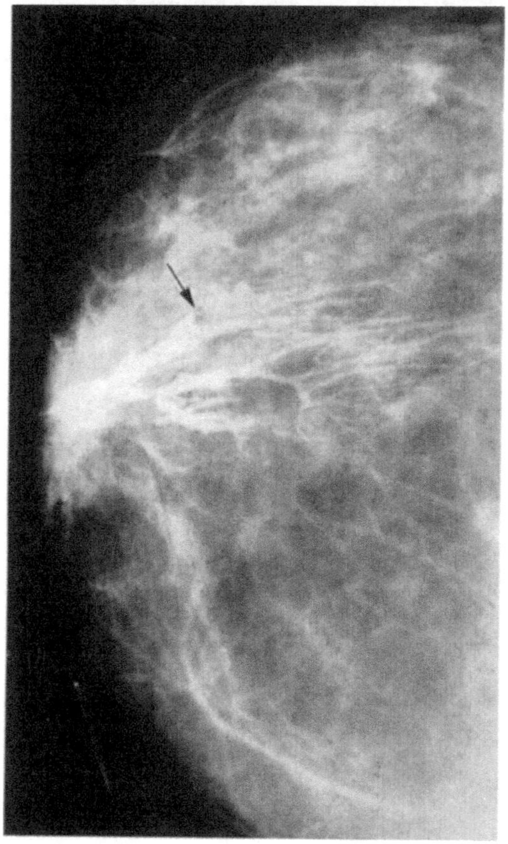

Fig. 15. Papilloma (arrow) in duct injected with contrast material (Renografin)

IV The Normal Breast

and is secreted in the same way. The substance is often referred to as "witch's milk." The condition usually disappears within a few days, but if it persists, true lactation acini are formed.

In some cases, the changes parallel those of secretory disease in adults. Even in these cases, postnatal mammary development seldom persists beyond six months of age. After six months, childhood enlargements can no longer be considered physiologic and must be classified with the pathologic hypertrophies. Rarely, postnatal hyperplasia persists beyond infancy, or regresses to return again later (Fig. 16).

2. The Adolescent Breast

The process of breast development is fundamentally similar in all girls, but it is subject to wide variations in rate and degree, with no exact correlation between age and development.

In the normal adolescent breast fibrous tissue predominates, and unless the subject is obese, only occasional islands of fat are seen. Nodules may be felt in some adolescent breasts, but they need cause no concern if one remembers the breast's normal lobular-like structure and tendency to irregular maturation. The possibility of fibroadenoma should be considered if one or more distinct nodules are felt, but it is usually advisable to withhold biopsy since malignancy is rare at this age. It is tragic to remove developing breast tissue needlessly, with the possible result of underdevelopment or deformation in the breast of an adolescent or young adult female (Figs. 17, 18).

If serial sections of adolescent breasts are examined, the irregularity of development in different parts of the same breast is striking. In some places there will be much greater subdivisions of the ducts than in others, and such areas persist through a number of serial sections.

The connective tissue of young breasts is always well developed and quite obviously of two kinds: the intraductal, belonging to the duct itself; and the interductal or perilobular. Interductal tissue is a supporting structure. Intraductal connective tissue is an integral part of the mammary gland.

3. The Adult Breast

Before embarking on a description of the normal breast, certain generally used terms should be clarified. Trabecula, stroma, parenchyma, and lobule are defined well in books, but when these words are applied to the breast in vivo there is considerable difficulty knowing just what they mean.

The breast, like other organs, consists of mammary tissue proper (parenchyma) and stroma. But in the breast, unlike other organs, the parenchyma is fibrous as well as epithelial. Grossly, it is impossible to distinguish the fibrous parenchyma from the equally fibrous stroma. Microscopically, the difference is obvious, but when a lobule undergoes involution it is replaced by fibrous tissue, merges with the stroma, and becomes indistinguishable from it. Possibly much of the adult stroma is formed in this way. Theoretically this "scar tissue" might be thought of as parenchyma, but it is nonfunctional.

When the ducts are distended, their outlines can be seen if interspersed fat is present, and each duct is part of the "trabecula." A trabecula actually consists of both stroma and parenchyma and in practice the two elements cannot be separated either grossly or radiologically. Since the term trabecula has been sanctioned by usage, it is retained.

The word "lobule" also gives rise to some ambiguity. A lobule is a group of ductules arising from the distal extremity of a duct. It must not be confused with the club-shaped terminal ducts found in the adolescent breast. Lobules are situated chiefly at the periphery and are most numerous at the base near the pectoral fascia, probably because of the rich blood supply there.

In the early 20s, the lobules are apt to be rather scanty and the breast is often partly of the adolescent type, especially in virgins. The virgin breast resembles the adolescent in great measure because there has not yet been large-scale proliferation and involution of lobules with fibrous replacement, as happens after pregnancy. During the menstrual cycle, the lobules undergo changes due to hormonal influence and they are not necessarily regular. Imperfect differentiation of ductules is common, and it is often difficult to decide at which stage of development a lobule may properly be so called. In some adults, because of hormonal imbalance, ducts may reach only the adolescent stage instead of developing into lobules, or a lobule may start to develop and instead of continuing to subdivide by proliferation at certain growing points, the entire duct wall may grow. This may result in a collection of cysts, which are large or small depending on the stage of development reached before the abnormal stimulus intervened and also upon its intensity.

In the late 20s and early 30s more lobules appear, and the difference between the parous and nonparous breast is not so obvious. The lobules are irregular in contour in the parous breast. In multiparae, there is a tendency to dilatation of prelobular ducts and the lactiferous ducts may also be dilated. Lobules attain their full development during lactation.

In the late 30s and in the 40s, many more irregularities are apparent in all women. The hangovers from an earlier age are joined by distortions due to premenopausal imbalance. During the menopause and for a year or two after it, irregular growth and regression may at times reach considerable proportions. The changes would in most cases be considered pathologic, but the line is not always easy to draw. Involution in these florid breasts may be expected about two years after the menopause.

Normal Breast Types. In view of these variables, it is obvious that it is difficult to classify breast patterns into distinctive types, but in general four normal breast types are recognized: 1. immature; 2. glandular; 3. involutional, and 4. atrophic.

1. Immature. In girls before the menarche, the gland shows an almost homogeneous opacity. In the few cases where fat is present, the trabeculae may be more easily distinguished, but usually they merge and their outlines cannot be seen. The immature breast, normal in adolescents, may persist in some women into the early 20s (Figs. 17, 18).

2. Glandular. The glandular breast is normally seen during the reproductive period. The lobules occupy the base and periphery of the breast. The subareolar area contains only lactiferous ducts and clusters of fingerlike offshoots. These are rudiments of Middendorp-Koenecke bodies which develop during lactation.

Radiographically, the principal density is found at the base and in well-developed breasts it is broad and rather fluffy. The trabeculae, which are wide and have ill-defined outlines, emerge from the base and course toward the nipple. In the subareolar area the lactiferous ducts merge to form homogeneous bands or fields which extend to the nipple (Figs. 19, 20).

3. Involutional. The involutional fibrous breast is seen following the menopause whether it be natural or artificial. Normally, it is characterized by gradual involution of lobules and relative increase in fibrous tissue of the trabeculae. In the majority of women, as the parenchyma diminishes, the adipose tissue increases (Fig. 21). The breast becomes flabby, but the total volume may remain the same or be increased or diminished, depending upon the nutritional status of the individual. In very thin subjects, intertrabecular fat is sometimes lacking and even the subcutaneous fat may be almost absent. The breasts then present a firm, compact core of mammary tissue in contradistinction to the flabbiness of fat-containing organs. Some postmenopausal glands exhibit fine nodularity, usually in the upper and central parts. Although frequently found, this type of fibrosis is not a normal condition, strictly speaking, but follows certain dysplasias.

As age advances, the parenchyma becomes more and more atrophied and the trabeculae correspondingly thinner.

4. Atrophic. In the atrophic breast, fat is usually deposited between the trabeculae, which become more and more attenuated. Sometimes the trabeculae are bunched together and appear on films as bands of varying widths surrounded by clear zones of fat. In very emaciated old women no fat may be present (Fig. 22).

The superficial veins are discerned with ease, especially in fat breasts. The arteries are visible when they become calcified.

When the radiologist becomes acquainted with the appearance of normal skin and venous structures, recognition of the early stages of inflammation or edema with engorgement of the venous complex with thickening of the skin becomes easy (Fig. 23).

4. The Breast in Pregnancy

Histologic examination reveals that the mammary gland undergoes changes very soon after conception. Apart from slight lobular hyperplasia, which would ordinarily pass unnoticed, the earliest detectable change is proliferation of the basal cellular layer of epithelium, particularly in the prelobular ducts and lobules. The lumina of the ductules are often so filled with cells that eventually they appear to be solid cords. Similar foci of proliferation and heaping up of cells are seen in the smaller ducts as well, and here also the lumen may be replaced by proliferating cells.

It must be stressed that although hyperplasia is an overall phenomenon, heaping up of cells occurs in scattered foci. The primitive basal cells in these foci are large, with big clear nuclei and prominent nucleoli. The cytoplasm is abundant. A little later, the differentiation into epithelial and myoepithelial cells can be discerned.

A rather heavy infiltration by mononuclear cells in lobules and around the ducts is a prominent finding in early pregnancy. As with other features, the infiltration occurs sporadically. In the third month of pregnancy, lobular development varies considerably in different parts of the same organ. If the clumps of slightly dilated club-shaped terminal ducts are examined under high power, it is seen that the epithelial cells are large and vacuolated and that the majority are loaded with fat. This is of interest because in the later months of pregnancy the intracellular fat often decreases. At term, many cells show few fat globules. The explanation may be that the fat is excreted into the ducts during the formation of colostrum.

Three to four months postconception, myoepithelial cells are abundant. They can be seen growing out in many places from the walls of the terminal ducts. In many, the cytoplasm is elongated and fibrillary. Others contain large globules of fat like those of the epithelial cells. In fully developed areas there are large lobules with well-formed acini in which practically all the cells are loaded with fat.

In the later months of pregnancy, as the lobules develop, a larger proportion of the myothelium is differentiated, but its essential characteristics are unchanged. The impressive hypertrophy of the myoepithelial cells at this time is a preparation for their ultimate function in lactation.

Roentgenographic detection of pregnancy before the third month is not usually possible. The overall density of the breasts is increased and the trabeculae are somewhat broadened, but on the X-ray film no distinction can be made at this stage between the immature breast, adenosis, and pregnancy. The first obvious changes can be seen at about three months' gestation. The glandular hyperplasia appears on the X-ray film as a gradually increasing density, and the trabeculae, which had been sharply defined, become fluffy, broader, and irregular in contour due to elongation and buckling (Fig. 24).

Some breasts, instead of adopting a trabecular pattern, will show irregular fluffy opacities which resemble adenosis except that they are more irregularly scattered throughout the breast. As the breast increases in size and density, it becomes rounded in shape, and the texture takes on a ground-glass appearance (Fig. 25).

With further development of the parenchyma, the trabeculae become more closely crowded (Fig. 26). The swollen lobules push into the subcutaneous layer of fat, forming densities with pyramidal contours, the apices pointing toward the skin. Later, these apices may become rounded or even flattened (Fig. 27).

5. The Lactational Breast

The earliest signs of lactational involution may be noted in young primiparae who are given stilbestrol immediately after parturition. Dilatation of lactiferous ducts may still be present but it is not the same as the distention of the subareolar area that occurs under the stimulus of suckling. The X-ray film shows that the ducts and sacculi are less crowded. The sacculi are small and are probably only visible because they are not masked by overdistended ducts (Fig. 28).

Following this stage, the lactiferous ducts narrow and are less tortuous. They decrease in size until involution is complete, although some slight dilatation often persists and may be considered normal for the multiparous breast (Fig. 29). When lactation ceases, the lobules shrink. The breast becomes less dense and the trabeculae reappear. In some cases of post-lactational involution the X-ray film shows a generalized haziness due to the breaking up of the lobules, infiltration by phagocytic cells, and edema. As involution proceeds, irregular scattered opacities resembling those of adenosis are seen (Fig. 30). These, too, finally disappear and the breast resumes its normal pattern.

In women who do not nurse, involution takes place in about two or three months. Judging from cases under our observation, if lactation has once been established the process appears to take longer and is more irregular. Irregularity of involution may be expected in cases where drying up of the secretion is accompanied by pain or nursing has been halted because of a breast lesion. Any form of hormonal imbalance may interfere with the normal process, but X-ray films taken before pregnancy and after involution show that in the absence of fresh hormone disturbance, the breast reverts to its former type.

6. Congenital Anomalies

1. Accessory Breasts. Supernumerary mammary organs or rudiments are very common. They are generally found along the milk line, but have been recorded on the cheek, neck, ear, trunk, upper arm, and thigh. The majority of accessory breasts in women occur in the axillae where they are nearly always bilateral. The nipple and areola are usually absent. Recognition on the X-ray film is easy once the possibility of the anomaly is borne in mind.

2. Anomalies of the Nipple and Lactiferous Ducts. Deformities of the nipple may be congenital. Inversion of the apex, or less commonly retraction of the entire nipple, may be present. Often the nipple is flat and fails to evert sufficiently to enable the infant to suckle.

A variable number of ducts, put by most authors at 15 to 20, normally opens onto the nipple. A lesser number may be present. Occasionally, there is a single duct. At times, ducts open on the areola as well as on the nipple.

Fig. 16. Bilateral uneven enlargement of breasts with no distortion of structural components in an 11 year old girl

Fig. 17. Normal breast of a 17 year old girl. The predominance of fibrous tissue accounts for the homogeneous density

Fig. 18. The adolescent breast. As the breast develops in late adolescence, the pericanalicular and periacinous hyperplastic proliferation in the subareolar area will occasionally be separated from the main body of the posterior breast by an area of fat. A palpable tumor at the site of the skin marker was a fibroadenoma

Fig. 19. Normal breast, 32 year old woman. The fields of glandular tissue occupy mostly the upper outer quadrant of the breast and spaces between the ill-defined trabeculae as they approach the nipple

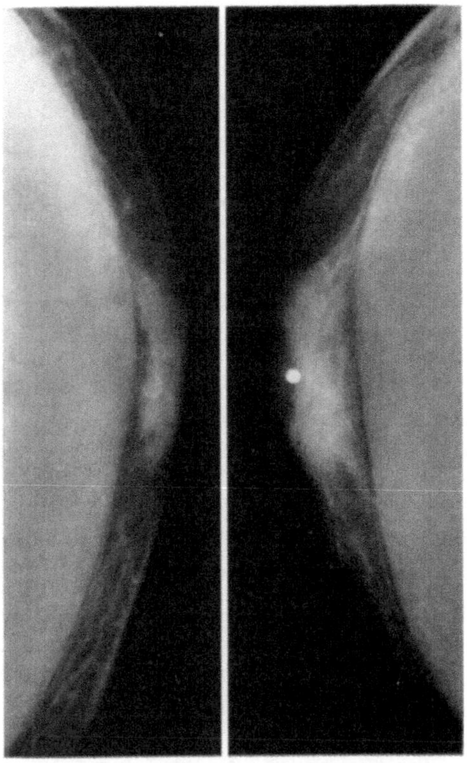

16

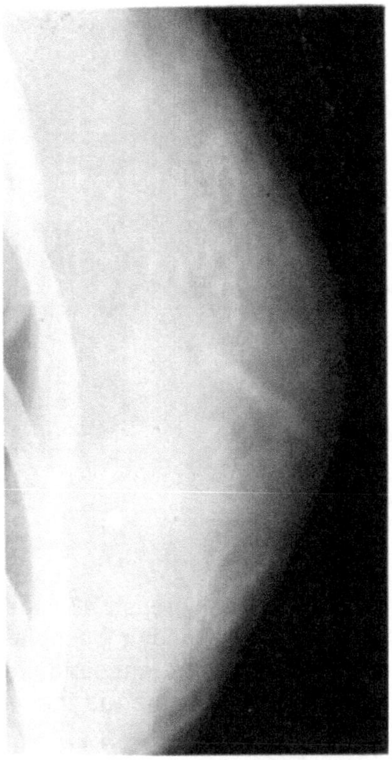

17

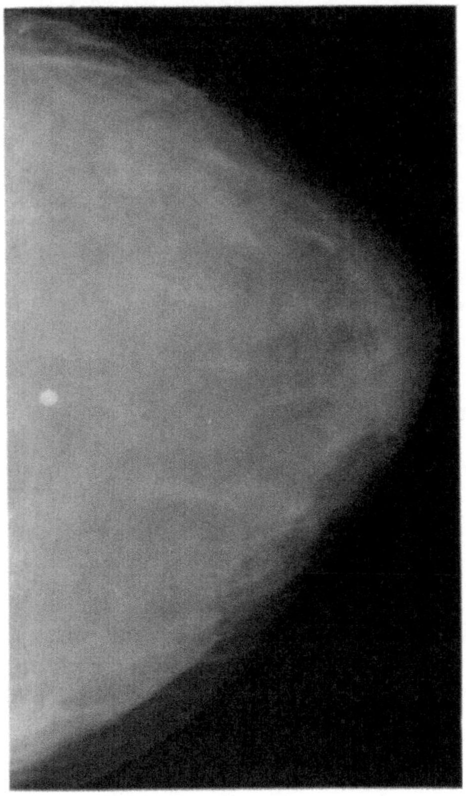

18

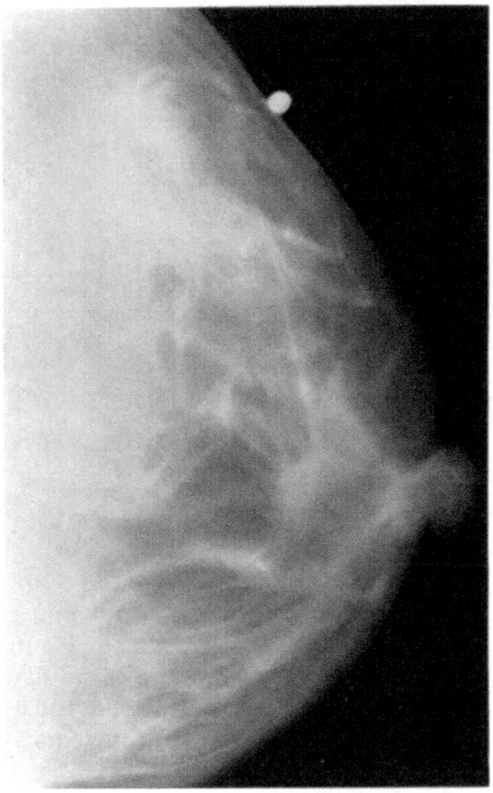

19

Fig. 20. Normal breast, 43 year old woman. The glandular tissue occupies chiefly the upper outer quadrant, and the trabeculae are bunched together as they approach the nipple

Fig. 21. Normal breast, 49 year old woman. Involution of the lobular components has occurred except in a small area of the areolar region. The trabeculae are fibrous

Fig. 22. Normal atrophic postmenopausal breast in a 58 year old woman. Complete involution and fibrosis of the glandular and ductal structures are clearly visualized by the fat replacement. The superficial veins stand out

Fig. 23. Normal atrophic breast in a 71 year old woman. The superficial veins and partially calcified arteries are clearly visible

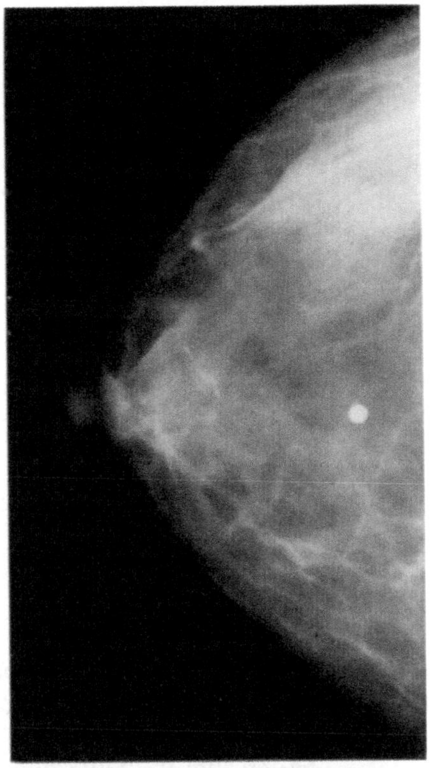

20

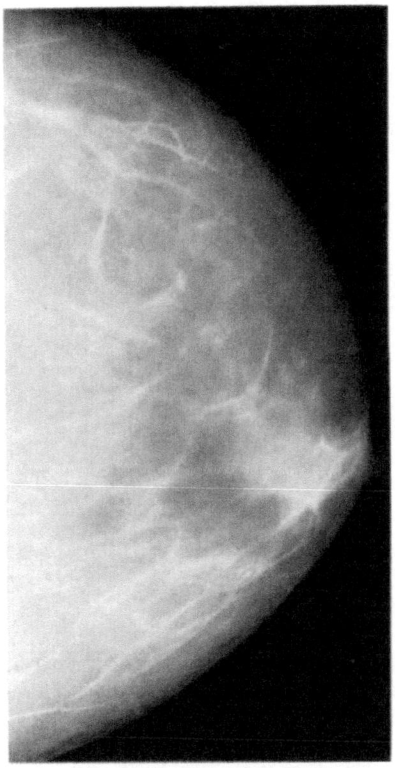

21

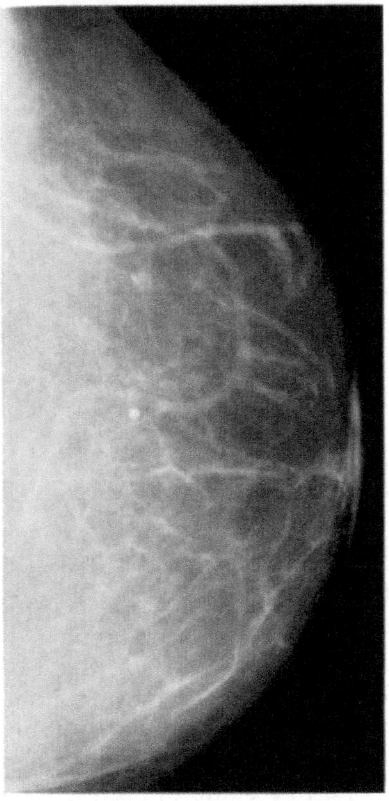

22

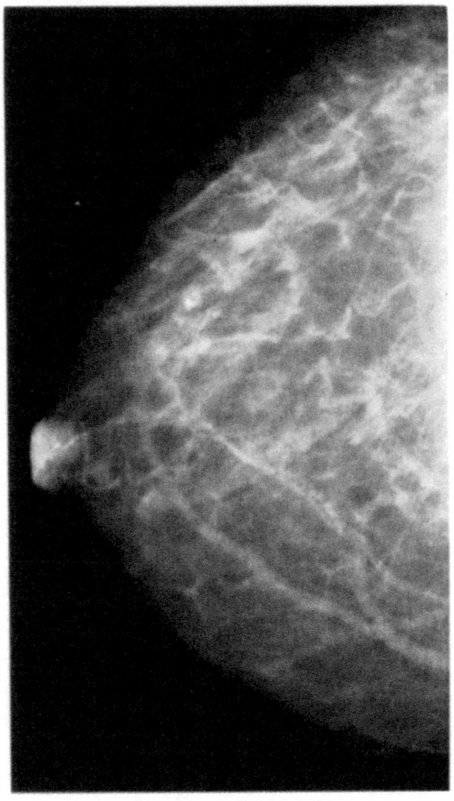

23

Fig. 24. Pregnancy, 4 months. Subareolar density with subjacent dilated, tortuous ducts leading to dense basilar lobular matrix

Fig. 25. Pregnancy, 5 months. The dilated, tortuous trabeculae merge with the dense lobular matrix to resemble mazoplasia fibrosa, so that a history and physical examination are needed to establish the diagnosis

Fig. 26. Pregnancy, 6 months. Dilated trabeculae conform with a history of gestation of 6 months' duration

Fig. 27. Pregnancy, 7 months. Dilated and tortuous ducts, dense lobular parenchyma, and prominent superficial veins are visible at this stage of pregnancy

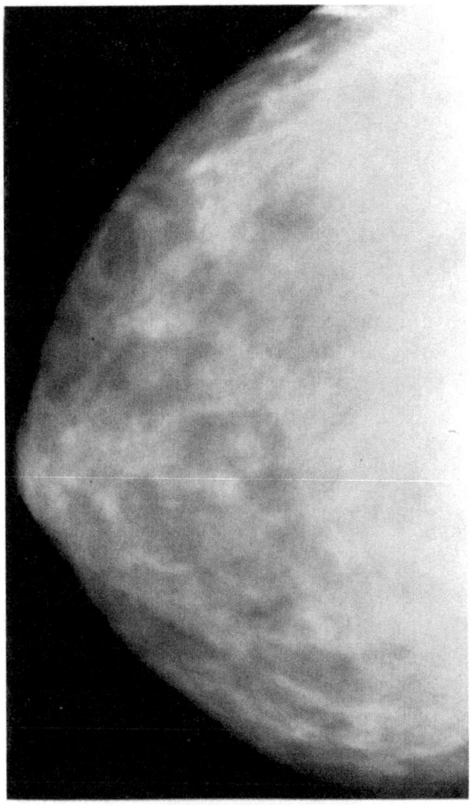
24

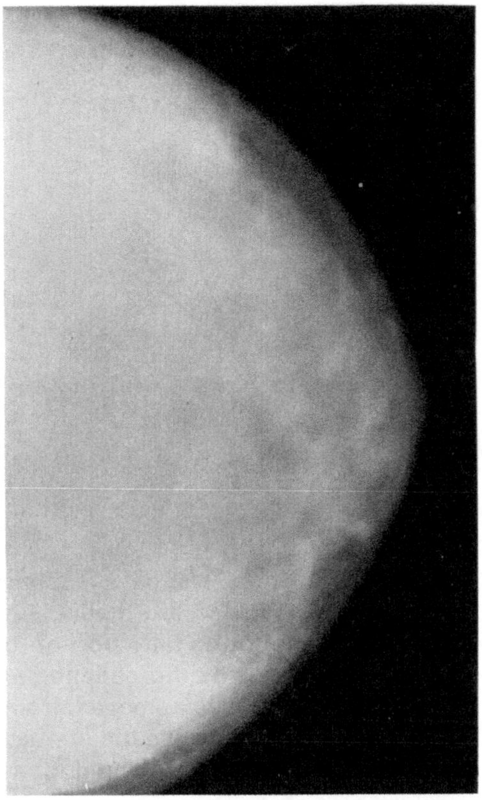
25

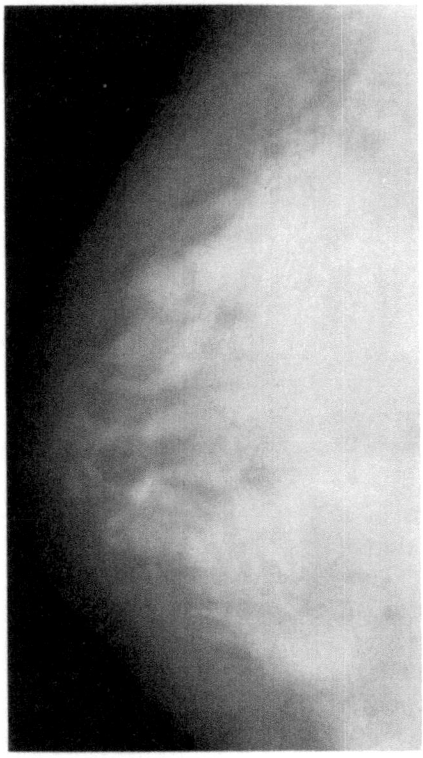
26

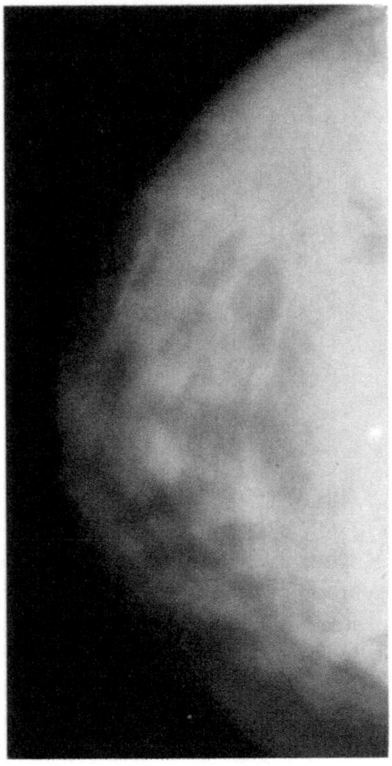
27

Fig. 28. Normal breast, 2 days postpartum. The dilated trabeculae are distinctly seen, especially in the lower fatty portion of the breast. Adenosis and a fibroadenoma were found in breast tissue removed from this 22 year old patient because the surgeon felt he was dealing with a "dominant mass"

Fig. 29. Postpartum breasts (6 weeks) in a 24 year old woman. The distended ductal system in the areolar area has not yet completely involuted, and in the presence of mazoplasia fibrosa the involution of the lobular system is not easily appreciated. A few dilated ducts can barely be discerned in the lower portion of the breasts

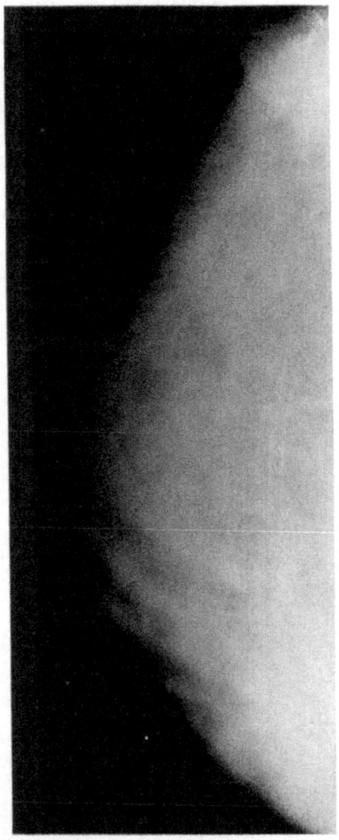

28

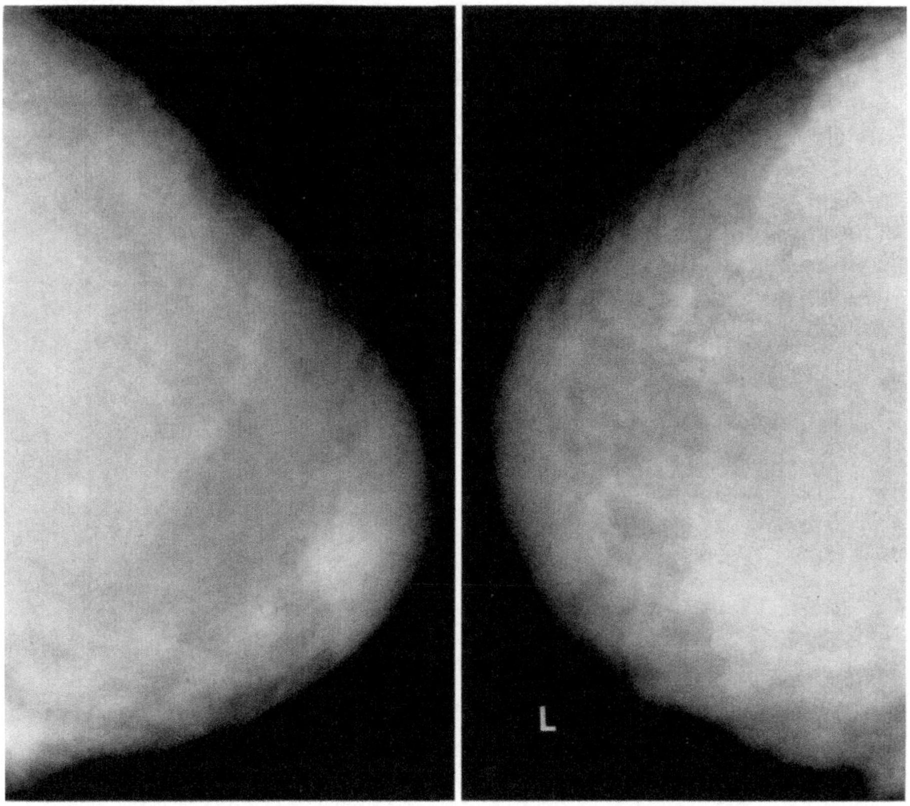

29

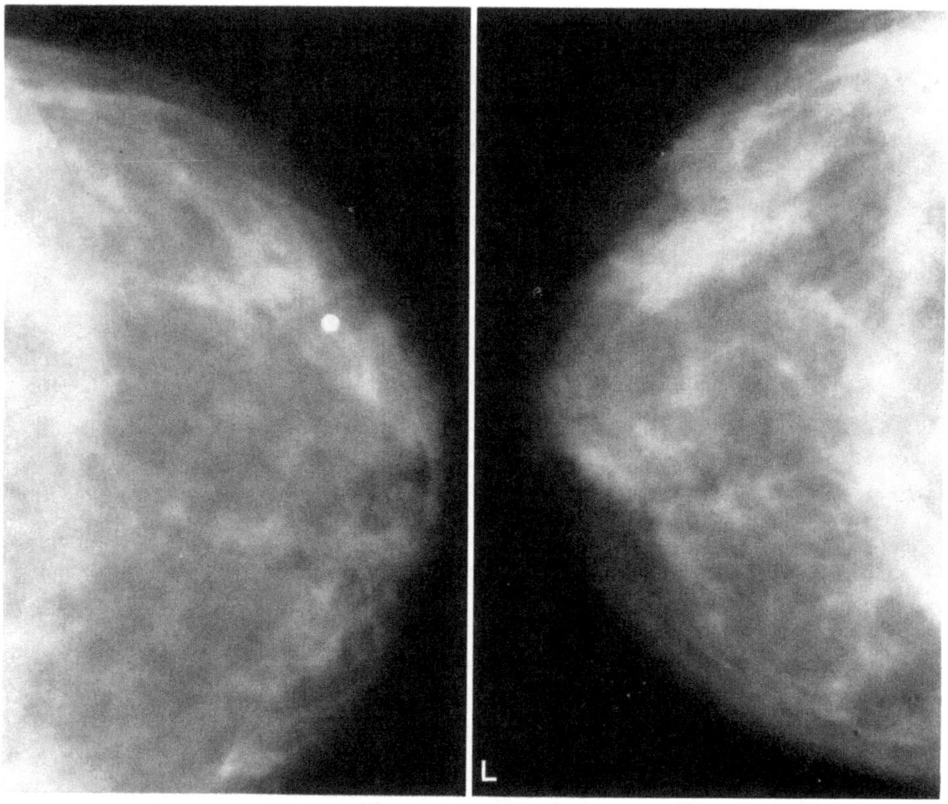

Fig. 30. Postpartum breast after 6 weeks of lactational involution. Some residual dilatation, elongation, and tortuosity of the ducts are visible. Lobular involution is almost complete. Only the pre-existing areas of adenosis remain, more prominent in the left breast. The surgeon thought a "dominant mass" was present in the right breast. No biopsy was performed, and the patient has remained well for 8 years

V The Dysplasias

1. History

Mammary dysplasia is a general term embracing benign lesions peculiar to the breast and essentially due to hormonal disturbance.

Noncancerous tumors of the breast were noted by Galen (A.D. 131—201). In more recent times Bellini (1730) described benign mammary tumors. In the 19th century Colles (1811) gave the first clear clinical description of dysplasia. He noted its connection with irregular menstruation and the disappearance of the tumors after pregnancy.

Sir Astley Cooper (1831) in his classic volume *Diseases of the Breast* speaks of "hydatiform" cysts. In his *Anatomy of the Breast* he describes changes in the feel of the breast during the menstrual cycle.

Benjamin Brodie (1846) laid a solid clinical and pathological foundation for what he named "serocystic" disease. His observations were confirmed by Reclus (1883). Histological observations were added by Schimmelbusch (1892). Prominent in the early part of the 20th century are the names of Aschoff, Semb, and Cheatle. German authors from 1890 onward linked some forms of dysplasia, especially abnormal secretion, with pelvic disorders. Moszkowicz (1927) noted uterine disorders and alterations in the sexual cycle in cases of mastopathy. Ingleby (1932) showed that cyclic changes occurred in fibroadenomas and postulated that these tumors were merely a local manifestation of the generalized disorders common to the mammary gland, especially toward the menopause.

Pathologically speaking, mammary dysplasia is essentially an abnormal interplay of epithelium and myothelium. It has no connection with bacterial inflammation. The term "mastitis" is a misnomer and should be dropped. "Fibrocystic disease" is a widely used term and as a descriptive label it fits many cases, but it offers little or no help in distinguishing between the varieties of dysplasias — a distinction which is often important from the prognostic point of view. Although much has been written on mammary cysts, very little has been said of the different *types* of cysts, and for this reason much of the voluminous work on the relation of cysts to carcinoma is valueless.

2. Classification

Classification of any group of disorders is valuable only insofar as it conforms to nosological entities. In other words, a classification must have clinical as well as roentgenographic and pathologic significance. There should be a clear clinical implication not only of diagnosis but of prognosis and treatment. An attempt must be made to distinguish physiologic aberrations from the strictly pathologic.

But breast lesions do not fit into absolute compartments. There is a certain amount of overlap between the physiologic and the pathologic and between the various types of dysplasias. No system therefore is entirely satisfactory, but so far as cyclic disturbances under the general heading of "mammary dysplasias" are concerned, the following simple, logical, and easily applied classification is proposed.

Classification of Mammary Dysplasias:

a) Hypertrophy and gynecomastia;
b) Adenosis;
c) Mazoplasia fibrosa;
d) Mazoplasia cystica;
e) Fibroadenoma;
f) Secretory disease (duct ectasia);
g) Epithelial hyperplasia, papillomatosis, and carcinoma in situ;
h) Mastopathy (Schimmelbusch's disease).

a) Hypertrophy and Gynecomastia

True juvenile hypertrophy is seldom seen before the age of 7 years. Thereafter, in little girls, hypertrophy without recognizable cause is fairly common. In boys, hypertrophy is rarely seen before the onset of puberty. Pathologic hypertrophy occasioned by tumors of the ovary, the adrenals, or the pituitary gland must be kept in mind.

On the X-ray film, the hypertrophied juvenile breast appears either as a rounded, circumscribed area of mammary parenchyma, or as an irregularly outlined opacity from which long strands extend toward the chest wall.

In adults, hypertrophy of the female breast is most often an abnormal continuation of adolescent development. Sometimes it has its origin in pregnancy or menstrual disorders.

Gynecomastia, or hypertrophy of the male breast, is quite common and usually without significance. It is due to hormonal imbalance and excessive circulation of estrogens. Hepatic dysfunction, which interferes with the breakdown of estrogenic substances, is an important etiologic factor, as is administration of estrogens to older men who have prostatic enlargement.

Attention has been drawn to mammary hypertrophy in cardiac patients following digitalis medication. Bilateral gynecomastia is common. In a small series, the X-ray film showed bilateral involvement in 22 of 34 cases, whereas clinically only nine cases of bilateral involvement were recognized.

Radiographically, the gynecomastic breast closely resembles that seen in juvenile hypertrophy. In the hypertrophy of puberty, the gland resembles that of adolescent adenosis (Figs. 31—36). In older men, strands of mammary parenchyma invade the surrounding fat as in mazoplasia fibrosa. These must not be mistaken for the tentacles of carcinoma. Hypertrophied trabeculae course in the expected directions from the nipple and cysts may occur. All the dysplasias can be found in gynecomastia (Figs. 37—42).

b) Adenosis

Mammary hyperplasia is a normal finding in the newborn, at puberty, and during the cycles of menstruation and pregnancy. Imitations and exaggerations of these processes are also found under conditions of hormonal imbalance. The boundary between normal physiologic changes and the entity called adenosis is therefore hard to draw. Essentially, adenosis may be defined as unencapsulated lobular hyperplasia.

Irregular parenchymatous hyperplasia is an extremely common finding in female breasts. X-ray studies show that the lesions are nearly always bilateral, although they may preponderate in one breast. The adenomatous foci may be confined to one area or scattered generally throughout the breasts. The most characteristic feature of adenosis and one that occurs in about one-half of all cases is variation in the size of the masses. In some cases, masses as large as several centimeters in diameter have been noted (Figs. 43—45).

Areas of adenosis appear as fluffy or blurred opacities, and breast trabeculae may be seen coursing through them. The margins may be sharp or curvilinear. Occasionally, apart from the trabeculae, an incompleted capsule is found, as though the lesion had set out to be a fibroadenoma but had not finished

the job. This is precisely what is seen in many pathologic specimens (Figs. 46—49).
In women with fatty breasts, the opacities are isolated between clear zones of fat. In generalized adenosis the films are dotted with fluffy opacities, sometimes confluent. Even with the use of the dissecting microscope it is often difficult to draw a line between early adenosis and normal lobules. But apart from such doubtful lesions adenosis may, in theory at least, be classified into four types of lobular dysplasia. The purpose of classification is to predict the outcome of the lesions (Figs. 50 to 52).
Type A is characterized by lobular hyperplasia with normal development of ductules. Microscopically, the lobules have a dense, bushy appearance and the ductules are lined by many more cells than usual. In places they push up the epithelium and may even occlude the lumen of the duct. In the prelobular ducts the hyperplasia is even more intense. It is logical that the myoepithelium should be exceptionally well developed in these ducts.
Type B presents lobules which consist of a few more or less dilated ductules. The lobules are numerous, but because they fail to form dichotomous branches their development is incomplete. Cystic dilatation occurs whenever the walls of a duct or ductule proliferate as a whole instead of at specific growing points. Microscopically, the affected lobules are seen as groups of small cysts.
Type C is nearly always found in the vicinity of a malignant tumor in young women. It must therefore be regarded with grave suspicion. The lobular hyperplasia in these breasts may be widespread, but there are no large cysts and the lobules consist of dilated ductules. The epithelium, especially that of the basal cells, may show proliferation, *but myoepithelial cells are inconspicuous or absent.* The essential factor seems to be a disturbance in the organization of the walls of the ductules. In these circumstances, *undifferentiated cells may accumulate within a duct.* If they do not degenerate and proliferation persists, the condition passes over into the type of epitheliosis which is a direct precursor of carcinoma.
Types A, *B*, and *C* cannot be differentiated on roentgenograms.
Type D is the sclerosing adenosis of Urban and Adair. The areas involved may vary in size from a centimeter or more in diameter to minute specks scarcely visible to the naked eye (Figs. 53, 54). In early stages, the microscopic section shows a mixture of epithelial and myoepithelial cells, the myothelium

preponderating. Later the nuclei are smaller and the myothelial cells develop long fibrous processes. Eventually they take collagen instead of muscle stain. The epithelial cells are few and degenerated, as in the normal menstrual phase.

Type D adenosis follows the rule that where myoepithelium is well developed the lesion is not likely to be precancerous. It does, however, mimic carcinoma very closely. In paraffin sections rows of myoid nuclei surrounded by fibrils are found and may be mistaken for epithelial invasion. Careful histologic technique coupled with experience is required if error is to be avoided.

In certain patients it has been possible to trace the development of adenomatous lesions over varying periods. Some of these masses disappear by a process similar to normal postmenstrual involution. Some disappear after pregnancy. Some, especially those of long standing, are replaced by fibrous tissue. Others develop into mazoplasia cystica, or form fibroadenomas.

Collateral evidence of resolution of the lesions is afforded by the long histories of patients with painful breasts in which lumps come and go and eventually subside at the time of the menopause. Most of the patients then have no further trouble. In elderly women, the X-ray film often reveals fibrous patches, usually bilateral and more or less symmetrical in distribution. The most likely interpretation of these would seem to be fibrosis following adenosis. The lesions might be thought of as quiescent. Unfortunately the facts do not always warrant this assumption (Figs. 55—60).

Another common form of fibrosis which follows involution of adenosis is hyperplastic fibrosis, commonly seen at or after the menopause. We have been able to trace its transition from adenosis to fibrosis on X-ray films and in pathologic specimens. While this type of fibrosis is not necessarily precancerous, it is intimately associated with certain forms of carcinoma.

Type B adenosis, which comprises about three-fourths of the cases seen, is definitely not a precancerous lesion. The same may be said of Type D. The one form of adenosis which may be dangerous is Type C. It is deceptively like Type B on superficial examination and can be recognized only by the scarcity or lack of myoepithelial cells. In cases of carcinoma, myoepithelial cells are rarely present in the tumor area. In microscopic sections where the diagnosis of malignancy is in doubt, the presence of well-developed or hyperplastic myoepithelial cells in the tumor indicates a benign lesion. *Their absence is strongly suggestive of carcinoma.*

The possibility of progression of benign dysplasias to a neoplastic state must not be overlooked. At present, it is generally accepted that carcinoma occurs four times as often in dysplastic breasts as it does in normal breasts, but we have much to learn of the type of dysplasia which precedes the malignant change. Perhaps the most important objective of classification is the distinction of intrinsically benign from potentially malignant states.

The fact that carcinoma is a possibility, albeit a remote one, emphasizes the need for a certain caution in dealing with adenosis. Although as a rule no treatment is necessary, patients with adenosis should be kept under observation. By far the best method is periodic mammography.

c) Mazoplasia Fibrosa

Cheatle coined the term "mazoplasia" to denote diffuse nodular painful breasts (from the Greek words "mazos," for breast, and "plassein," meaning to form). He believed it to be an entity "sui generis." His description and illustrations show that adenosis, especially Type B, is included in his syndrome. Mazoplasia was also described by Semb (1928) under the name "fibroadenomatosis simplex (microcystica)." Cheatle's work of the 1930s should not lightly be forgotten. Our interpretations have changed with time, but Cheatle's observations, descriptions, and illustrations may still be studied with profit. The term "mazoplasia," which simply means hyperplastic breast, is retained, although with some qualifications of its meaning, as a fitting tribute to a great man.

Pathologically, the gross appearance of the breast is fairly characteristic. The gland may be small and tough and often feels nodular, but when the nodules are cut down upon there is no obvious lesion. The cut surface looks normal. In both slicer and paraffin sections the outstanding feature is hyperplasia of the fibrillary (intraductal) zone which lies immediately beneath the epithelium of the ducts. The duct presents a collar of fibrillary tissue many times the diameter of its lumen. This may cause compression atrophy of the epithelium, with narrowing or complete obliteration of the lumen.

In other ducts the lumen proliferates to some extent, and these ducts will show mild dilatation. There is considerable diminution in the number of lobules. In their place one finds groups of club-shaped ducts. Their general conformation simulates the pattern of terminal ducts in the adolescent breast. Under the dissecting microscope the contrast between the closely packed ducts of the adolescent gland and the sparse thickened ducts of mazoplasia is obvious.

Focal fibrillary hyperplasia of the intraductal tissue, if it continues, leads to fibroadenoma of the intracanalicular type which often accompanies mazoplasia.

In early studies of the mammary gland by roentgenography we were struck by a group of cases in which the breast was uniformly dense and homogeneous. Comparison of the films with the pathologic sections showed that we were dealing with mazoplasia of the type described by Cheatle, or mazoplasia fibrosa of our classification (Figs. 61—64).

The condition is most often seen in women before the age of 30. As in all dysplasias, the lesions may be general or focal, and are practically always bilateral. Fibroadenomas, single or multiple, are very common (Figs. 65, 66).

The nodules of mazoplasia fibrosa must be distinguished from areas of adenosis and from cysts. Radiographically, the breast in mazoplasia fibrosa closely resembles the adolescent or immature breast and may be indistinguishable from it. Both show the same uniform density, but in mazoplasia fibrosa the subcutaneous margin of the gland may be bosselated. If the lesion is localized to one quadrant, the smooth "ground glass" opacity will be confined to that area. The coexistence of fibroadenomas might be expected to confirm the diagnosis, but since these tumors are also commonly found in adenosis and mazoplasia cystica, this sign cannot be relied upon (Fig. 67).

d) Mazoplasia Cystica

Mazoplasia cystica is a form of dysplasia which combines adenosis and cysts with intraductal fibrosis and, often, fibroadenomas. It has its onset most often in the 30s and 40s. Increase in intraductal connective tissue is an important and probably fundamental component of the disorder.

Many women complain of a sudden onset of pain and the appearance of a mass. This history occurs too frequently to be ascribed merely to the patient's imagination. Generalized pain with swelling is the rule in women with mazoplasia cystica, but in contradistinction to adenosis, variations in the size of the mass are rarely noted. Waxing and waning of the tumor are probably due to accompanying adenosis rather than to the cysts themselves. On the whole, the cysts tend to increase in size as well as in number. We have never been able to verify disappearance of a cyst before the menopause other than by evacuation of its contents.

The cysts are found with diminishing frequency after the menopause and few persist after 60 years of age. Cysts in mazoplasia are generally multiple and usually bilateral.
Cysts vary in size from microscopic dimensions to those occupying a large segment of the breast, but only those more than 0.5 cm in diameter can, as a rule, be seen on an X-ray film. On a satisfactory film, they appear as well-defined opacities with a smooth outline. Isolated simple cysts are usually spherical; conglomerate and loculated cysts are either oval or have irregularly scalloped borders (Figs. 68—72).
As with tumors, cysts are more distinctly visualized on a background of fat. Fortunately for radiologic diagnosis, the majority occur after 25 years of age when fat begins to be a normal component of the breast. There is little difference in the degree of density between cysts and breast parenchyma, but the uniform density of a cyst helps to distinguish it from the trabecular structure of breast tissue. Bloody fluid or hemosiderin in cysts increases their density. A clear space or halo is sometimes seen around cysts as well as around fibroadenomas. However, since some circumscribed carcinomas also show a clear peripheral zone, this sign cannot be relied upon to determine diagnosis.
A second important distinction is the type of scalloping of the border. Multiple and multilocular cysts show notches at the points of overlap. When clearly outlined, the notches are angular. Notches are also seen in carcinoma, but they are rounded. The diameter of cysts as measured on the film is usually greater than the diameter measured on the patient. In carcinoma the reverse is true (Figs. 73—78).
Multiple cysts are frequently bilateral even when the patient limits complaints to one breast. In the absence of cysts, adenosis may be expected in the contralateral organ. Solitary cysts are usually unilateral (Figs. 79, 80). To find a single cyst of the mazoplastic type is unusual, although they do occur. Large apocrine cysts are occasionally seen. Very often a single large cyst is found to be inflamed. If the inflammation is severe, an origin other than mazoplasia should be considered. A differential diagnosis between cyst and fibroadenoma cannot always be made on the X-ray film (Figs. 81, 82). The point will be discussed under fibroadenoma.
Pathology and Pathogenesis of Cysts. The most obvious, if not the most important, features of mazoplasia cystica are the cysts. Cysts are common in the breast and differ in their characteristics according to the type of dysplasia which has engendered

them. The principal varieties, apart from the common mazoplastic type, are apocrine, secretory, and papillary. Pseudocysts are occasionally seen, as in some cases of fat necrosis.

Apocrine cysts are to be expected since mammary parenchyma and apocrine sweat glands are derived from the same anlage. Small apocrine cysts occur in the breasts of practically all women over the age of 30 and need scarcely be thought of as pathologic. Often small papillae project into the cysts. The myoepithelial cells are extremely large and well developed and are similar to those of normally situated apocrine glands.

Although secretory disease is characterized by dilatation of ducts, secretory cysts large enough to be clinically obvious are the exception rather than the rule.

Papillary cysts are easily confused with mazoplasia cystica both clinically and radiographically. It seems likely that the papilloma has its origin in a duct and that the growth of tumor tissue, together with secretion from the hyperplastic epithelial cells and hemorrhage from broken or degenerated papillae, causes cystic distention of the duct.

Apart from the necessity of differentiating them from other conditions, large simple cysts of mazoplasia have no significance. More important is the adenosis which is practically always present and which precedes cyst formation. In the vast majority of cases, good cell differentiation is present and the myoepithelium is abundant in the neighboring fields of adenosis. The adenosis may be of Types A, B, and D, none of which is dangerous. Only if Type C were found, especially if accompanied by intraductal hyperplasia, would there be any question of a precancerous condition. Unfortunately, when cancer does arise in these breasts it is apt to be in areas of adenosis away from large cysts.

An all too popular treatment for patients with large cysts is to drain or remove them. It is useful to verify whether the cysts have collapsed after withdrawal of fluid and to check on the presence of any other lesions which might have been masked by the cyst. Mammographic examination after the injection of an amount of air less than the fluid withdrawn has a double advantage. It verifies the success of the operation and the absence of intracystic growth (Figs. 83, 84).

e) Fibroadenoma

Fibroadenomas have been given many names. A few reflect some theory of origin, but most are merely descriptive. Since these tumors originate from the mammary parenchyma the term "adenoma" is strictly accurate. "Fibro-" understood as an adjective is in order because of the propensity of the myoepithelium to form fibrous tissue.

With a few exceptions fibroadenomas arise during the period of sexual activity. The incidence reaches its peak between the ages of 20 and 25 years. The chief symptom is the presence of a freely movable mass. In most cases the tumor is solitary, but two or more are not uncommon. Occasionally numbers of tumors are seen.

Since fibroadenomas consist of tissue resembling that of the normal mammary gland and of about the same density, in the dense breasts of young women they are especially difficult to discern.

The tumor is seen as a sharply defined, round, ovoid, or slightly bosselated opacity. Often a clear halo is seen around it. Some fibroadenomas are only partly outlined. This means that the mass is only partly encapsulated, a common feature in recent growths. Another exception to the sharp margin is found in menstruating fibroadenomas. Their outlines are often fuzzy due to intense engorgement and edema. Cysts within the tumor as well as mucoid degeneration, seen in so many fibroadenomas, do little to change the X-ray appearance (Figs. 85 to 92).

Calcification, which is rather common in long-standing tumors of elderly women, is readily recognized by its bizarre appearance. The plaque-like deposits are easily distinguished from the fine grains of calcium seen in carcinoma and still more easily from the larger, more widespread areas found in late secretory disease and fat necrosis (Figs. 93, 94).

The differential roentgenologic diagnosis of fibroadenomas would be a simple matter were it not for their close resemblance to cysts. Both fibroadenomas and cysts show smooth sharp margins. Cysts are apt to be circular, but so are some fibroadenomas. A halo is not diagnostic since a clear space occasionally surrounds a cyst. Cysts are more often multiple, but a conglomeration of cysts may mimic a bosselated fibroadenoma. Fibroadenoma is the more likely diagnosis if the breast is that of a young woman, and in practice considerations of age, history, mode of onset, and the like are often helpful.

Fibroadenomas are quite frequent in breasts with carcinoma, but the distinction between the sharp smooth outline of the fibroadenoma and the spiculations of the carcinoma is ordinarily easy to make. If difficulty arises, the question may be settled by comparing the measurements of the tumor in the patient and on the film. The measurements of the carcinoma are smaller on the film than in the patient, while those of the fibroadenoma are usually larger.

The earliest fibroadenomas are seen in conjunction with some other form of mammary dysplasia, such as mazoplasia fibrosa, or in an unencapsulated area of lobular hyperplasia (adenosis). The rapid growth of the breast at puberty is often attended by foci of irregular proliferation. With the termination of the adolescent period most of the irregularities become absorbed into the general lobular pattern of the breast. If abnormal proliferation continues, the surrounding connective tissue becomes compressed and forms a capsule around the area.

During pregnancy and lactation some tumors grow rapidly. Others, although the epithelium undergoes alteration, show very little overall increase in size. Some tumors lactate and secretion may persist in them even after the breast as a whole has returned to the nonpuerperal state. After the menopause the fibroadenomatous tissue is often hyalinized and sometimes calcified.

Rarely, there is an outburst of myoepithelial and epithelial hyperplasia in the tumor and a giant fibroadenoma (cystosarcoma phyllodes) is formed. The majority of giant fibroadenomas occur about the time of menopause. Such tumors are occasionally malignant and may have an alarming sarcomatous appearance under the microscope.

Authors have tried to classify fibroadenomas according to their histologic appearance, but detailed classifications such as this implies have few, if any, uses and may erect barriers where none exist. To make a separate classification for each of the types would obviously be absurd. In tumors which originate in areas of adenosis, variations are present from the start and are even more accentuated when aggregations of abnormal lobules are added to the original mass.

Each part of a tumor may proliferate in a different way. In one and the same tumor may be represented the lesions of mazoplasia cystica and fibrosa; adenosis Types A, B, and D; intraductal hyperplasia; papillomatosis; and myoid hyperplasia with fibrosis. To add to the confusion, normal cyclic changes may be expected. These are most evident at the periphery of the tumor. Besides proliferation, degenerative changes are present in all but very recent tumors. Edema and mucoid degeneration, hyalinization, and calcification are common. Epithelial necrosis occurs in the massive shedding that is sometimes associated with menstruating tumors. Larger areas of necrosis result from sudden interference with the blood supply. Adipose tissue may be included in a fibroadenoma, but actual fatty degeneration is unusual.

Bizarre features, occasionally met with in human mammary tumors, have misled observers into coining names such as chondroma, osteochondromyxoma, etc., thereby implying a different type of growth and harking back to the so-called "mixed" salivary gland tumors described by older pathologists. Of course, salivary gland tumors and myothelial mammary growths have much in common.

Carcinoma is hardly ever discovered arising in a fibroadenoma. Proliferation of epithelial cells is seen occasionally in fibroadenomas and accompanies hyperplasia of the tumor as a whole. But even in large and active tumors there is a strong tendency for differentiation to myothelium rather than epithelium.

Sarcomas, while rare, originate in fibroadenomas more frequently than in other breast structures. Perhaps "sarcoma" is a misnomer, since the tumor arises from immature myoepithelial cells. The differential diagnosis between sarcoma and giant fibroadenoma (cystosarcoma phyllodes) is often difficult. Sudden growth accompanied by pain in a fibroadenoma which has been quiescent for years should arouse suspicion (Figs. 95 to 99).

In summary, it may be said that careful histologic appraisal of many fibroadenomas yields strong evidence that, although epithelial proliferation may occur pari passu, in most of them the myothelial stroma predominates. The statement that the common form of fibroadenoma is a myothelial tumor is therefore justified.

f) Secretory Disease (Duct Ectasia), Plasma Cell Mastitis, Fat Necrosis, Mammary Abscess

Secretory disease is a form of mammary dysplasia characterized by the secretion of milklike substances in a nonpregnant, nonpuerperal breast. The condition has long been known and has been described sporadically under various names, such as varicocele tumor of the breast, comedo mastitis, mammary duct ectasia, and the like. Its common sequel, plasma cell or chemical mastitis, has remained largely unrecognized except in the rare generalized form. In recent years, roentgenographic studies combined with serial sections of entire glands have established that secretory disease and plasma cell mastitis are one nosological entity and clarified much that was previously obscure.

Although secretory disease is the direct cause of chemical mastitis, better known as plasma cell mastitis, it is never inflammatory in its inception and may run its entire course without inflammatory complications. The term "comedo mastitis" is therefore incorrect and moreover substitutes a purely descriptive term for an etiologic cognomen. Although cysts occur, the ducts are often uniformly dilated rather than strictly cystic. As in mazoplasia cystica, the cysts are not fundamental; they are secondary to hyperplasia of all the components of the duct wall. Secretory disease may engraft on any of the dysplasias and is rather frequently seen with mazoplasia cystica.

In secretory disease distention of the lumen by products of secretion is a prominent feature. Here, if anywhere, blocking of the ducts by thick, inspissated secretion might plausibly be invoked to account for the dilated ducts and the occasional cysts.

Actually, in secretory disease there is proliferation of both epithelium and myothelium. The proliferation is followed by differentiation of the epithelium into secretory cells and the myothelium into fibrous tissue. Because of more complete differentiation, cell proliferation ceases sooner than in mazoplasia. Hence there is less growth of the duct wall, the dilatation of the lumen is never as great as in advanced cases of mazoplasia cystica, and cysts are not formed to the same extent.

X-ray studies have shown that secretory disease is nearly always bilateral. In the absence of complications, many patients are asymptomatic. The inference is that secretory disease is not in itself harmful. Symptoms, when they appear, are generally unilateral and the majority of clinical cases show at least minimal plasma cell mastitis.

The history differs in many respects from that which obtains in other forms of dysplasia. The age of onset is difficult to determine because manifestations may show themselves only after years of quiescence. When symptoms do appear the patient is usually alarmed and seeks advice promptly. The age at which symptoms are discovered varies from the early 20s to the 70s. Nearly all cases occur in married women.

The chief symptoms in the order of their diagnostic importance are nipple discharge, nipple retraction, tumor, and pain. The first two are seldom present together because the fibrosis which causes retraction is apt to compress the ducts beneath the nipple and block the exit of secretion. Either may be unilateral or bilateral.

Nipple discharge occurs in about 40 per cent of cases as compared with 5 per cent for nipple retraction. Secretion may be intermittent or continuous. In uncomplicated cases in young women the discharge resembles milk. Some patients give a history of recrudescence of lactation after they had stopped nursing. Usually the secretion ceases, to return months or years later. Pregnancy is not necessarily a factor. Lactation in virgin breasts is a well known although rare clinical phenomenon.

In older women the discharge is thick or inspissated and is apt to be discolored gray or yellow. Occasionally a serous or frankly bloody discharge is seen, but repeated examination reveals the usual opaque secretion. In plasma cell mastitis it is reddish brown, green, or even black. The colors are due to degenerated blood which oozes from ulcerated surfaces in the ducts. Bright red discharge is unusual.

Retraction of the nipple takes place gradually over a longer period of time than is the rule in carcinoma. Bilateral retraction when not congenital is strongly indicative of secretory disease.

The X-ray appearance, although highly characteristic, will vary with the age of the patient and the length of time the disease has been present. The film is apt to show dilated ducts beneath the nipple resembling those of pregnancy. The ducts of older women are often irregularly dilated and have a beaded appearance, easily confused with papilloma. Longstanding fibrosis around the lactiferous ducts is discerned as an opacity shaped like a truncated cone with the apex at the nipple (Figs. 100—102).

Pain is not characteristic of secretory disease per se, although some women complain of a drawing sensation and bilateral fullness which is relieved by nipple discharge. Pain is usually an indication that *plasma cell mastitis* has supervened. A typical history is one of slight trauma, insufficient to cause damage in a normal breast, followed a short time thereafter by pain and then by a tender mass. The skin may be reddened or occasionally discolored. The sequence indicates rupture of an inflamed duct wall with extravasation of blood and discharge of the contents into the surrounding tissue. A reaction is set up akin to fat necrosis. Traumatic fat necrosis, also a form of chemical mastitis, is excluded if the trauma is but slight. In both conditions, the pain and redness subside in a few days and the mass becomes smaller.

When plasma cell mastitis is also present, ill-defined flame-shaped shadows spread from the fibrous area toward the base of the breast (Figs. 103, 104). Generalized plasma cell mastitis betrays itself by indistinct smudgy opacities which may be unilateral or bilateral (Fig. 105). They vary greatly in extent and numbers. The diagnosis is helped by seeing accompanying signs of secretory disease on the X-ray film. In the absence of such signs the differentiation from other lesions may be impossible.

A few small calcific deposits in the region of ducts affected by secretory disease of some duration are a fairly common finding on correctly exposed films. These deposits are tubular in the ducts and spherical in the lobules. The tubular casts of calcification vary in length and diameter with their location and with the type and extent of the dilatation of the ducts. The lobular casts vary in number, size, and location. Many are so small as to appear to be solid dots of calcification, but the larger casts have radiolucent centers, and so we tend to call these deposits "epithelial pearls" (Figs. 106—108).

More spectacular is extensive calcification of ducts occasionally seen in longstanding cases in elderly women. Rarely, there may also be irregular calcified patches similar to those sometimes found in healed fat necrosis. These probably indicate an old focus of plasma cell mastitis which is pathologically a similar lesion. It is obvious that however startling the roentgenologic appearance in these cases, the lesion is quiescent and surgical intervention is not required.

Differential Diagnosis. Secretory disease must be differentiated from carcinoma, papilloma, intraductal hyperplasia, other forms of mammary dysplasia, papilloma, intraductal hyperplasia, fat necrosis, and abscess. Onset with pain, a tender mass, and discharge from the nipple indicates plasma cell mastitis. The mass in acute cases gradually becomes smaller. The greatest difficulty arises when an elderly woman discovers a hard painless lump indistinguishable from carcinoma on palpation. There may be no nipple discharge or, to make matters more confusing, the patient may give a history of a bright bloody discharge which ceased before advice was sought. Roentgenographic examination is then mandatory.

Surprisingly, in some of these cases no tumor is seen on the film. On the other hand, if an opacity is present it will tend to be larger than the mass as measured clinically. A carcinoma would be smaller and more dense. The margins would be more sharply defined than in plasma cell mastitis. The tentacles in carcinoma usually cut across the line of the trabeculae. The extensions of plasma cell mastitis spread along the trabeculae. Examination of the other breast would show secretory disease. Clinically, papillomas are confused with secretory disease because of the discharge which may occur in both. As in secretory disease a mass may or may not be present. Pain is unusual in papilloma.

Intraductal hyperplasia of the precancerous type is extremely hard to recognize without radiographic help. The X-ray film usually shows irregularly dilated ducts and sometimes fine non-polarized calcifications. The calcifications in secretory disease are tubular, ovoid, or spherical and aligned with the long axes of the ducts. The fact that they are most often situated in the wall of the duct and not in the lumen as in hyperplasia gives them a characteristic contour well seen in advanced lesions. A transverse view of a calcified duct shows a sharply defined deadwhite ring with a clear central lumen, resembling the so-called epithelial pearls, mentioned previously. Seen longitudinally, the duct appears as a cylinder with open ends.

Fat necrosis produces a cell reaction similar to that of plasma cell mastitis. This is to be expected since fat necrosis is a feature of both conditions (Figs. 109, 110).

Breast abscess is a fairly common complication of the puerperium. It can also be seen apart from the gestational cycle and even occasionally beyond the menopause.

The older, more complex classifications of mammary abscess are open to objection on various grounds. A simple division of abscesses into those that are superficial and those that are intramammary seems satisfactory.

a) *Superficial abscesses* are usually due to a cracked nipple, an infected Montgomery gland, or a skin infection. The cause is usually self-evident. The abscess seldom affects the gland itself, so there is no need to elaborate its pathology and roentgenography.

b) An *acute abscess* appears on the film as an irregular density, often with flame-shaped extensions. At first, and in rapidly spreading lesions, the boundary is indistinct (Figs. 111, 112). Localization of the abscess is shown by the development of sharp margins resembling those of a cyst (Fig. 113). Encapsulation is apt to be incomplete for some time when broad tentacles are seen to emerge from the abscess margin.

An important sign which often helps in differential diagnosis is edema of the skin. Thickened skin is seen on the film in all active lesions if they are large. If the lesion is small and deep-seated, the cutaneous edema may be absent and the abscess will be more difficult to diagnose. Distended veins are a feature of the acute stage; they persist as long as the infection is active (Fig. 114).

c) The *chronic* stage of an abscess, especially in nonpuerperal women, is difficult to distinguish from a cyst both clinically and mammographically. The outlines of a chronic abscess are sharp. In the absence of pertinent history, an obsolescent lesion would probably be mistaken for a cyst; but if inflammation is still present in the surrounding tissue, portions of the circumference will appear slightly blurred. Edema of the areola and surrounding skin is a feature of all forms of subareolar abscess. The nipple may actually be retracted, but more often only appears to be so because the swelling pushes up the adjacent tissues while the nipple itself is anchored by the lactiferous ducts (Figs. 115, 116).

Healing may take place in a breast abscess, as elsewhere in the body, by fibrous replacement. The pus is slowly absorbed and the abscess cavity is replaced first by granulation and then by fibrous tissue. At this stage, X-ray diagnosis is extremely difficult. In fact, the patternless fibrous tissue forming part of the healing abscess is usually impossible to distinguish from nonspecific fibrosis or even cancer.

d) *Recurrent Abscess and Mammillary Fistula.* Recurrent abscess may be the result of inadequate treatment. There is, however, one form, named mammillary fistula, in which recurrence is almost inevitable unless the condition is rightly understood and proper surgical measures taken. In general, the history is that of an abscess in the subareolar area which was incised but which healed only with difficulty. After months, even years, a fresh exacerbation occurs with formation of a fistula. Excision of the fistula is not usually effective, but cure follows saucerization of the lesion.

In mammillary fistula infection follows stasis of secretion in a lactiferous duct. The first abscess is sometimes associated with lactation, but more often the cases are nonpuerperal and are a complication of secretory disease. Stagnant secretion is a good culture medium, and in secretory disease the liability to abscess formation may be increased by ulceration in the wall of the duct and discharge of contents into the surrounding tissue. The area of chemical mastitis thus produced is vulnerable and invites the lodgment of bacteria which gain access to it from the skin.

The X-ray film of mammillary fistula shows a retracted, sometimes edematous nipple partly surrounded by a thickened fold of skin. The fistula is best shown by injection of opaque material. The prodromal stage of mammillary fistula may be recognized on the X-ray film by the presence of dilated lactiferous ducts in the abscess region. The duct ectasia may be puerperal but is more often due to secretory disease. In all cases of subareolar abscess, dilated ducts should be looked for.

Although acute puerperal abscesses admit of ready diagnosis, the same is by no means true of the nonpuerperal form. A good clinical history is essential. Without it, an abscess may be mistaken for hematoma, fat necrosis, secretory disease (when accompanied by cysts), plasma cell mastitis, adenosis, mazoplasia cystica, fibrosis from scar tissue, and carcinoma.

Differentiating abscess from plasma cell mastitis is important and often difficult. To open and drain an area of chemical mastitis is to invite infection. Neglecting an abscess may result in a spread of cellulitis. Where doubt exists, the differential diagnosis must be made on clinical grounds. The initial fever, pain, and swelling decrease in chemical mastitis; they increase in abscess. But enormous veins surrounding a lesion which appears benign requires the exclusion of an abscess before a diagnosis of cyst or adenosis or even plasma cell mastitis can be made.

Confusion between abscess and carcinoma occurs only rarely, but their occasional resemblance sets a trap for the unwary. Abscess is characterized by rapid onset of pain, but this may happen also in inflammatory carcinoma. Tentacles are fewer in abscess than in carcinoma. Spicules are not an obvious feature. The presence of minute calcified particles emerging from a tumor is proof of malignant growth.

g) Intraductal Epithelial Hyperplasia, Papillomatosis, and Carcinoma in Situ

Intraductal epithelial hyperplasia is often considered precancerous. In point of fact, most often the condition is benign. On the other hand, the reverse proposition is certainly true: most carcinomas do have their origin in intraductal proliferation. Hence careful study is indicated in all cases of this disorder.

Grossly, all stages of ductal dilatation are encountered, depending on the amount of epithelial proliferation within the ducts. Some degree of ectasia is always present. Well-developed papillomas cause focal distention, and where they are multiple the ducts are characteristically beaded. Epithelial hyperplasia without true papilloma may cause irregular dilatation depending on its severity and the extent of the lesion. In many cases of irregular dilatation a mixture of unorganized cell proliferation and papilloma is encountered.

Papillomas have no counterpart in the normal mammary gland. In this they differ from the dysplasias. Fibroadenomas are called tumors, but are in reality focal dysplasias.

Papillomas betray their presence by nipple discharge, often intermittent and usually bloody. As a rule the blood is bright red. When blood is not present the discharge is serous. A tumor may or may not be felt. Other forms of intraductal hyperplasia may also be signaled by bloody nipple discharge. Sometimes hyperplasia, benign papillomas, and malignant papillomas are found in close juxtaposition in the same duct.

Contrast mammography may be used with considerable success in the diagnosis of papilloma (Fig. 117). A single intraductal mass may be accurately outlined, and with suitable instruments an intraductal biopsy may be taken. In the hands of a competent operator the procedure is safe and need not cause pain.

An X-ray diagnosis of papilloma is possible in most uncomplicated cases even without contrast mammography, although it is more difficult. On the roentgenogram a single papilloma will produce an opacity in the course of a duct. In multiple papillomas the film shows beaded varicose ducts leading to the nipple. In most cases the ducts are clearly discerned. They might, however, be confused with similar tortuous ducts seen in secretory disease. Both conditions may show a collar of homogeneous opacity beneath the nipple, but in secretory disease fibrosis is more marked (Figs. 118—122).

When a papilloma is accompanied by a collection of fluid, it is referred to as an "intracystic papilloma." When these lesions become malignant, they are called "intracystic papillary carcinomas." In either case, the lesion appears to be benign because of its smooth, sharp contours and margins. However, when notching occurs and comet-tail extensions issue from the periphery, the possibility of cancer is suggested (Figs. 123 to 125).

Replacement of the evacuated fluid with air can uncover the presence of the solid papillary growth inside the air-containing cyst.

Intraductal hyperplasia, while not invariably recognizable on the X-ray film, can be suspected in many cases and sometimes a definite diagnosis can be made. The larger ducts are dilated and of irregular caliber; definite beading is likely to be associated with papilloma. But the most significant sign, although not always present, is calcification. The calcifications resemble those seen in duct carcinoma. They may occur in tiny clusters or in rows. Their detection requires sharp eyesight and meticulous examination of the film, especially since they may occur away from a palpable mass and other lesions are apt to attract the attention of the radiologist.

Sometimes small deposits or clusters of microcalcifications may be found widely scattered in both breasts. The finding is alarming at first as indicative of widespread carcinoma; but the absence of symptoms, signs, or the occurrence of a tumor during the course of repeated examinations over months or years allays fears of the supervention of cancer (Fig. 126). We prefer to advise diagnostic resection to rule out carcinoma in situ.

Precancerous Hyperplasia, Carcinoma in Situ. There is at times a massive proliferation of cells which are uniform, not increased in size, and of normal nuclear pattern, but which show no tendency to organization. In some cases, these cells probably degenerate and cause no further trouble. In others, the cells may show some lack of uniformity, and in still others all degrees will be found, up to the atypical cells of carcinoma in situ. A very careful search must be made for the existence of a small carcinoma.

Another form of carcinoma in situ resembles carcinoma in everything except infiltration of the surrounding tissues. Groups of ducts are lined by a collar of rather uniform carcinoma cells which make no attempt to organize. The lumen is occupied by necrotic material, often with small foci of calcification. Carcinoma of this type grows extremely slowly and may remain in situ for a very long time.

Carcinoma in situ is clinically benign. Until growth invades the adjacent structures it does not metastasize. It is the last stage of intraductal hyperplasia before frank carcinoma develops.

Occasional minute calcifications are seen in benign papillomas, but fairly numerous calcifications, especially in the absence of a palpable tumor, suggest carcinoma in situ. If the presence of a few small calcifications is accompanied by disruption of breast structure, malignancy — whether intraductal or extraductal — is suspected, but differentiation between benign proliferation, precancerous proliferation, carcinoma in situ, and frank carcinoma may be impossible.

In the presence of a localized abnormal breast pattern, with no similar condition in the opposite breast, the X-ray film is then of service in designating the site for biopsy, a mandatory procedure in these circumstances whether or not the lesion is palpable.

b) Mastopathy (Schimmelbusch's Disease)

The term mastopathy is reserved for breasts excessively involved with multiple dysplasias. When the breast shows predominance of one type with only minor variations, the pathologic designation is assigned to the predominant lesion. Since different areas in the breast are involved in various kinds of dysplasias, a paraffin section is not usually sufficient to establish a complete diagnosis. The entire breast must be studied. Clinical examination is also not very satisfactory. In contrast, the radiologist is able to see everything mirrored on the X-ray film.

Roentgenographically, mastopathic breasts present features associated with adenosis, mazoplasia fibrosa, mazoplasia cystica, fibroadenoma, secretory disease, cysts of various origins, and fibrosis consequent to healing of some of the lesions. The changes are excessively scattered irregularly throughout different portions of the breast, and may involve one breast, but usually both.

In the older patient, fibrosis due to healing of some lesions is nearly always a conspicuous feature. It may be of any type but is usually nonspecific. If there is much fat in the breast, the fibrosis is essentially atrophic. If the breast is dense and compact, the fibrosis is hyperplastic and excessive. Thus, one must be wary in dealing with these dense, hyperplastic breasts, especially in the 6th and 7th decades, when a small cancer may not be detected readily in them (Figs. 127—133).

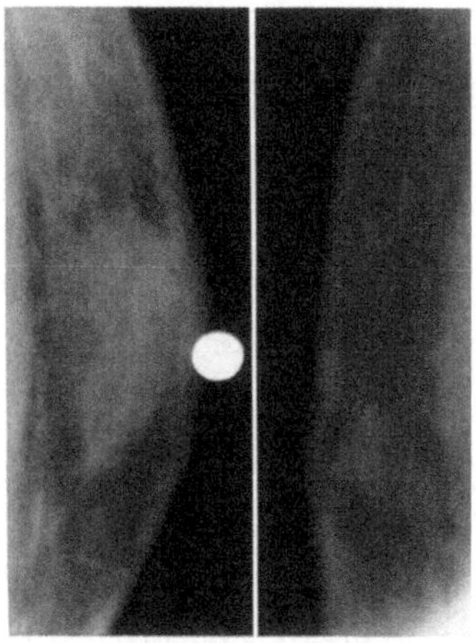

Fig. 31. Gynecomastia. The mazoplasia may be so dominant on one side as to appear unilateral

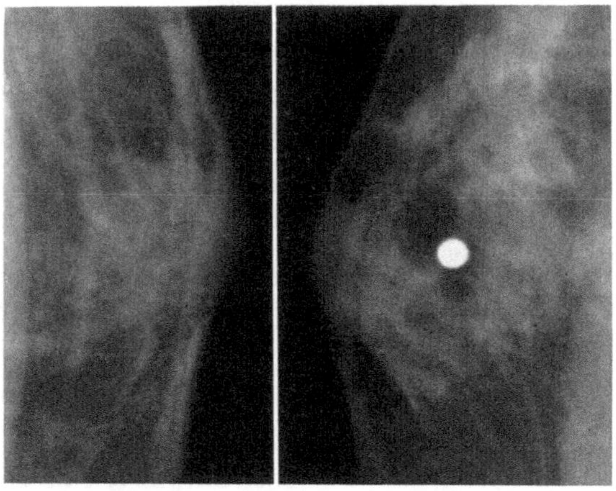

Fig. 32. Bilateral gynecomastia in a 24 year old patient. Pain was present in the left breast in the area under the skin marker. Proliferative ductal structures with flame-like peripheral margins are common to gynecomastia in young patients

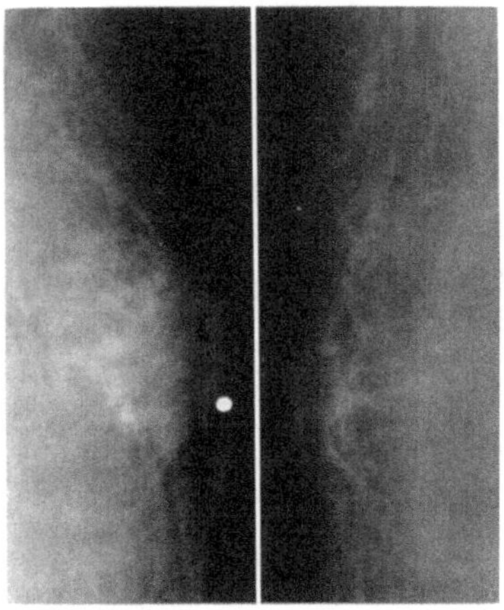

Fig. 33. Gynecomastia. Normal architectural hyperplasia is more advanced in the right breast of this 38 year old male than in the left

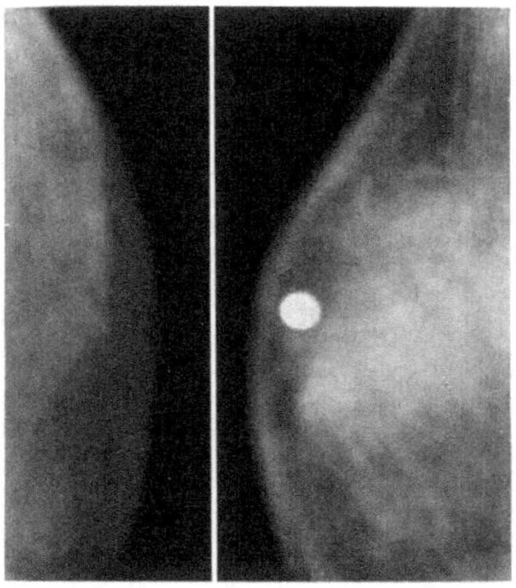

Fig. 34. Gynecomastia. Patient 49 years of age with mass in left breast under skin marker. Density and outline of breast tissue resemble that of mazoplasia fibrosa of female adolescent, but because male cancer can have this appearance, biopsy may be necessary

Fig. 35. Gynecomastia. The swelling of the breasts in some cases of gyneco-mastia seems mainly to be limited to increased arborization of ducts in a fibrillar matrix

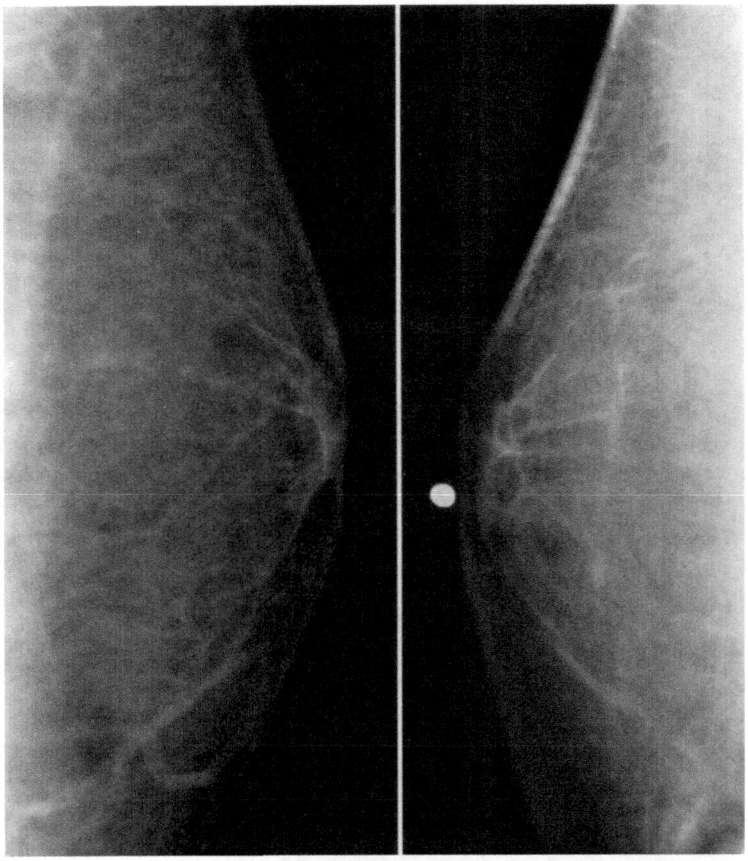

35

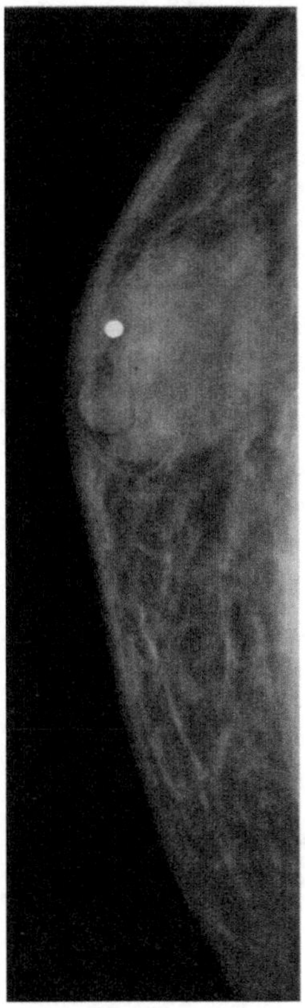

36

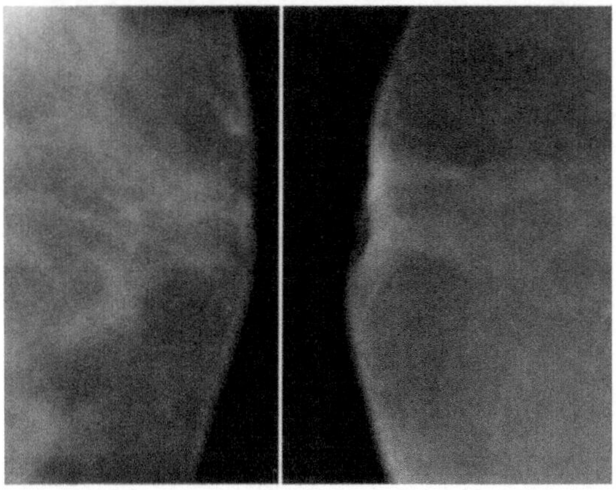

37

Fig. 36. Gynecomastia. The mazoplasia of gynecomastia may be uniformly dense and well circumscribed. The margins may undulate, resembling adenosis, fibroadenomas, or cysts, all of which may be present

Fig. 37. Gynecomastia. Predominantly one-sided ductal proliferation in a 57 year old male. In this type of dysplasia, resembling duct ectasia, the risk of failure to detect a cancer is negligible even though the patient is 57 years old

Fig. 38. Gynecomastia in a 64 year old man. The dense breast tissue, circumscribed except for a few peripheral strands, suggests mazoplasia fibrosa of adolescence. A biopsy is always advisable in this age bracket to exclude an obscured carcinoma

Fig. 39. Gynecomastia. The circumscribed hyperplasia is more pronounced on one side in this 66 year old male two years after prostatectomy. Only resection can establish the absence of an obscured cancer

Fig. 40. Gynecomastia. The mazoplasia of gynecomastia of the left breast of a 67 year old man resembles that of the normal female pubertal breast. When breast enlargement occurs after the age of 55 years, a diagnostic resection is always advisable since cancer can easily escape detection

Fig. 41. Gynecomastia and cyst. While gynecomastia is usually simply mazoplasia fibrosa, the cystic form of mazoplasia may occasionally be encountered and, rarely, larger isolated cysts, as in this instance

Fig. 42. Gynecomastia may be secondary to chronic administration of digitalis

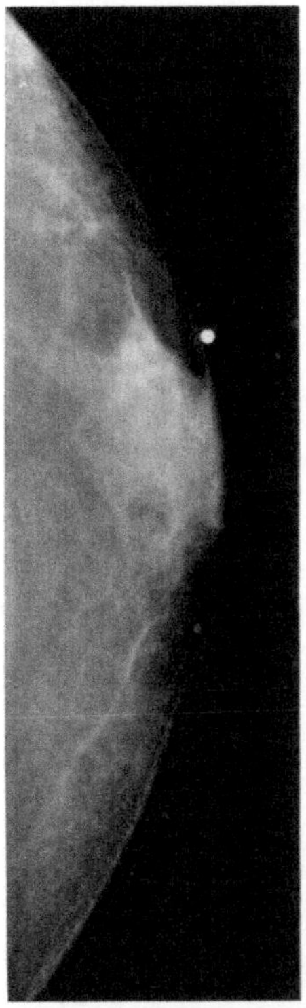
38

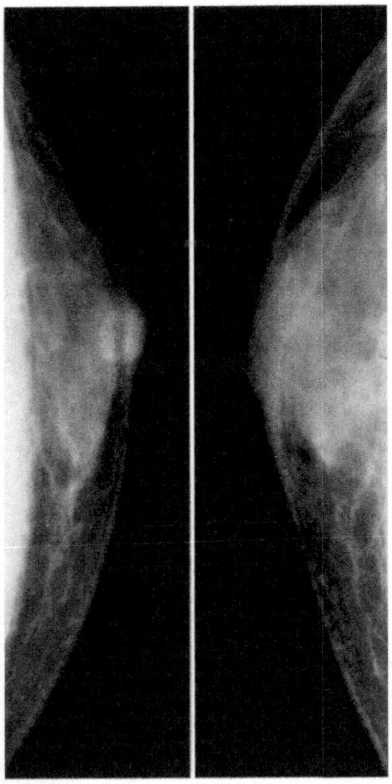
39

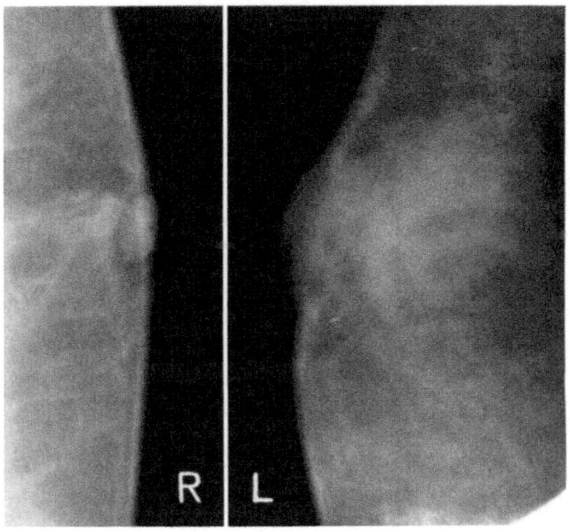

40

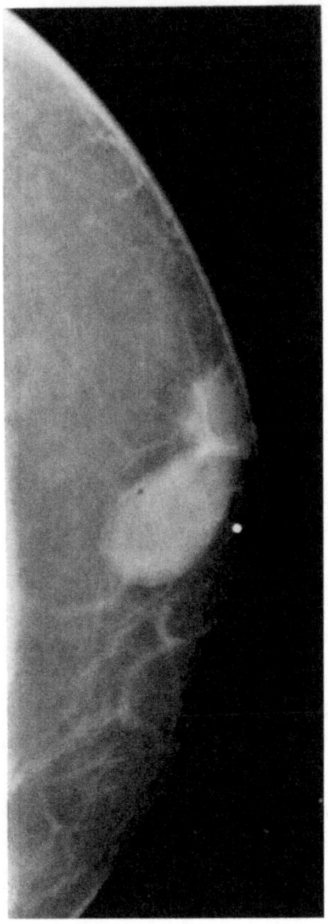
41

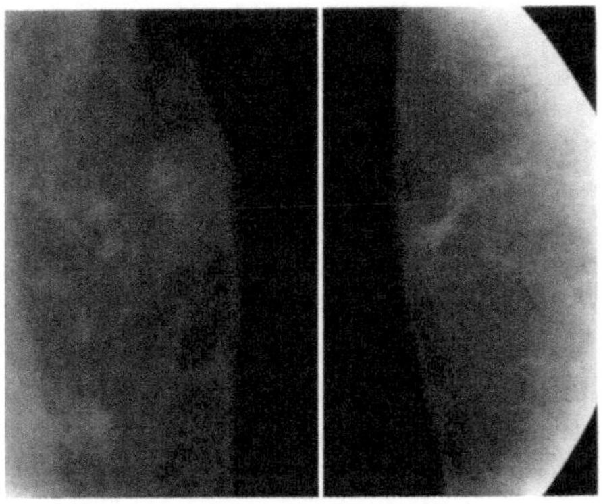
42

Fig. 43 A and B. Lateral view (A) and cephalocaudad view (B) of left breast of an 18 year old girl with secretion from both nipples. A more or less homogeneous density made of whorl-like patterns in an adolescent suggests adenosis. Fibroadenomas, some of which may be actively secreting, are occasionally found in such breasts

Fig. 44. Adenosis. In the early adult period of lobular growth, adenosis develops, crowding into the bases of Cooper's ligaments in the subcutaneous zone. The encapsulated anterior margins of lobules then become serrated, as in this 27 year old woman

Fig. 45. Adenosis. Whorls of homogeneous densities suggest adenosis. The possibility of an obscured cancer in such tissue in women over 30 years of age must be kept in mind, and a biopsy is warranted if the patient localizes symptoms or a palpable mass is present

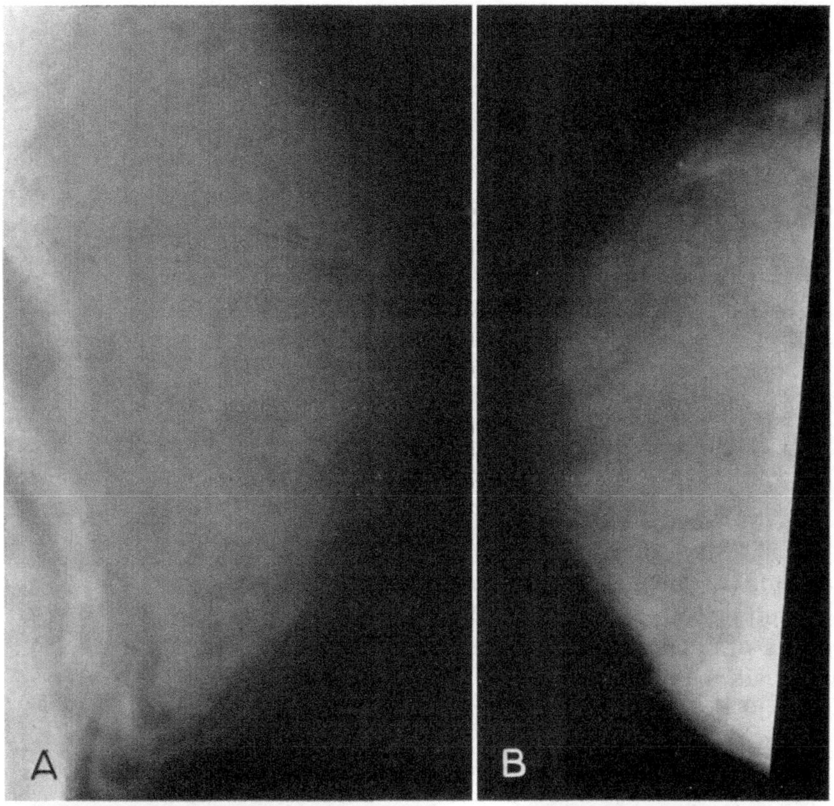

43

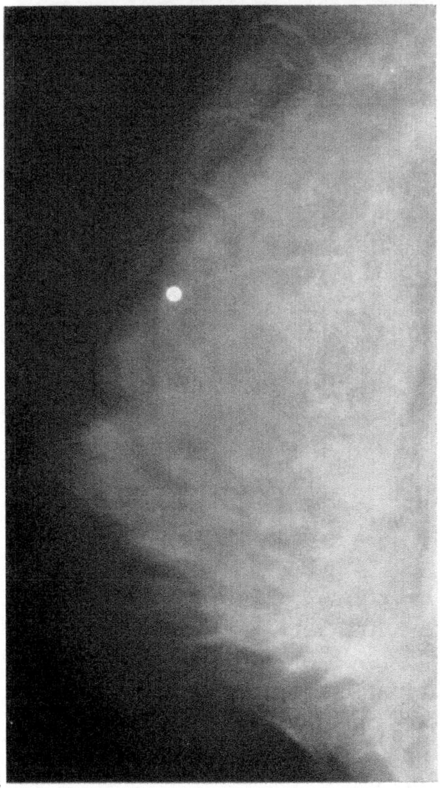
44

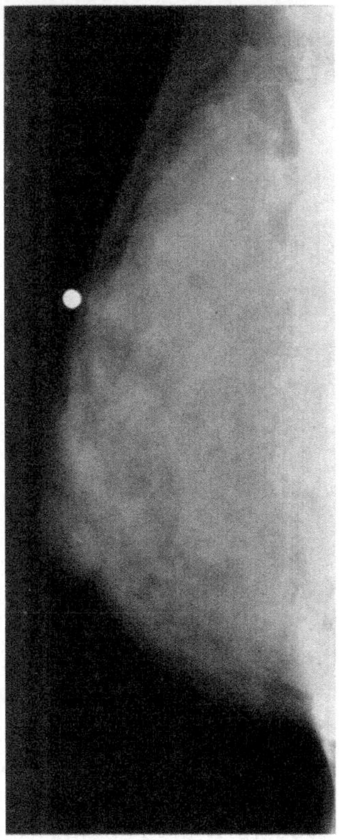
45

Fig. 46. Adenosis. As women pass through the third decade of life, whorls of tissue of homogeneous density appear in the intertwined peripheral ductal systems. In these fields of adenosis, fibroadenomas (arrows) or cysts may appear, and will only become evident if there is sufficient perifocal fat to afford contrast

Fig. 47. Adenosis. In the mature adult, fat invasion of the breast separates islands of poorly defined homogeneous densities of adenosis. Fibroadenomas and cysts may be interspersed, and cancer may lurk in such breasts without being readily detected

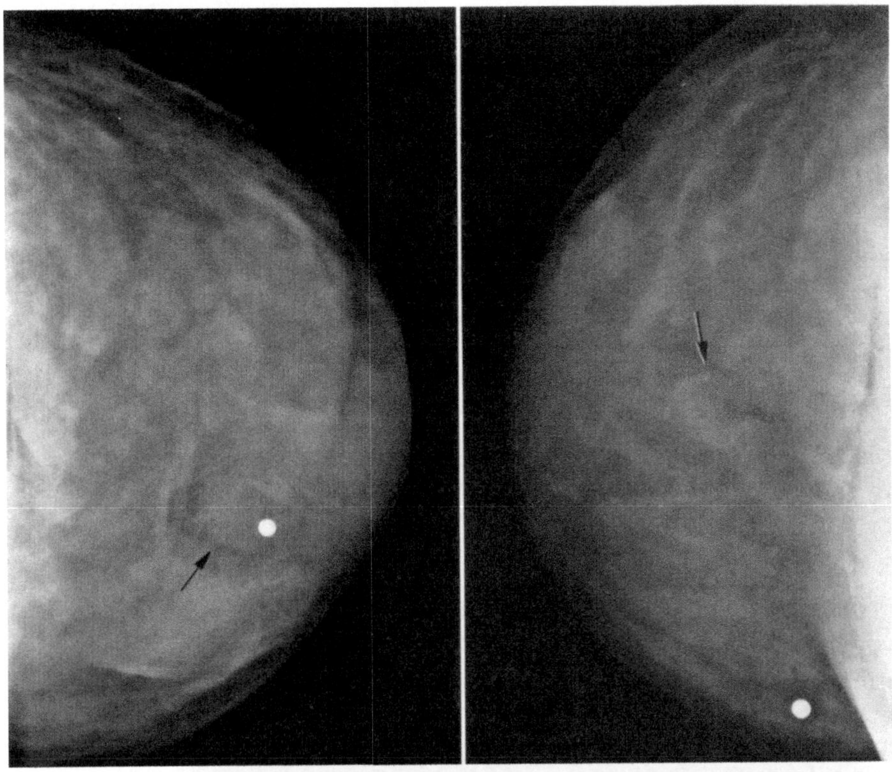

46

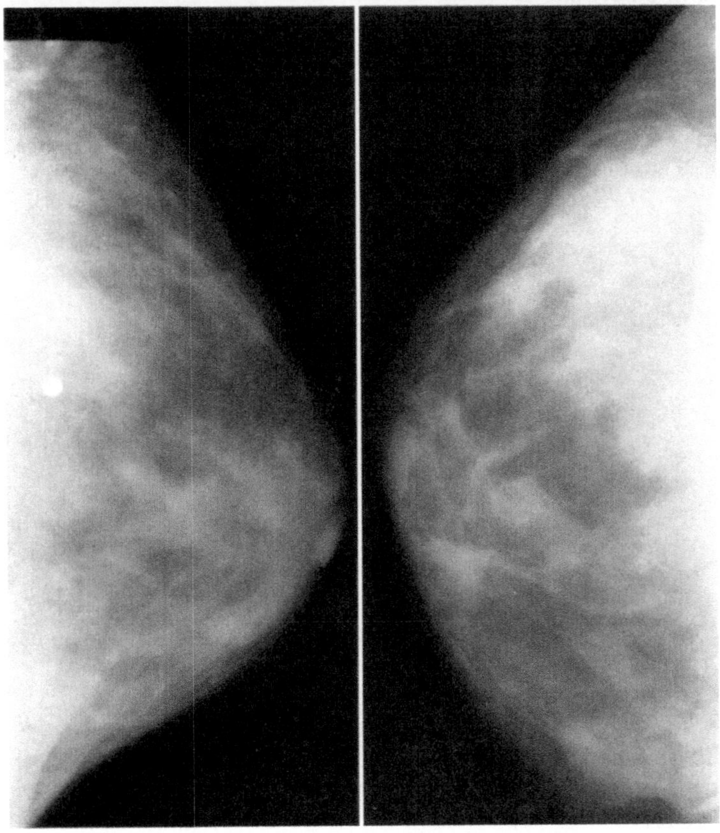

47

Fig. 48. Adenosis. Scattered, poorly defined zones of homogeneous density mark the presence of adenosis. The tendency to margination suggests increased fibrosis and sclerosis

Fig. 49. Adenosis. Irregular zones of homogeneous density make up the structural components, and where the borders are smooth and sharp, fibrous contraction and sclerosis are occurring (arrows). A large cyst is present in the upper part of the left breast

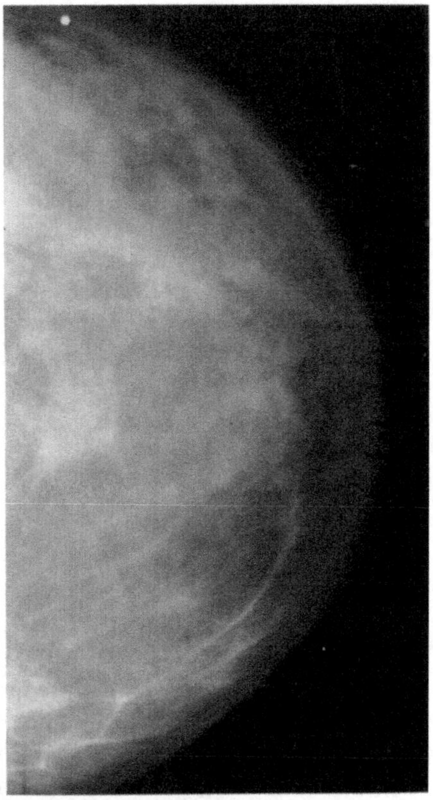

48

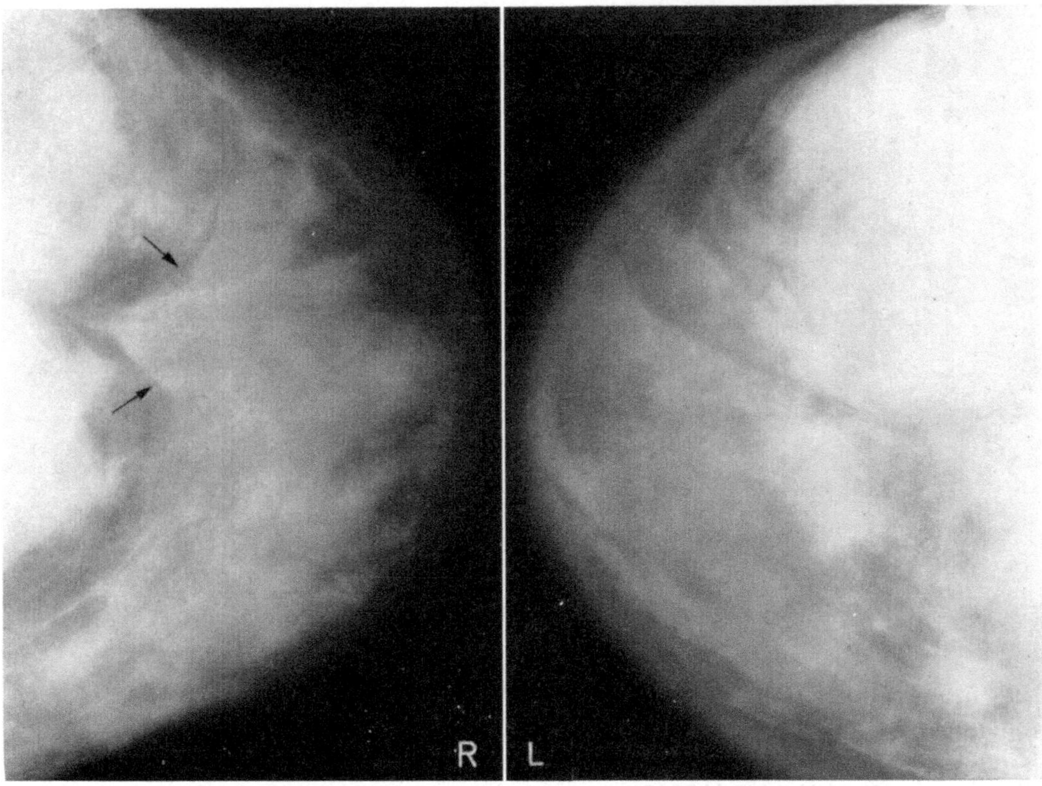

49

Fig. 50A and B. Adenosis. Lateral (A) and cephalocaudad views (B). When residual adenosis of the menopause involves chiefly the anterior breast, the fibrosis with traction on surrounding tissues may come to resemble infiltrating duct cell cancer

Fig. 51. Adenosis. The residual zones of adenosis encountered at times in postclimacteric women may be irregularly outlined and may resemble cancer

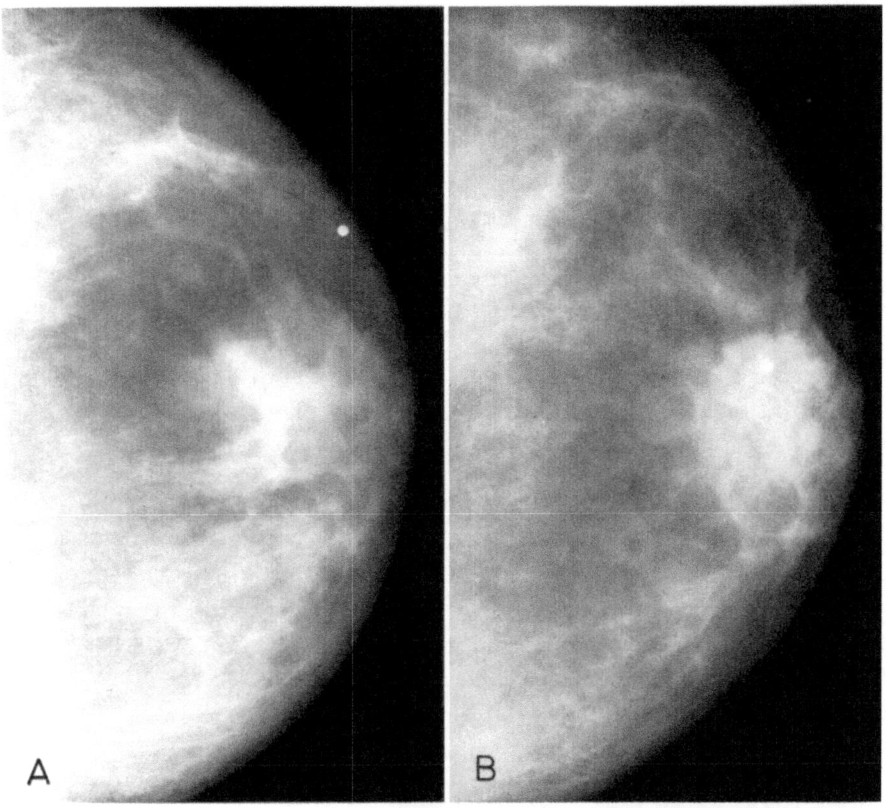

50

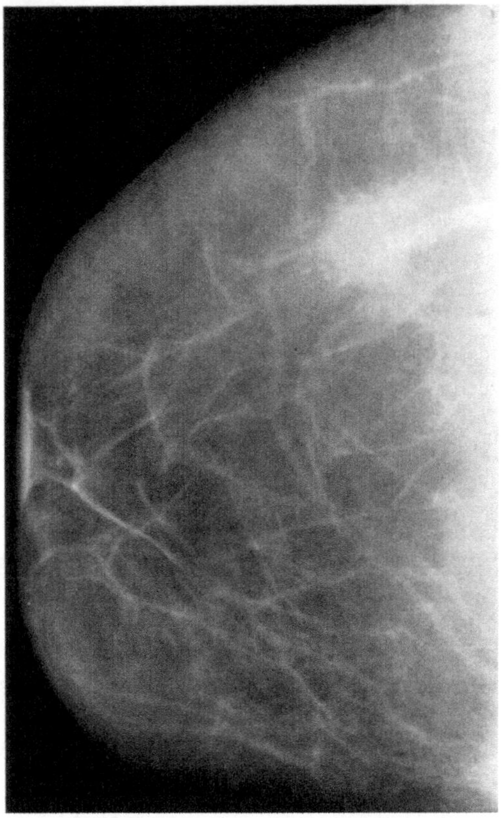

51

Fig. 52. Adenosis. When adenosis is associated with ductal epithelial hyperplasia, the ductal trabeculae are prominent in the anterior breast while the homogeneous densities of adenosis are more pronounced in the posterior breast region

Fig. 53. Adenosis, Type D (sclerosing adenosis). Arrows point to straightened margins due to beginning fibrous contraction of patches of adenosis which, on section, revealed prominence of myoepithelial cells in the tissues. As fibrous involution increases, the density and contraction increase, resulting in full-blown "sclerosing adenosis"

Fig. 54. Adenosis. Patches of adenosis with homogeneous density are irregularly distributed. Some denser areas with sharper outlines are due to sclerosing adenosis (arrow)

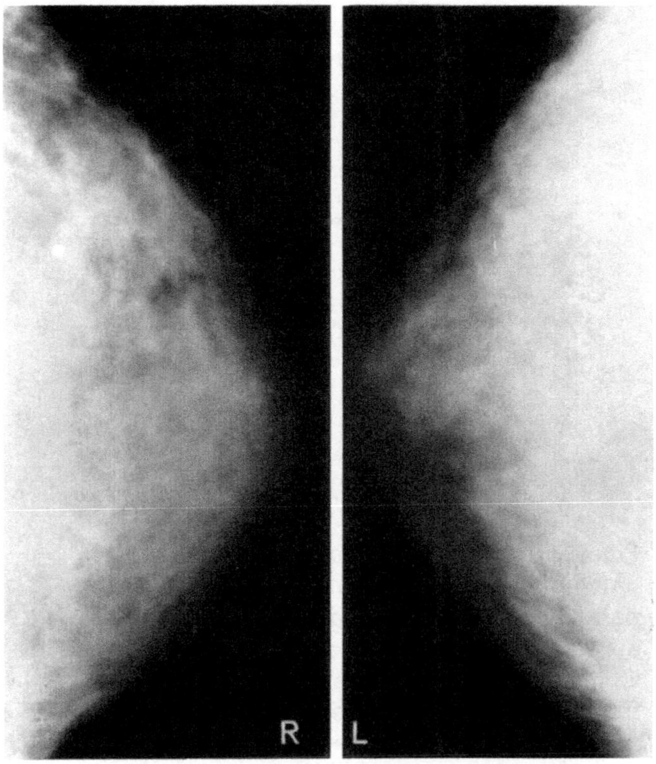

52

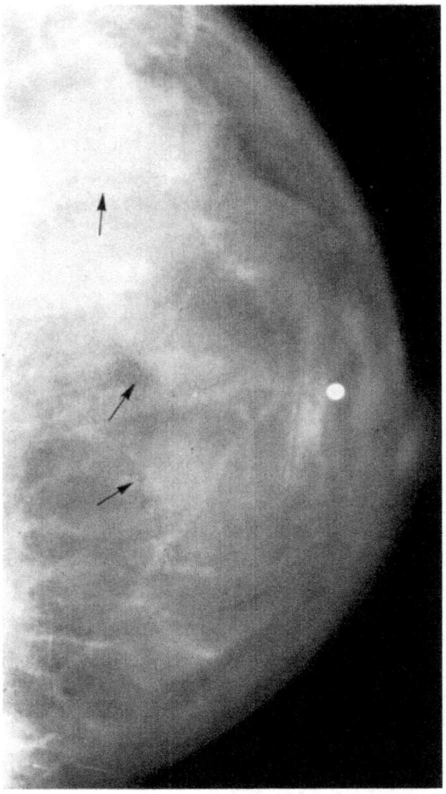

53

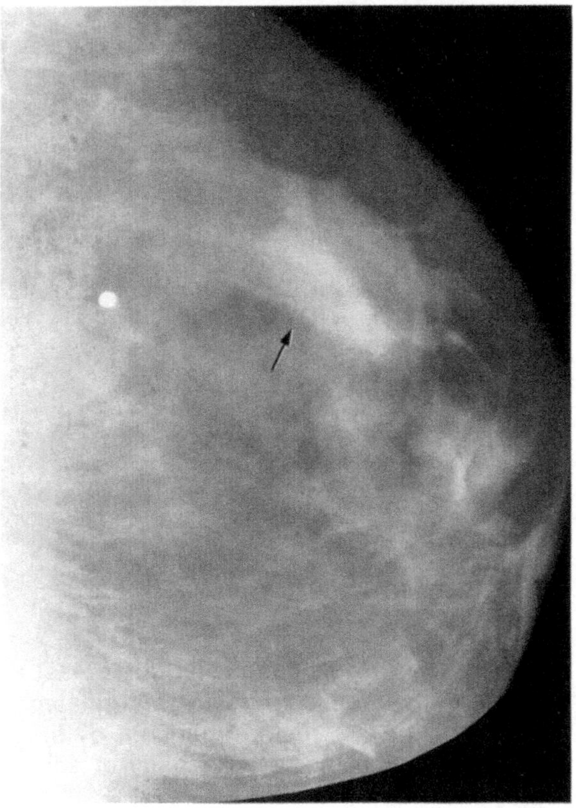

54

Fig. 55. Sclerosing adenosis, left breast. A patch of adenosis, denser than average and partially circumscribed (at site of skin marker) was mistaken for a cancer by palpation. Compare the denser adenosis due to contracting fibrosis of this breast with the adenosis of the opposite (right) breast

Fig. 56. Sclerosing adenosis, right breast. Compare the dense, partially marginated density of the sclerosing adenosis of the right breast with the usual density of adenosis as seen in the left breast

55
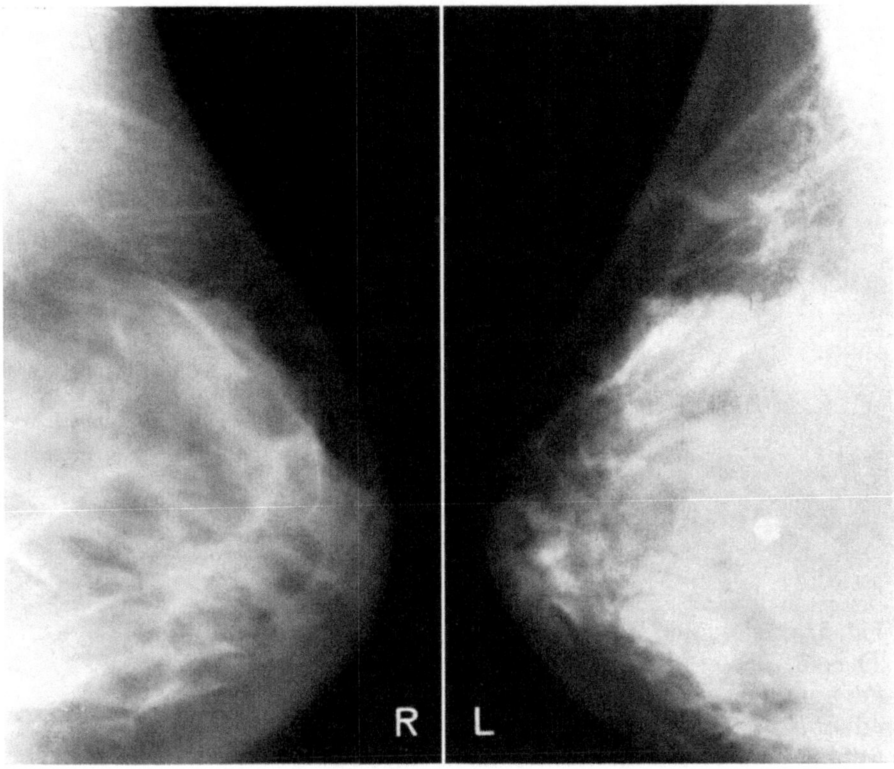

56
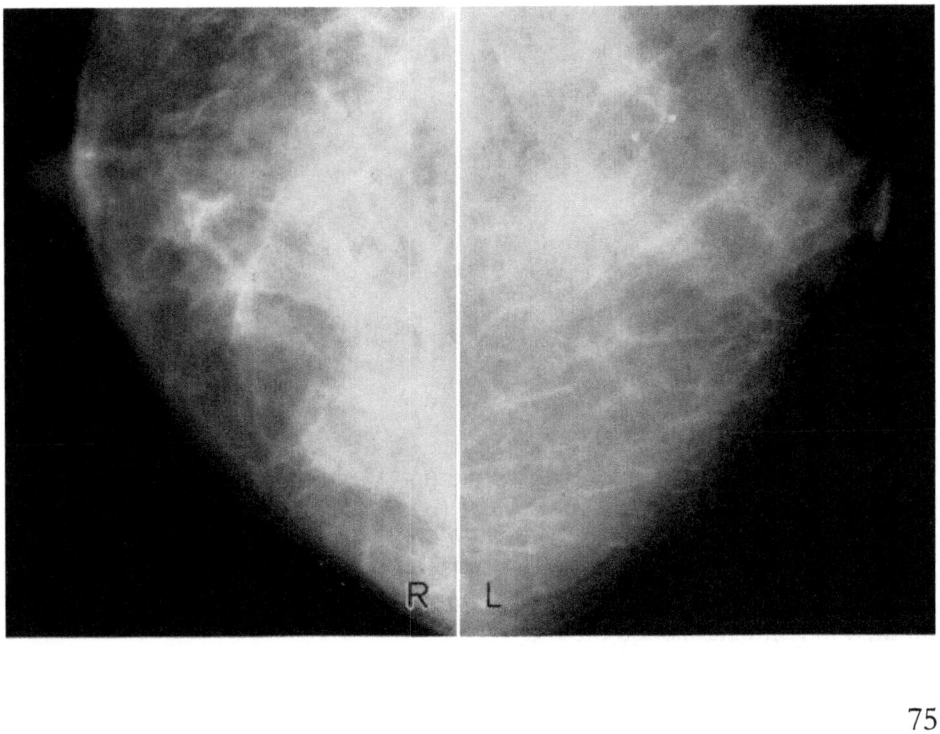

Fig. 57. Sclerosing adenosis, right breast. The increased densities in the areas of adenosis (arrows) as compared with the adenosis of the left breast are the result of fibrosis and contraction of tissue

Fig. 58 A and B. Sclerosing adenosis. Lateral view (A) and cephalocaudad view (B). Proliferative fibrosis of sclerosing adenosis is seen in the upper outer quadrant, where the homogeneous density, sharply marginated in (B), establishes the diagnosis

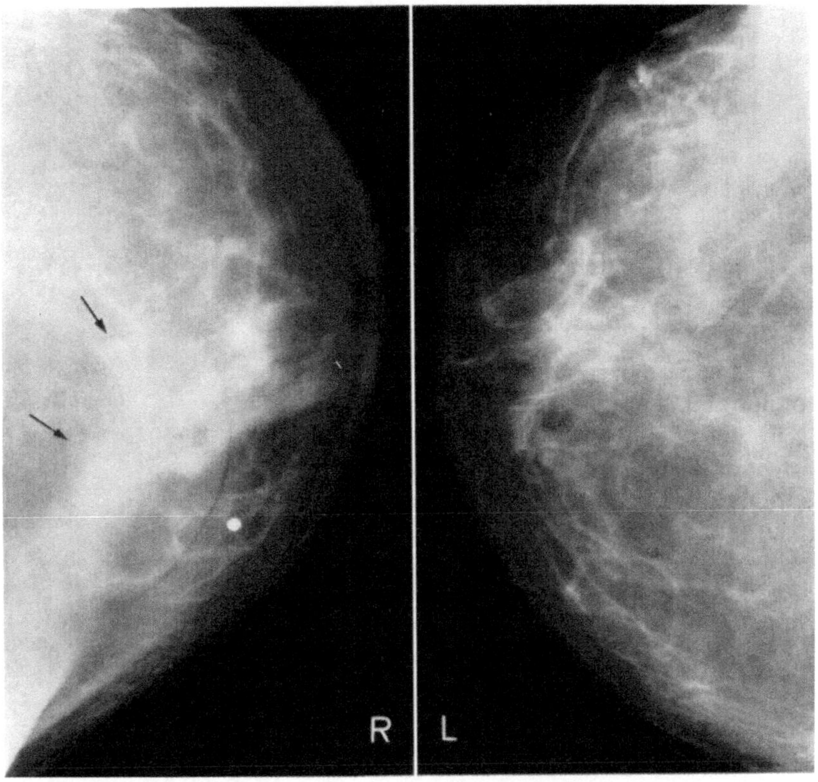

57

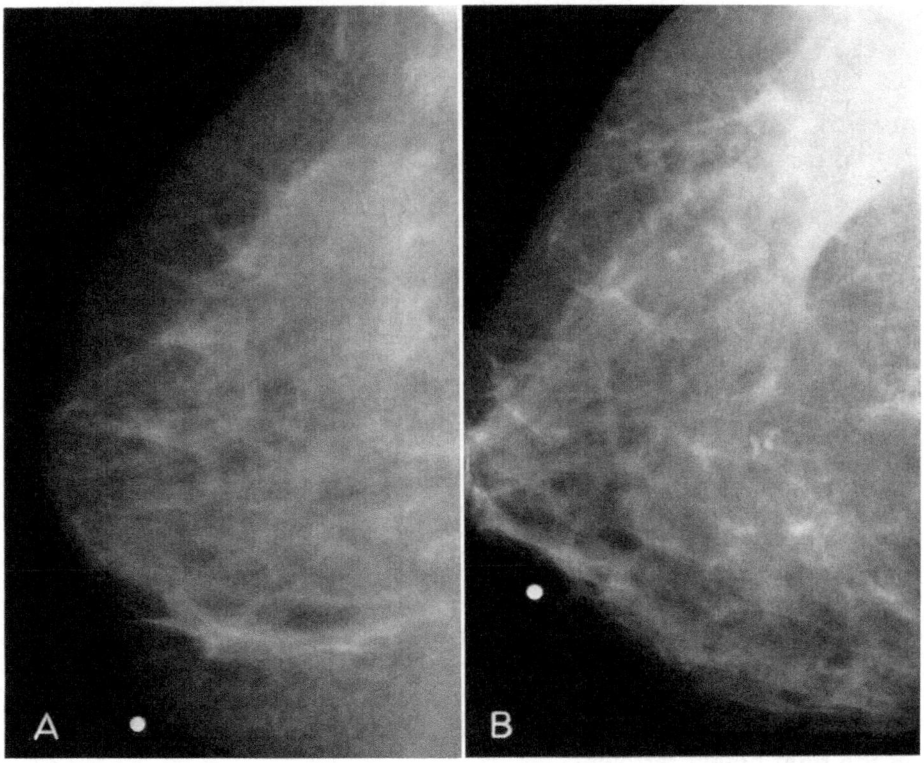

58

Fig. 59. Sclerosing adenosis. When fibrosis of lobular elements rather than involution persists beyond the menopause, detection of cancer may be difficult by physical examination. A mass was palpable under the skin marker in the breast of this 82 year old woman, but it was not dominant, and no evidence of cancer was found by the pathologist in an area of sclerosing adenosis

Fig. 60. Sclerosing adenosis. A firm, palpable mass at site of skin marker in left breast was thought to be a cancer. The sharp, smooth border of a homogeneous density (arrow heads) suggested fibrous or sclerotic adenosis to the roentgenologist, and was confirmed by the pathologist. Similar small patches of sclerosing adenosis are present in the right breast (arrows)

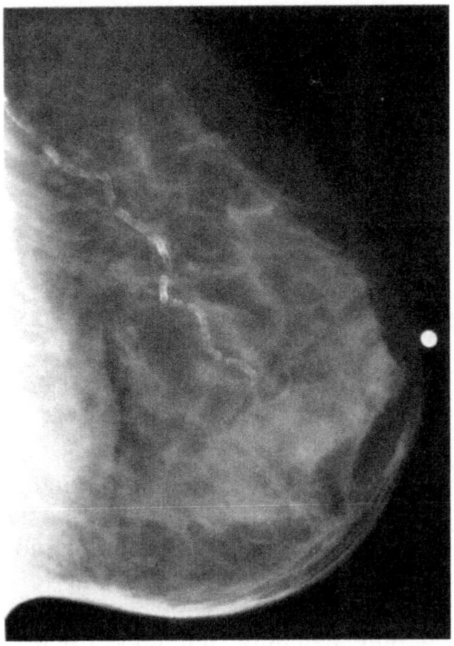

59

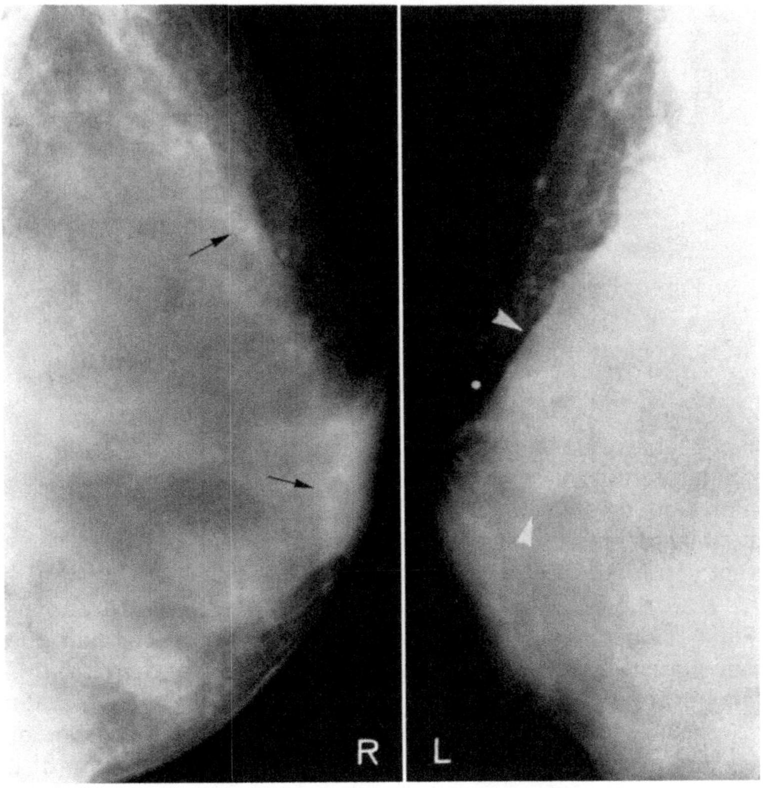

60

Fig. 61. Mazoplasia fibrosa. During adolescence, the hyperplastic pericanalicular and acinar fibrillar tissue is so extensive as to merge into a matrix of homogeneous density. As the ducts branch and form acini, fibroadenomas may develop. These might become palpable, but they are not visible on the X-ray film, being submerged in the fibrillar matrix. Such lesions are almost uniformly benign

Fig. 62. Mazoplasia fibrosa. A flat, homogeneous density with smooth contours impinging on the subcutaneous fat layer is the usual appearance of this condition in adolescents and early in the third decade. In the case of this 23 year old woman, the hyperplastic trabeculae are separated by invaginating columns of fat

Fig. 63. Mazoplasia fibrosa. The proliferative ductal structures nearer the apex of the gland become visible as they are separated by the increasing fat content of the breast in this young adult

Fig. 64. Mazoplasia fibrosa. The broad trabeculae streaming backwards into the base of the breast comprise the ducts with their excessive proliferation of pericanalicular, fibrillar, and intraductal epithelial tissue

Fig. 65. Mazoplasia fibrosa. The thick, dense trabeculae due to proliferation of epithelial and myoepithelial duct cells are clearly seen when separated by the fat digitations in the anterior breast. A fibroadenoma is present at the site of the skin marker

61

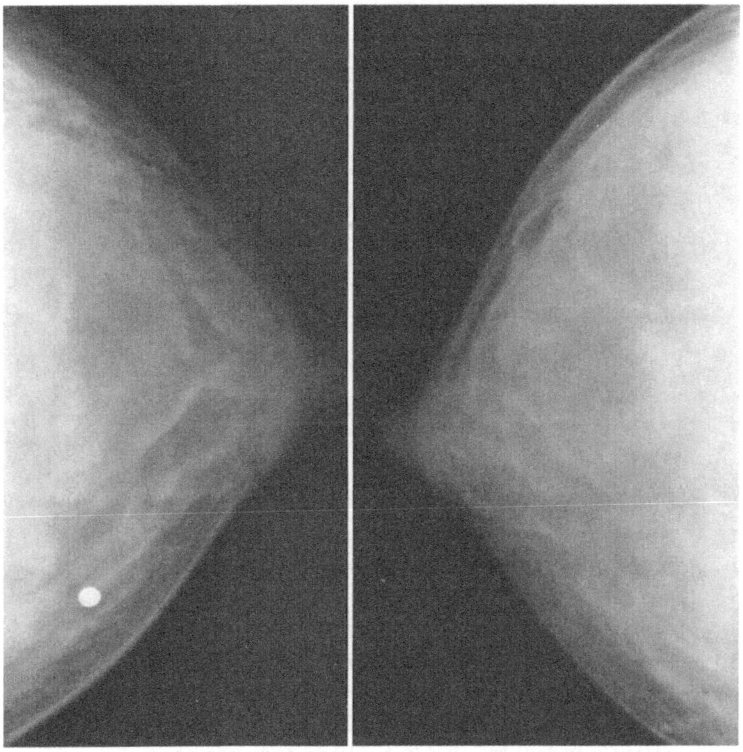
62

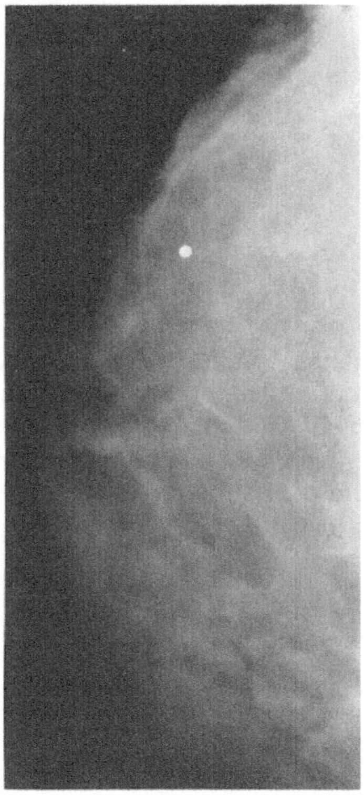
63

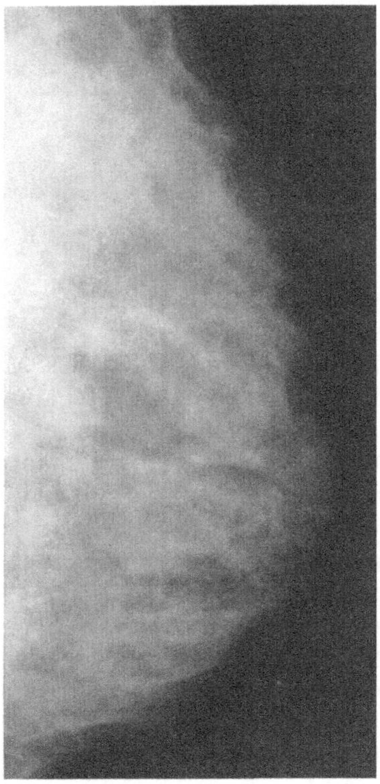
64

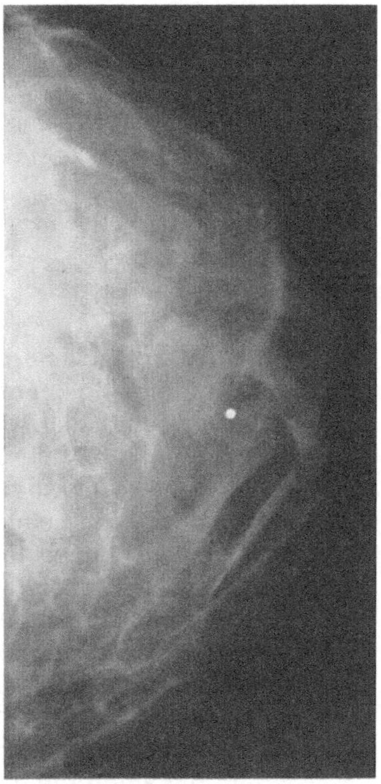
65

Fig. 66. Mazoplasia fibrosa. The thickened ducts due to overgrowth of epithelial and myoepithelial cells comprising the trabecula may be seen intertwined more clearly in older women whose breasts contain moderate amounts of fat. This 32 year old woman had four children whom she nursed. Some fields of adenosis are visible in the upper, outer quadrants, and two fibroadenomas are discernible (arrows)

Fig. 67. Mazoplasia fibrosa. The hyperplastic proliferation of the epithelial and pericanalicular myoepithelial cells of mazoplasia fibrosa may rarely be confined to the duct system due to retarded branching and development of the acini. When this abortive development persists throughout adulthood, the extensive branching of the duct system stands out in almost anatomical relief if the surrounding fat is uniformly distributed. Some mazoplasia cystica was also present in the breast of this 48 year old patient, but the cysts were microscopic in size and were strung out along the ducts

Fig. 68. Mazoplasia cystica and isolated cysts. Many ducts with bulbous cystic dilatations are visible. An isolated ovoid cyst is present. This was palpable and clinically aroused suspicion of cancer

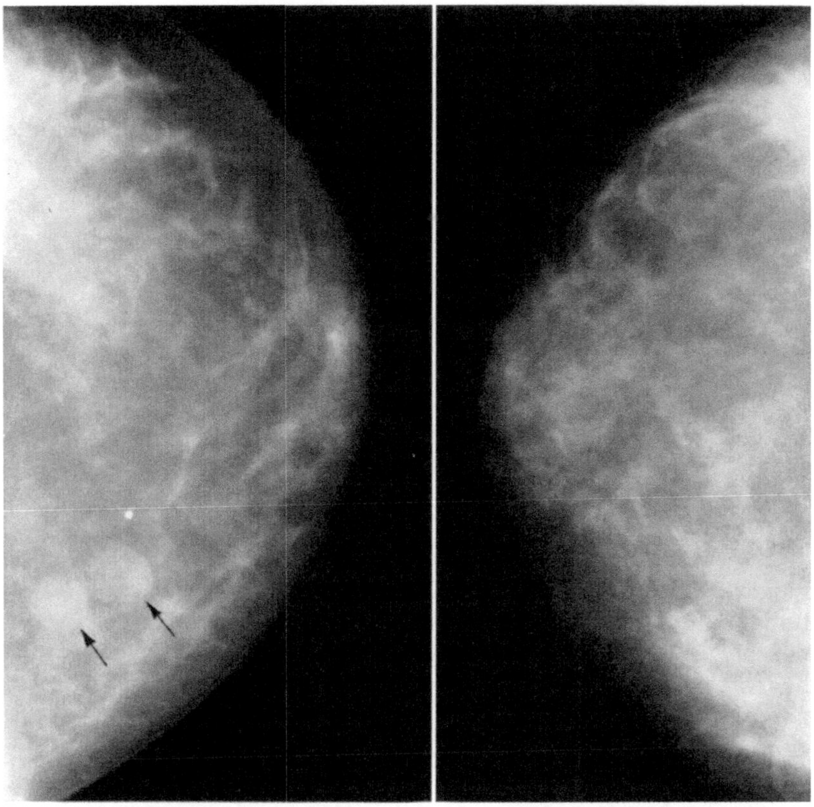

66

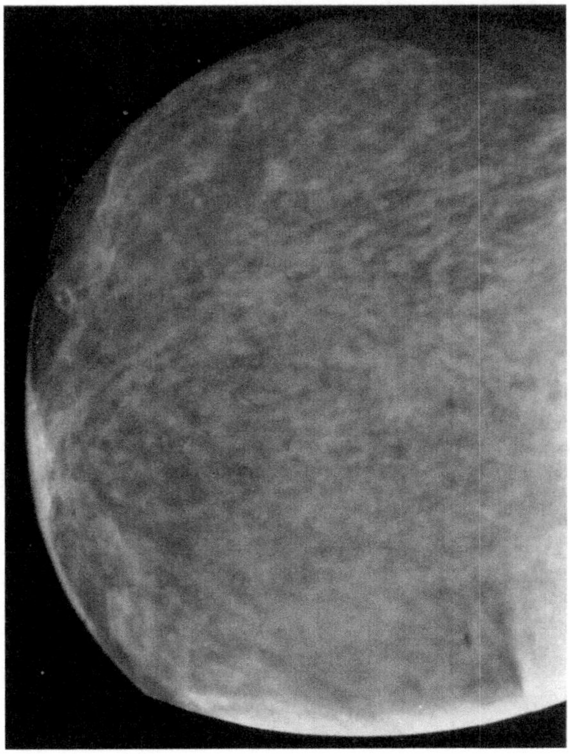

67

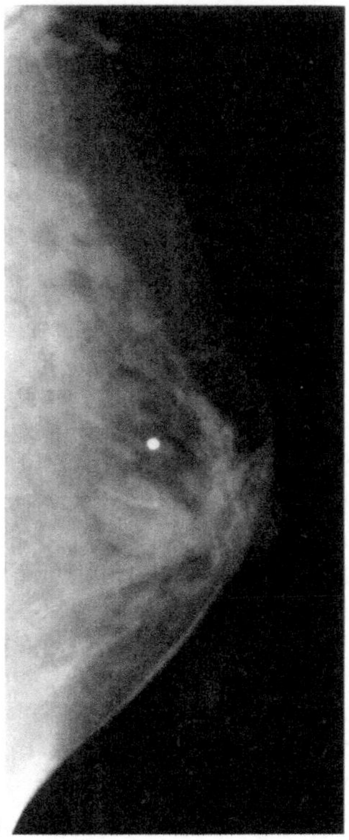

68

Fig. 69. Mazoplasia cystica. The palpable tumor under the skin marker (arrow) is sharply outlined and smoothly contoured. It was a cyst, indistinguishable from a fibroadenoma. In the upper area of the breast a zone of sclerosing adenosis is visible

Fig. 70. Mazoplasia cystica with a large, isolated cyst. The smoothly contoured wall of the cyst is apparently sinuous, undulating, and notched, so that its appearance simulates a bosselated fibroadenoma or a circumscribed cancer. The absence of perifocal edema, skin thickening, and vessel turgescence, and the age of the patient (35 years) are factors favoring a diagnosis of a benign lesion, especially since the character of the lesion's border is probably modified by the field of mazoplasia by which it is surrounded

Fig. 71. Mazoplasia cystica. This form of mazoplasia may fail to undergo normal involution and persist into the 6th decade, as in the case of this 53 year old woman. The presence of cysts may not be easily recognized in fields of adenosis

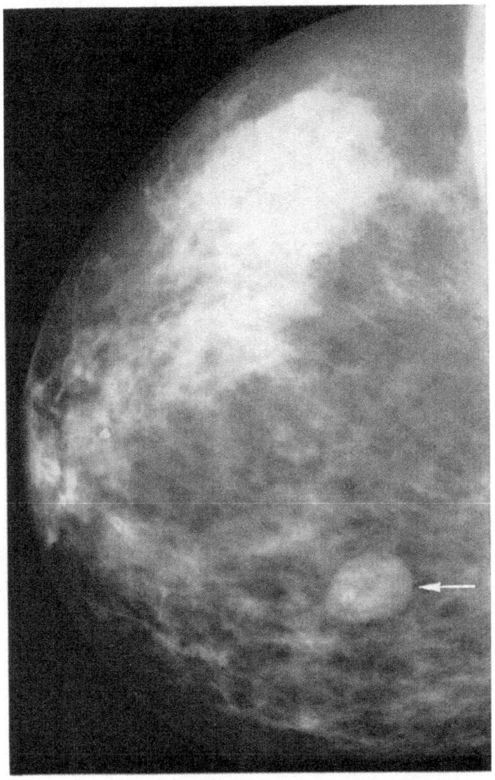

69

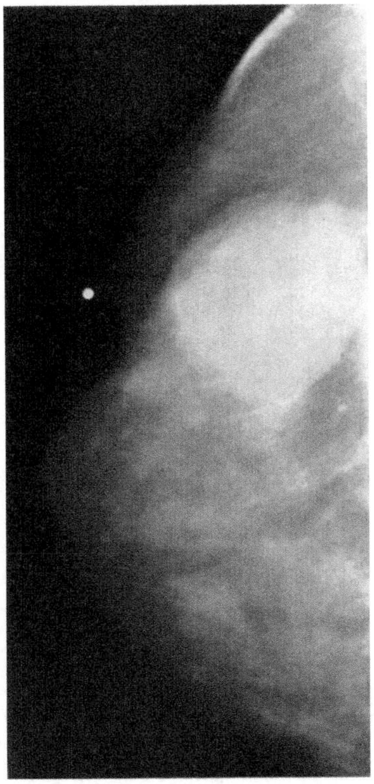

70

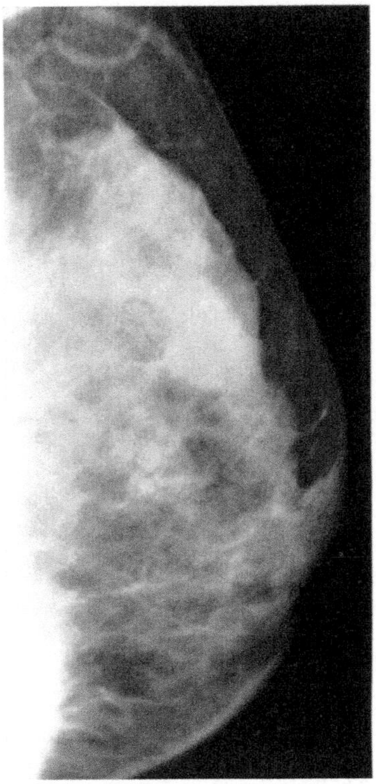

71

Fig. 72. Mazoplasia cystica, late stage. Residual cysts are visible in both breasts of this 45 year old woman after much resolution and involution of mazoplasia

Fig. 73. Mazoplasia cystica. Ovoid and compressed cysts are scattered throughout the breast

Fig. 74. Mazoplasia cystica. The outlines of multiple cysts are clearly visible because the perifocal tissue is predominantly fatty

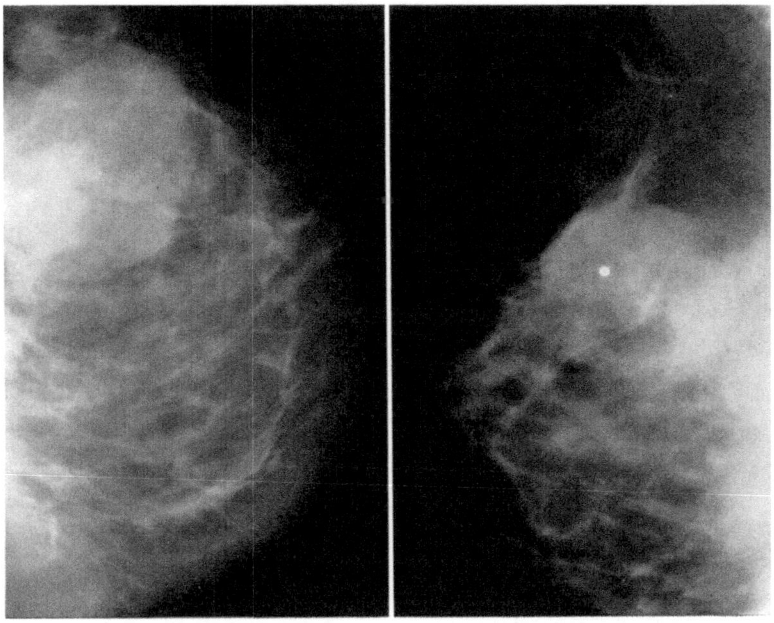

72

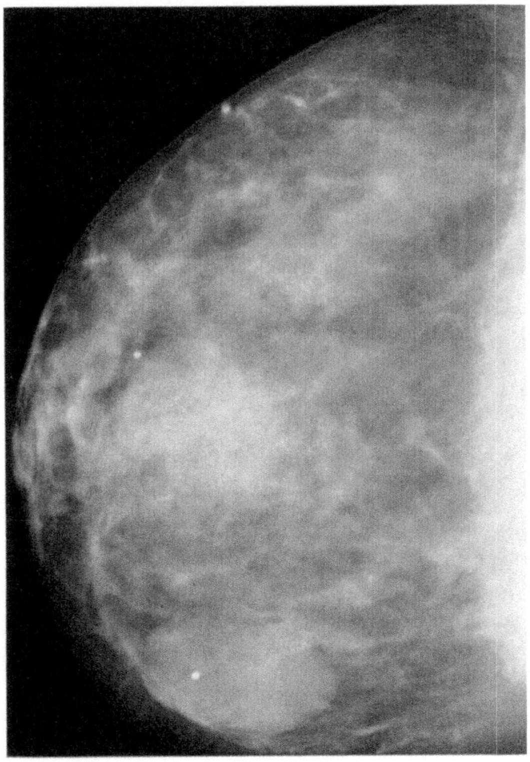

73

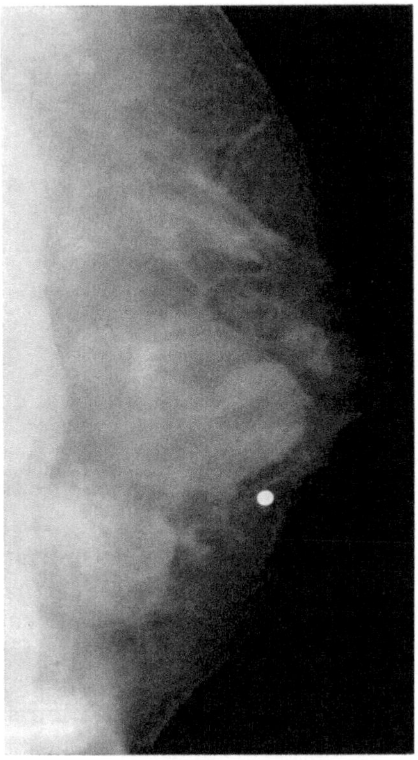

74

Fig. 75. Mazoplasia cystica. In the rarer forms of this dysplasia, the entire breast may be occupied by large cysts

Fig. 76. Mazoplasia cystica. A firm, fixed, palpable mass in the left breast under the skin marker was thought to be a cancer, but its smooth, sharp margins indicate a cyst or fibroadenoma. Adenosis is visible in the opposite (right) breast and the sharp posterior limits suggest fibrosis characteristic of sclerosing adenosis

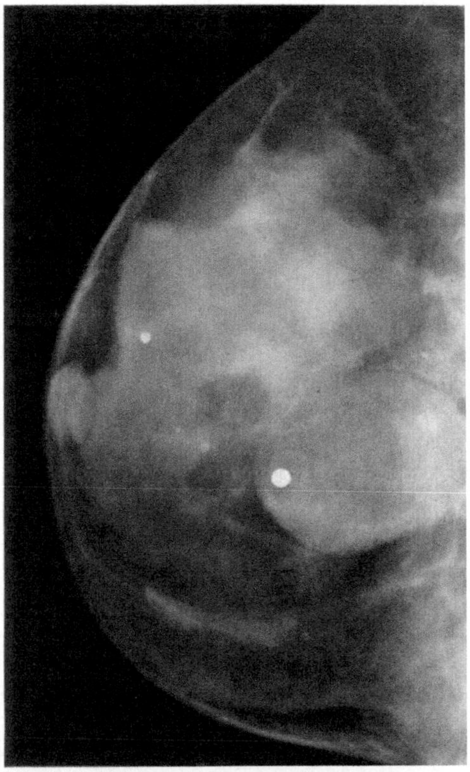

75

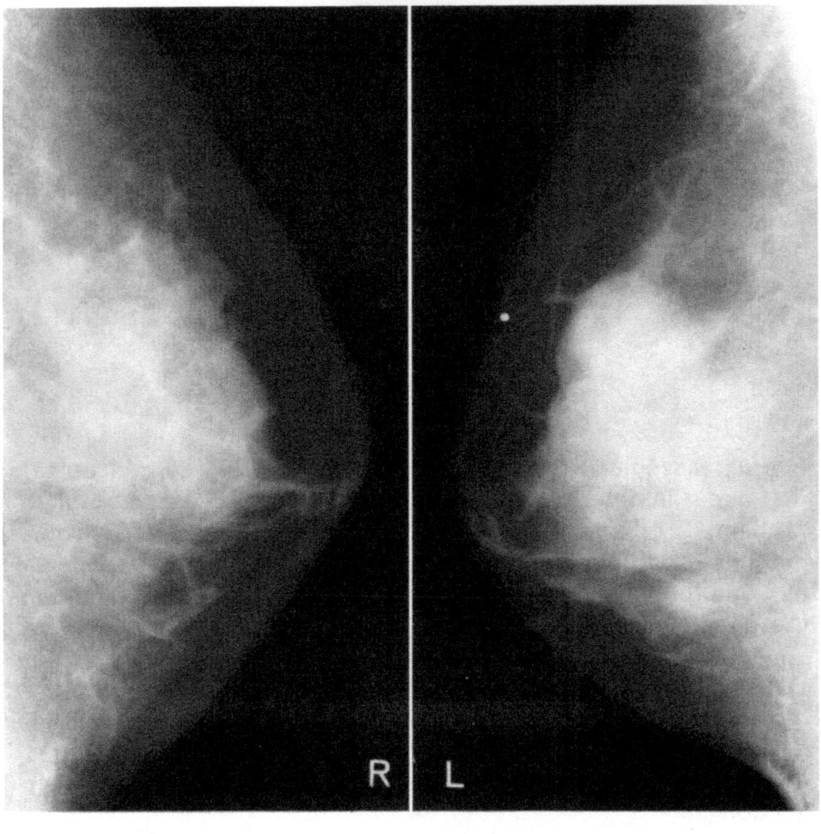

76

Fig. 77. Mazoplasia cystica. Multiple cysts ranging from 1—8 cm in diameter occupy most of the breast. Portions of their outlines are obscured because of overlapping

Fig. 78. Mazoplasia cystica. In some phases of mazoplasia cystica, large cysts may be so numerous that they occupy almost the entire breast. However, the phenomenon is rare

Fig. 79. Mazoplasia cystica. Isolated cysts that occur in older women pose diagnostic problems. When portions of the cystic margins are submerged in perifocal densities due to mazoplasia fibrosa or adenosis, the possibility of a scirrhous or medullary cancer cannot be excluded. Some reliance can be placed upon the absence of surrounding edema or disruption of structural patterns, but the wisest procedure to follow in these cases is to advise diagnostic resection

Fig. 80. Mazoplasia cystica. A sharply outlined, smoothly contoured lesion in the breast of a woman in the 4th and 5th decades is usually a cyst. It resembles a fibroadenoma and must also be distinguished from a circumscribed cancer. All accessory diagnostic measures should be employed, and only biopsy can be regarded as the ultimate diagnostic recourse in cases of doubt

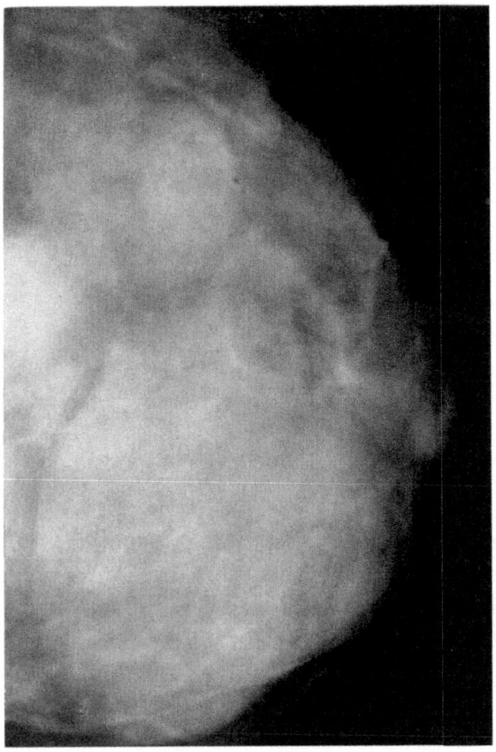

77

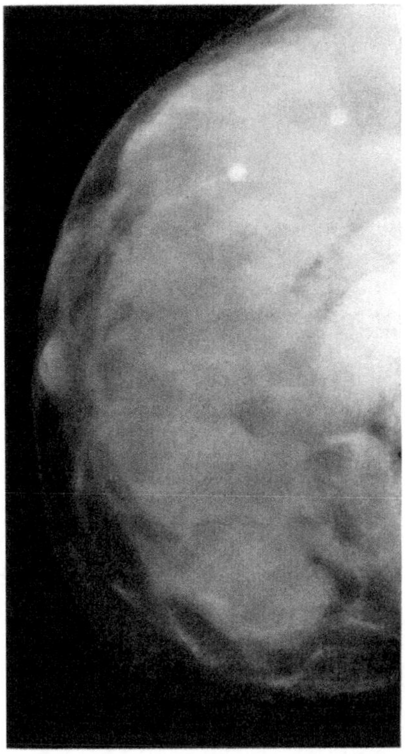

78

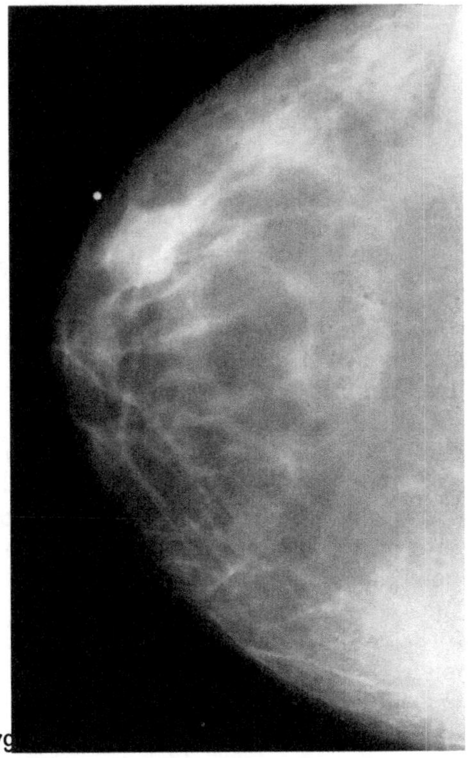

79

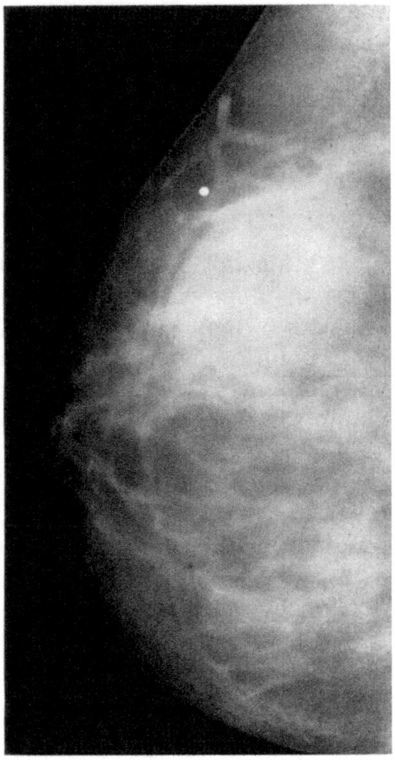

80

Fig. 81. Mazoplasia cystica. Inflammation may involve cysts of all sizes. When a large, isolated cyst becomes inflamed, the perifocal edema blurs details, as in cancer, making differentiation difficult

Fig. 82. Mazoplasia cystica. When inflammatory reaction and edema occur around an isolated cyst, they can so blur and distort the marginal details as to preclude distinguishing the lesion from a cancer. Resection for diagnostic purposes would be the safest procedure to follow

Fig. 83. Mazoplasia cystica. When isolated cysts in older women become large and, because of their smooth contours, there is little doubt of their cystic nature, many surgeons aspirate them to establish the diagnosis. We prefer resection, both for diagnosis and therapy. Only in this way can the presence of a papilloma or a cancer in or near the cyst be eliminated. Rarely, a surgeon can be induced to replace the aspirated fluid with air so that a re-examination of the air-filled cyst can be done. This helps to exclude the presence of an intracystic cancer and is a technique routinely adhered to by Professor Charles M. Gros of Strasbourg

Fig. 84 A and B. Mazoplasia cystica
A
The diagnosis of cysts was based on the smooth contours of the lesions behind the nipple
B
Air which replaced the aspirated fluid from one cyst reveals a series of cysts ranging from 5—14 mm in diameter, all probably associated with the same duct system

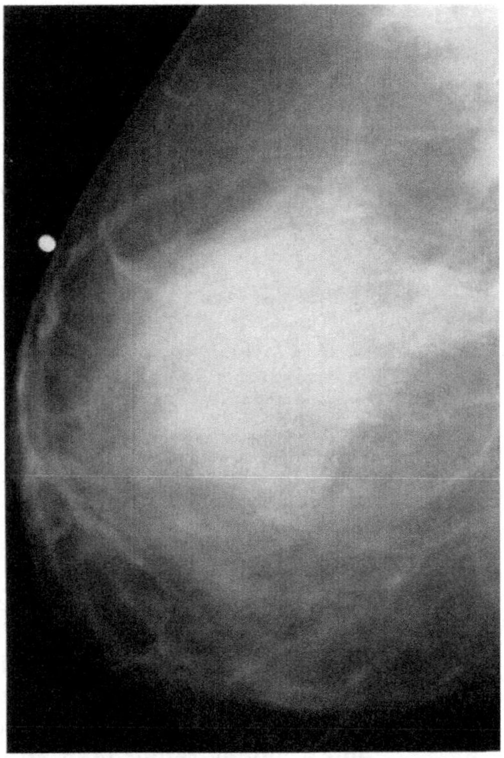

81

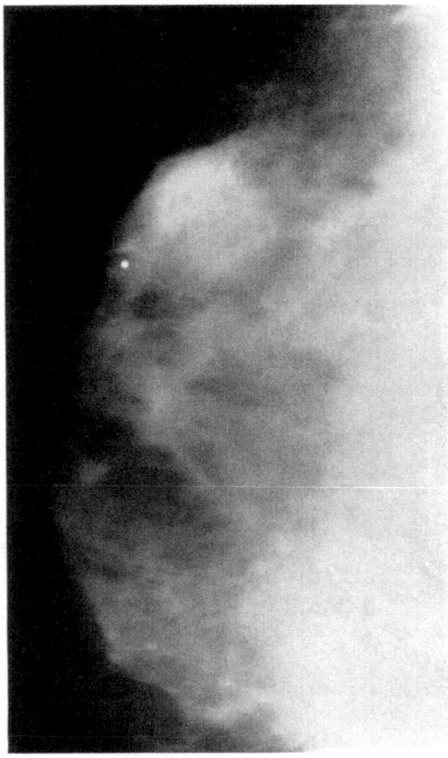

82

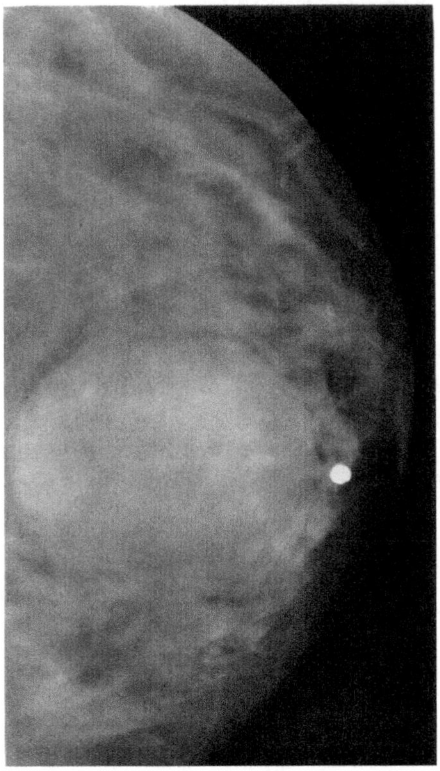

83

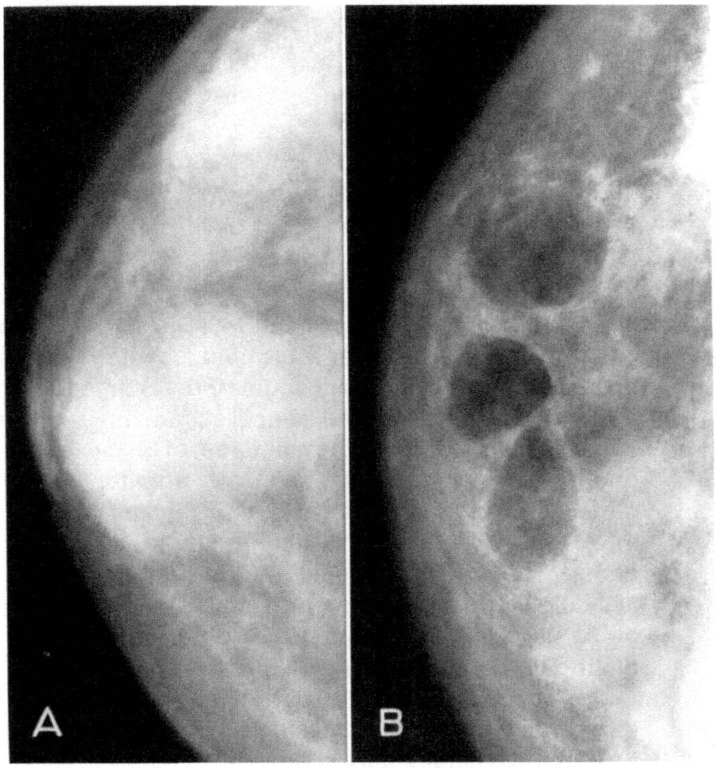

84

Fig. 85. Fibroadenomas. In areas of adenosis, the margins of fibroadenomas may be difficult to see

Fig. 86. Fibroadenoma. When these lesions occur in an area of adenosis, only portions of their margins may be visible. The diagnosis is therefore in jeopardy. If the patient is under 35 years of age, periodic re-examination at 6-month intervals is advisable. Over 35 years of age, the risk becomes greater, and a biopsy rather than an expectant attitude is desirable

Fig. 87. Fibroadenomas. These lesions can assume various shapes: globoid, ovoid, bosselated, notched, or angulated. Scirrhous and circumscribed cancers can assume similar shapes. The absence of secondary signs, such as perifocal edema, distortion of structural details, and thickening of the skin, helps to distinguish these benign lesions from cancer. When plaquelike calcifications are also present, to which these lesions are prone, the differential diagnosis becomes easier. Fibroadenomas and cysts can appear so much alike that to differentiate them is usually impossible and, fortunately, usually only academic

Fig. 88. Fibroadenomas. Globoid or ovoid masses with smooth contours which occur in women under 30 years of age are usually fibroadenomas, especially in the presence of mazoplasia fibrosa and adenosis, as in this case

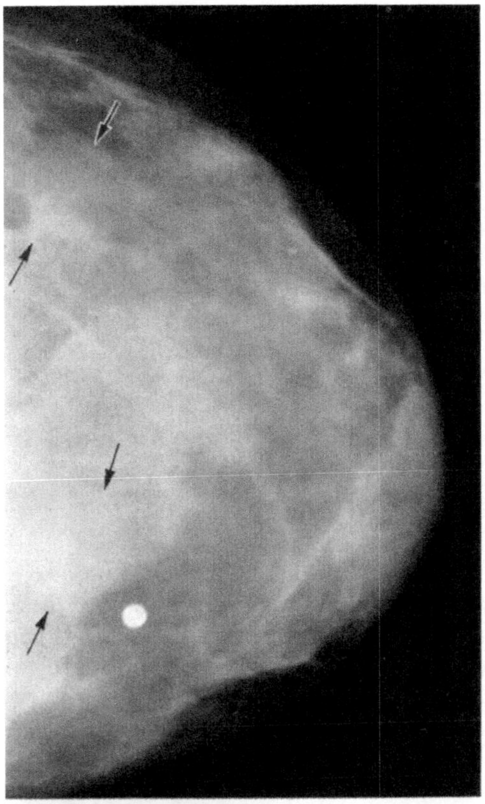

85

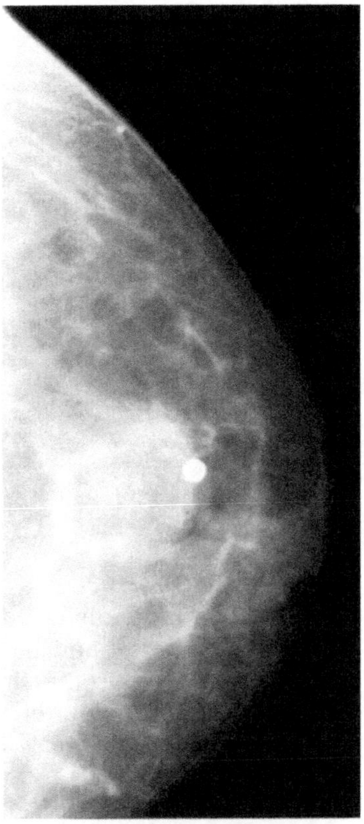

86

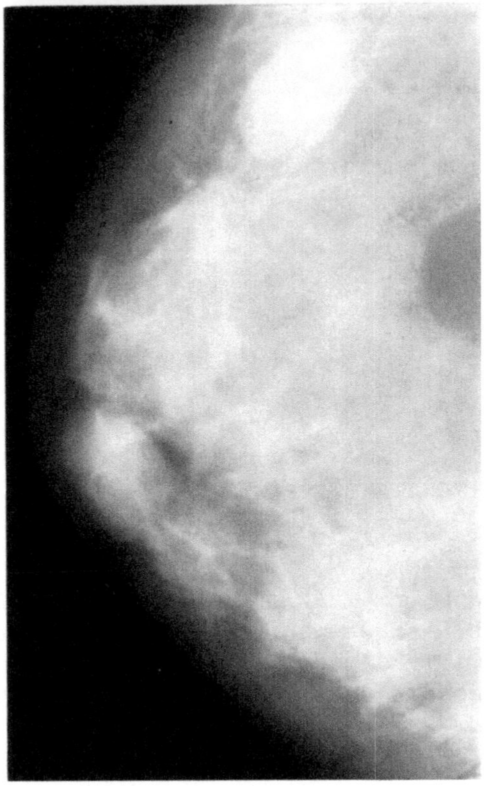

87

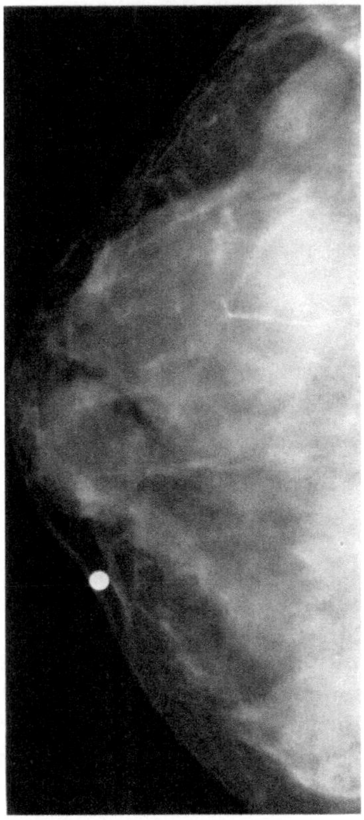

88

Fig. 89. Fibroadenomas. One lesion is sharply marginated and smooth in contour (upper arrow). The other has blurred margins due to the surrounding dilated hyperplastic ducts (lower arrows) of mazoplasia fibrosa

Fig. 90. Fibroadenoma. An isolated, smoothly contoured lesion in a postmenopausal breast may be a fibroadenoma, but its removal is advisable to rule out cancer

Fig. 91. Fibroadenoma. A smoothly contoured lesion not associated with disturbance of the perifocal structures is usually a fibroadenoma or a cyst, but when the margins are sinuous or notched, cancer must be ruled out by biopsy

Fig. 92. Fibroadenomas. Multiple lesions of various shapes have smooth contours. The notch in one (arrow) resembles that often seen in circumscribed cancer

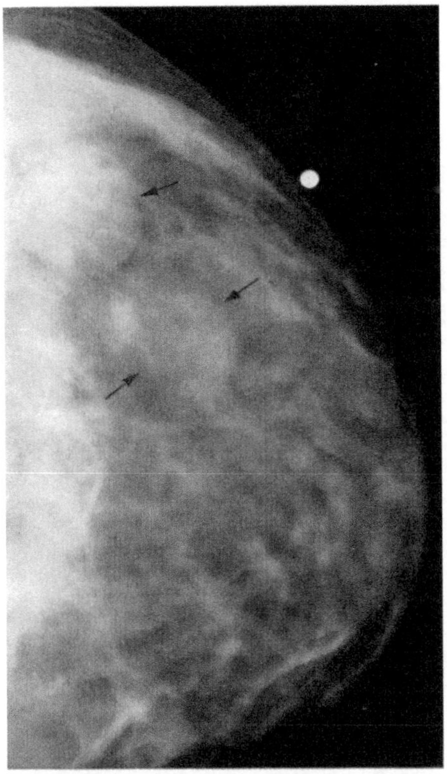

89

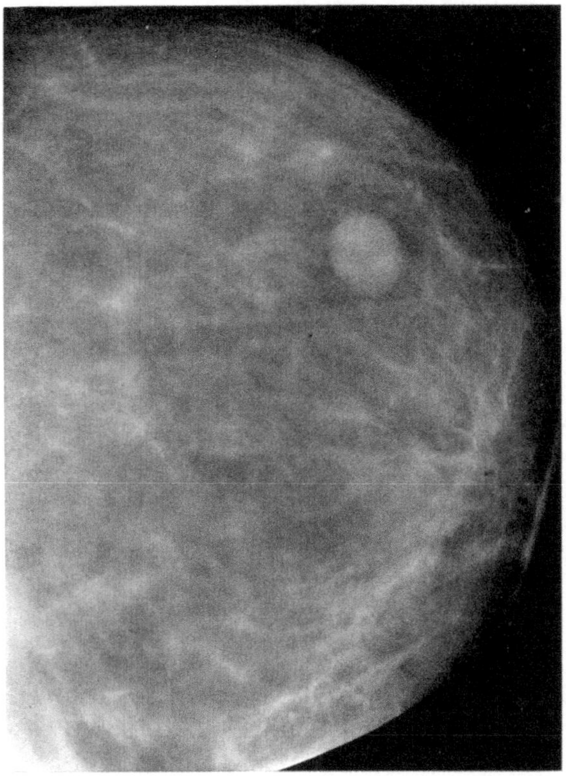

90

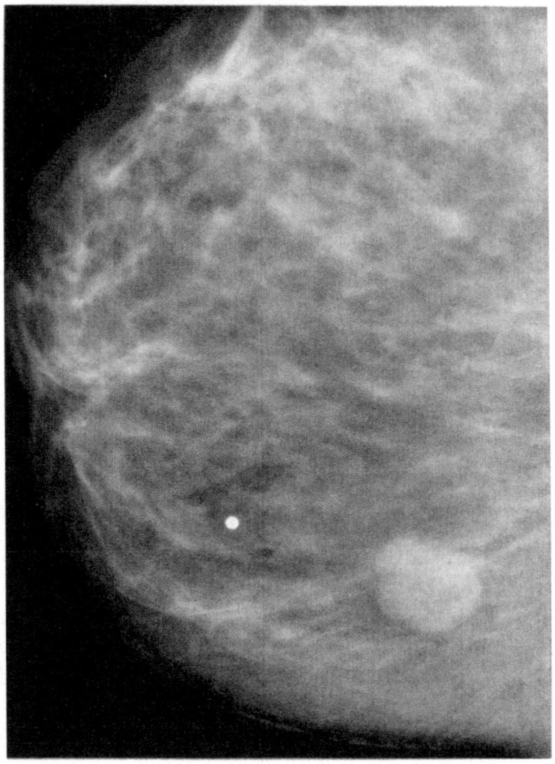

91

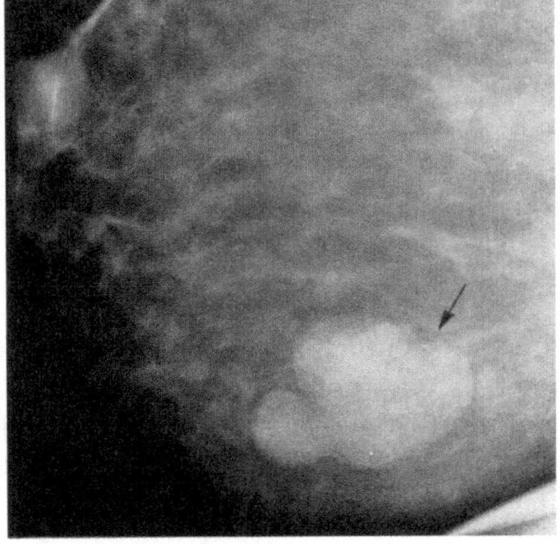

92

Fig. 93. Fibroadenomas. Many smoothly-contoured fibroadenomas are present, some with plaque-like calcifications

Fig. 94. Fibroadenoma. Plaque-like calcification may be extensive, even in a large lesion. (This example was furnished by Doctor Jack Widrich, Miami Beach, Florida)

Fig. 95. Cystosarcoma phyllodes. A sharply outlined, smoothly-contoured, rapidly growing mass, especially if partially coated by plaque-like calcifications, should raise the diagnostic possibility of a giant fibroadenoma

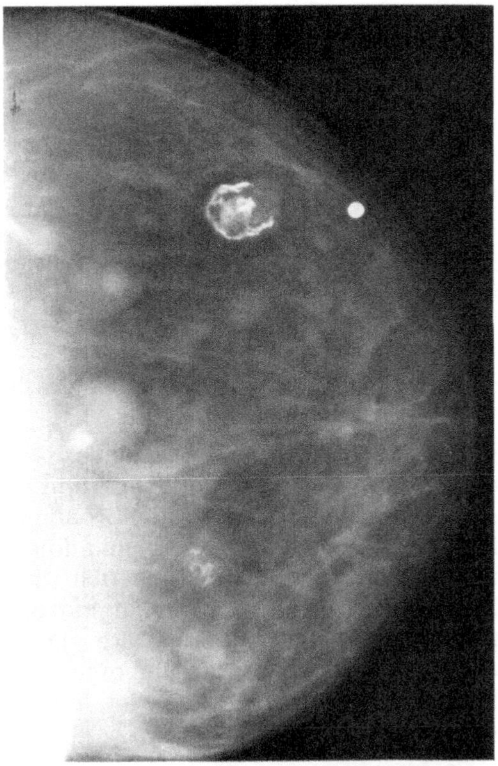

93

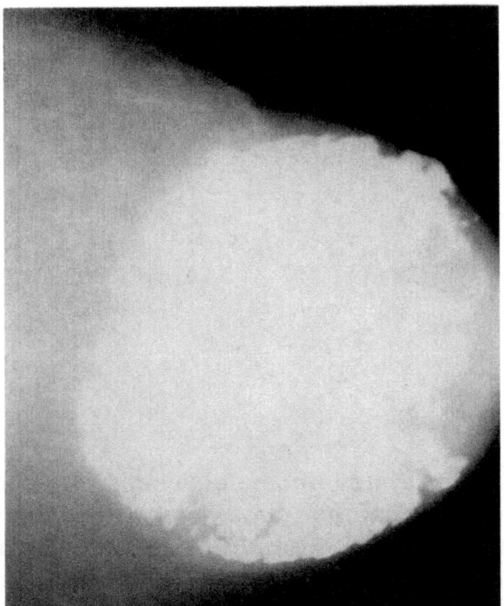

94

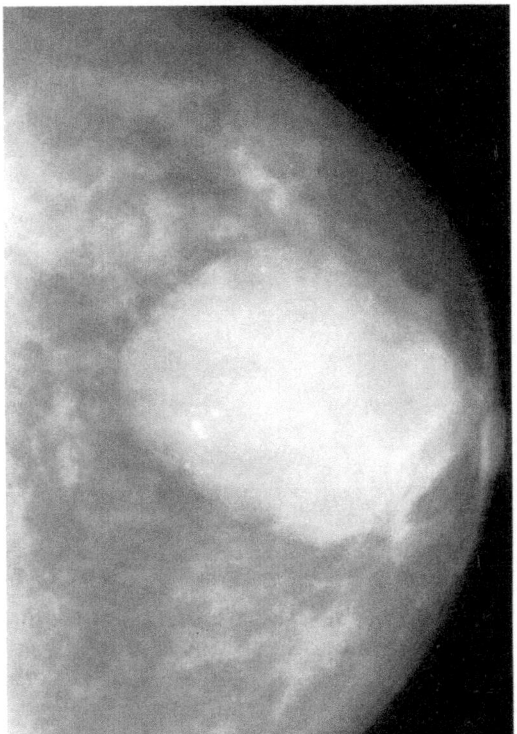

95

Fig. 96. Cystosarcoma phyllodes. In a 13 year old girl, rapid enlargement of the right breast suggested a growing giant fibroadenoma. Fibroadenomas often occur in adolescent mazoplasia fibrosa, as is seen in the left breast. Since the densities of mazoplasia fibrosa and a fibroadenoma are similar, in the absence of fat, fibroadenomas cannot be seen. They might, however, be readily palpable, as in this case

Fig. 97. Giant fibroadenoma. A large dense mass with smooth contours occupies the lower two-thirds of the breast of a 16 year old girl. Growth was rapid

Fig. 98. Cystosarcoma phyllodes. A rapidly-growing, sharply circumscribed mass, particularly in the 4th and 5th decades, may be a giant fibroadenoma or cystosarcoma phyllodes, and some of them may be malignant, as in this case

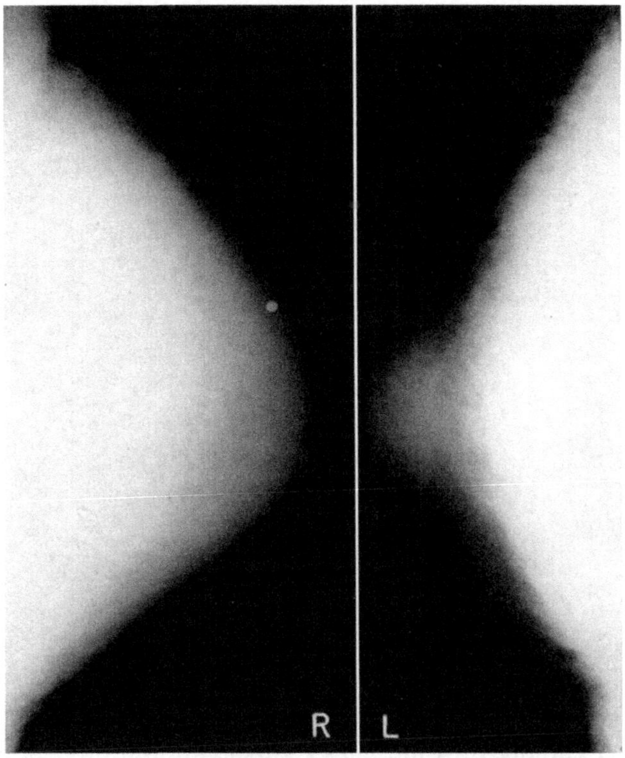

96

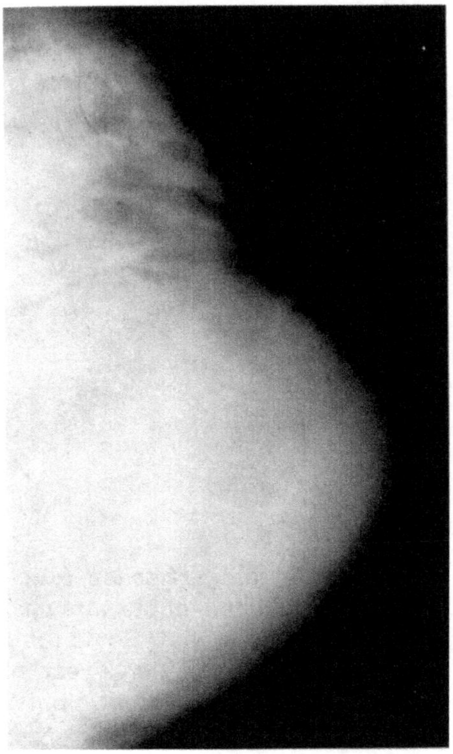

97

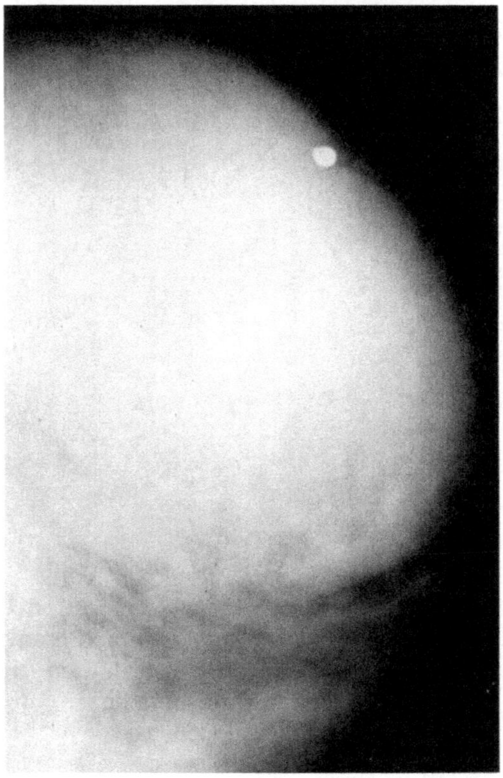

98

Fig. 99 A and B. Cystosarcoma phyllodes
A
A rapidly growing mass observed during a 3-month period virtually occupies the entire breast of this 42 year old Negress

B
Four months after a simple enucleation, another recurrent mass was removed from the residual breast tissue in the region of the axillary tail (arrow)

Fig. 100. Secretory disease. Secretion from the nipple of the breast of this 43 year old woman is associated with dilated ducts (arrows), so-called duct ectasia

Fig. 101. Secretory disease (duct ectasia). Numerous dilated ducts stream almost to the base of the breast. Some lobular proliferation is present. This 42 year old patient complained of intermittent nipple secretion for years

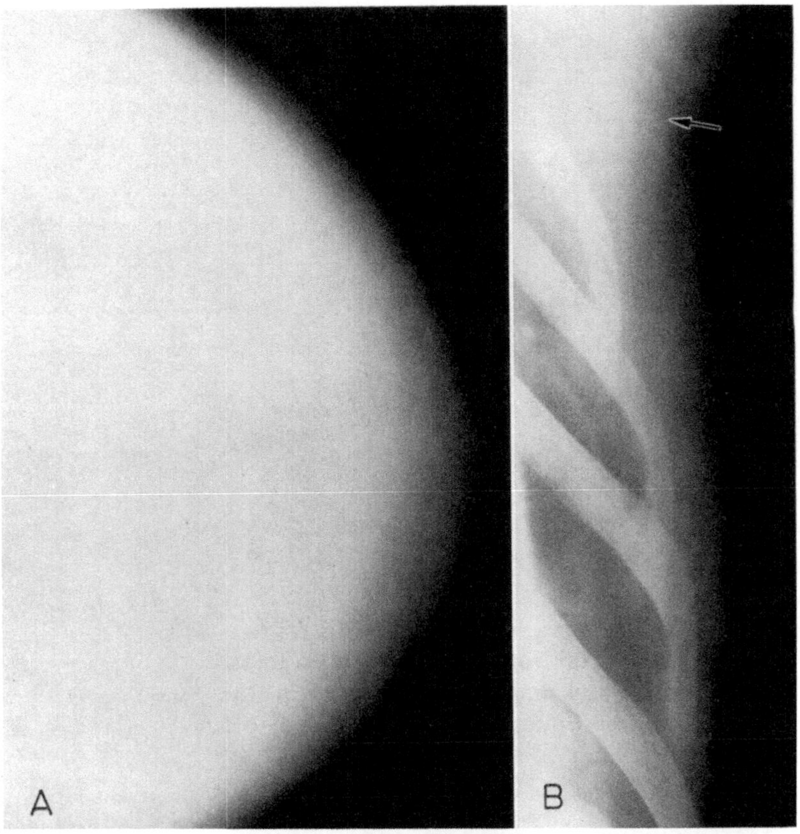

99

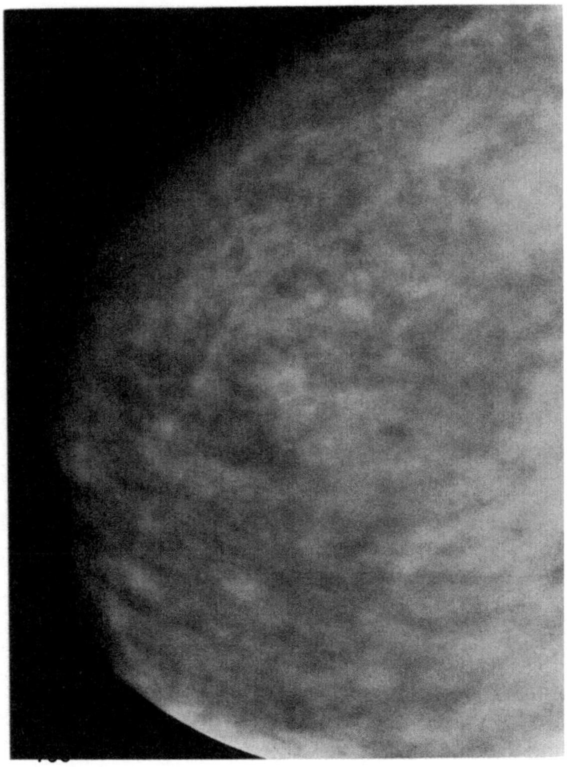

100

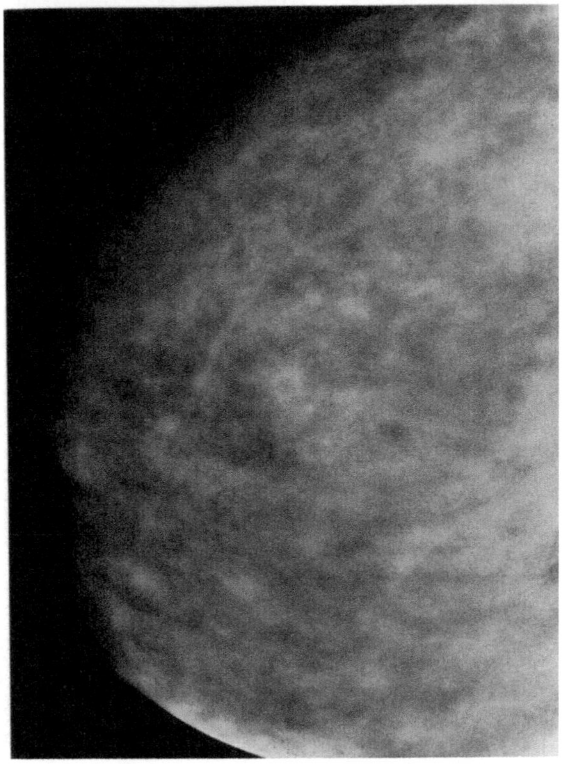

101

Fig. 102. Secretory disease. Fibrous trabeculae, often with retraction of the nipples, and particularly marked on the right in this case, may be encountered in cases of old healed secretory disease

Fig. 103. Plasma cell mastitis, right breast. Fibrous ductal involution of old healed secretory disease often results in a localized zone of density behind a *retracted* nipple. The occurrence of a recently palpable mass in the right breast suggested cancer, but plasma cell mastitis was found. The left breast is less extensively involved

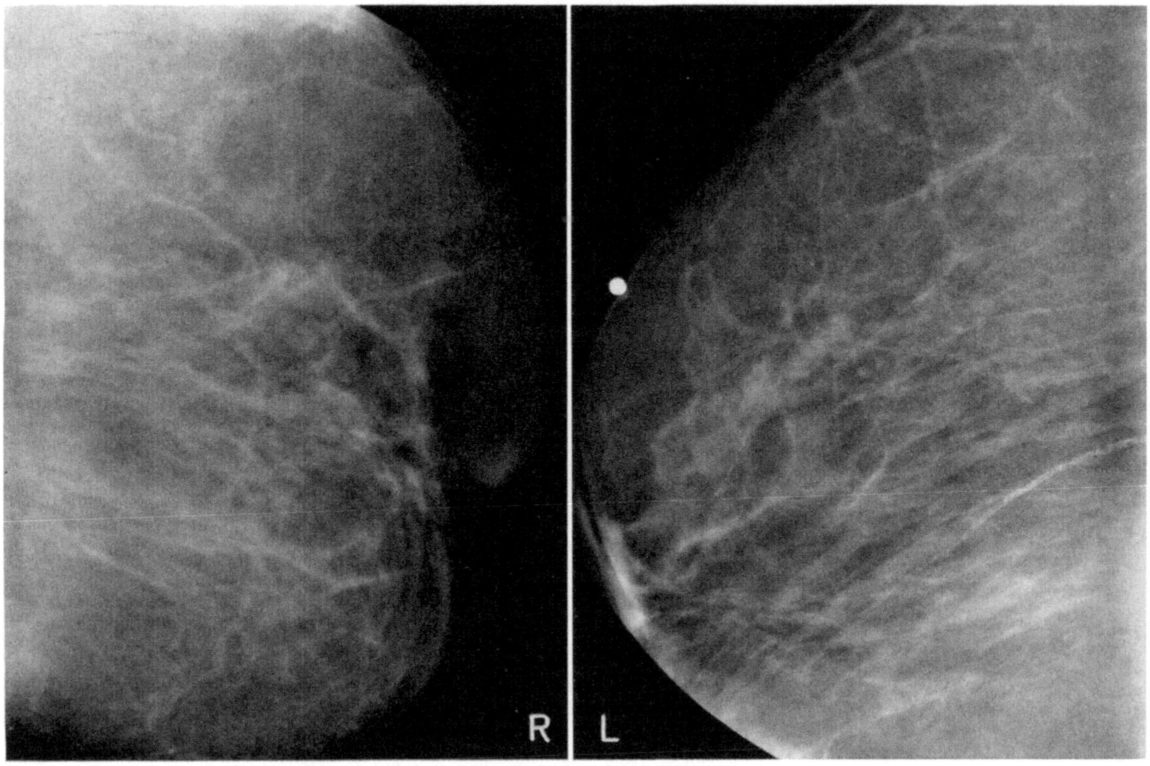

102

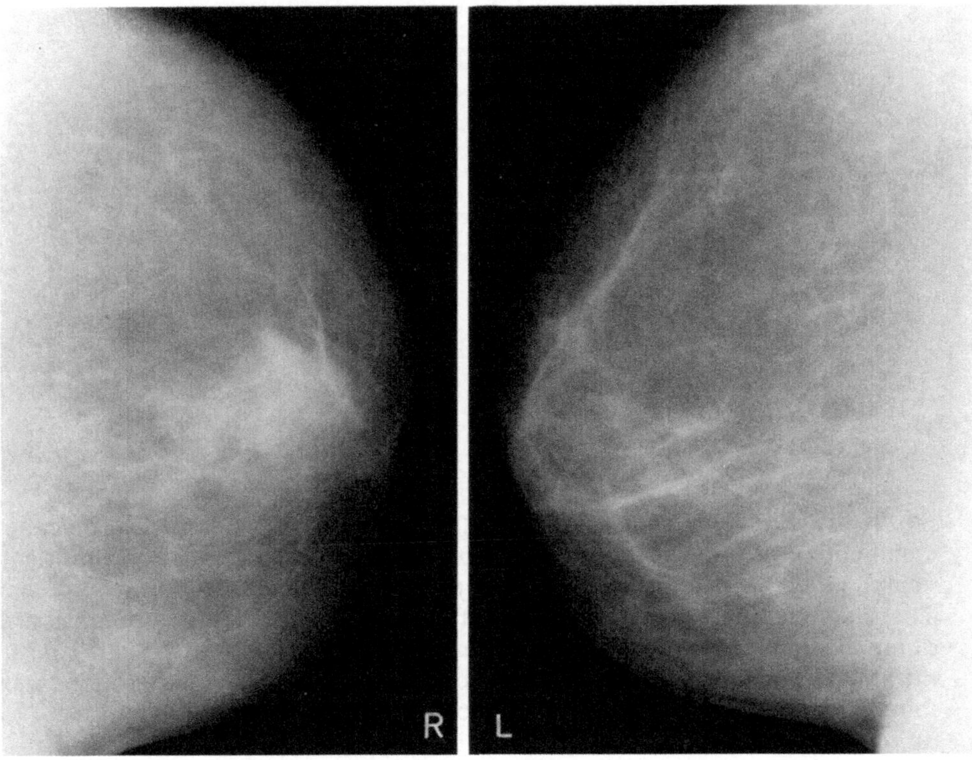

103

Fig. 104. Plasma cell mastitis. A palpable mass in a woman with nipple discharge was suspected to be cancer. An ill-defined uneven density in these circumstances suggests the possibility of plasma cell mastitis, however, and was confirmed by the histologist

Fig. 105. Plasma cell mastitis. A localized swelling occurred suddenly in the areolar area of the breast of an 88 year old woman. It seemed inflammatory, but the possibility of cancer could not be eliminated. The process gradually improved after 3 months' time on conservative management. A diagnostic resection was done, however, and plasma cell mastitis was found

Fig. 106. Secretory disease. Tubular, linear calcification is present as the result of old healed duct ectasia or secretory disease. The distended, tortuous, smoothly outlined ducts behind the nipple are the result of intraductal epithelial hyperplasia and papillomatosis with plaque-like calcification of an intraductal papilloma (arrow)

Fig. 107. Secretory disease with calcifications. Tubular, cylindrical calcifications of the ducts and ovoid, spherical calcifications of the lobules forming "epithelial pearls" are noted in the terminal aspects of secretory disease (duct ectasia)

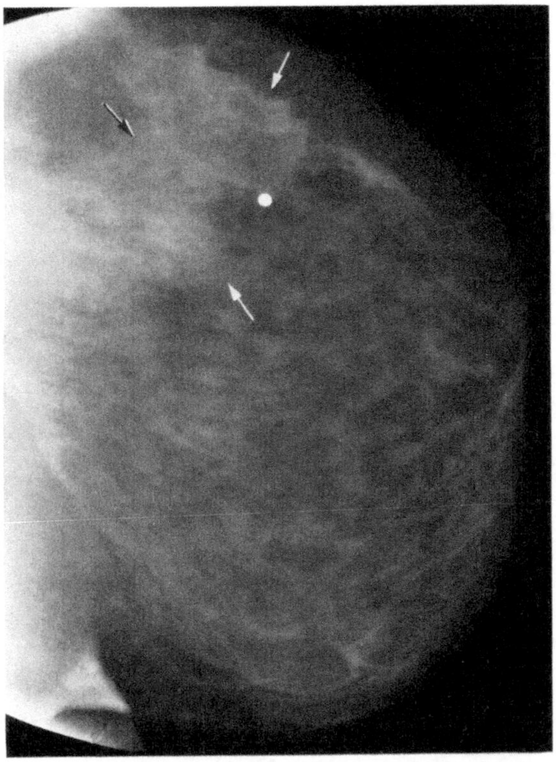

104

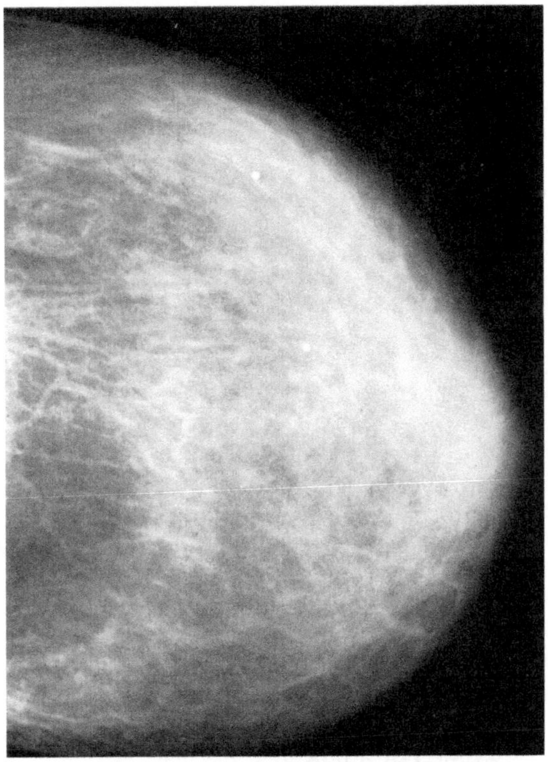

105

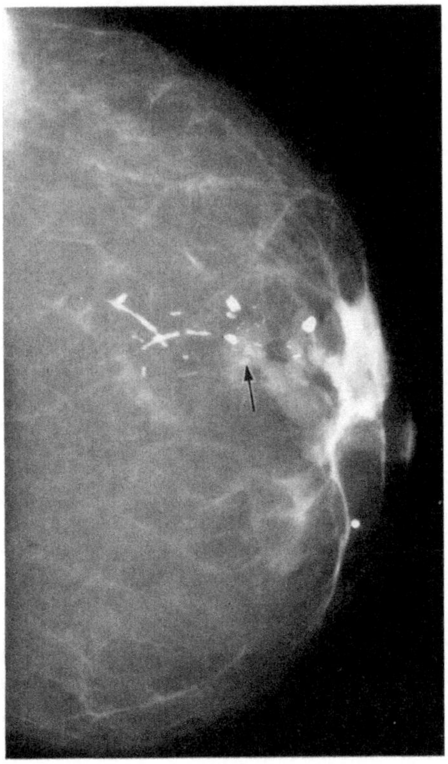

106

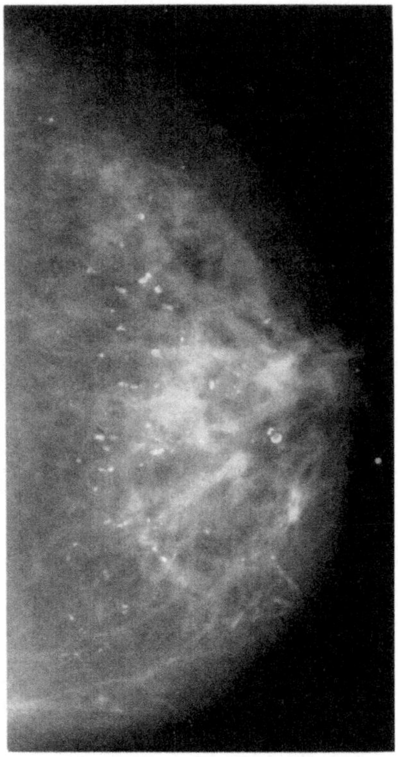

107

Fig. 108. Duct ectasia (secretory disease) with calcified "epithelial pearls." Disseminated spheroid-shaped particles of various sizes with smooth, calcified rims we have designated "epithelial pearls" occurring in lobules in the presence of duct ectasia. In this postmenopausal breast of a 60 year old woman are seen many residual patches of adenosis and scattered segments of dilated ducts

Fig. 109. Fat necrosis. When fatty tissue degenerates, usually as the result of an inflammatory process, the residual fibrosis (under skin marker) may simulate a cancer

Fig. 110. Fat necrosis. A palpable cyst under the skin marker misled awareness of a patch of fat necrosis nearby (arrow)

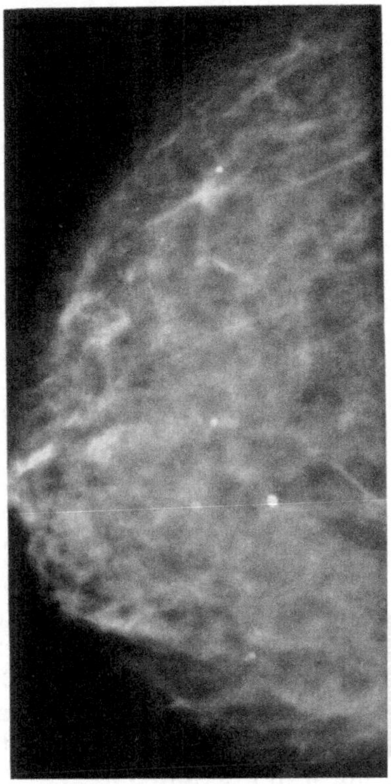

108

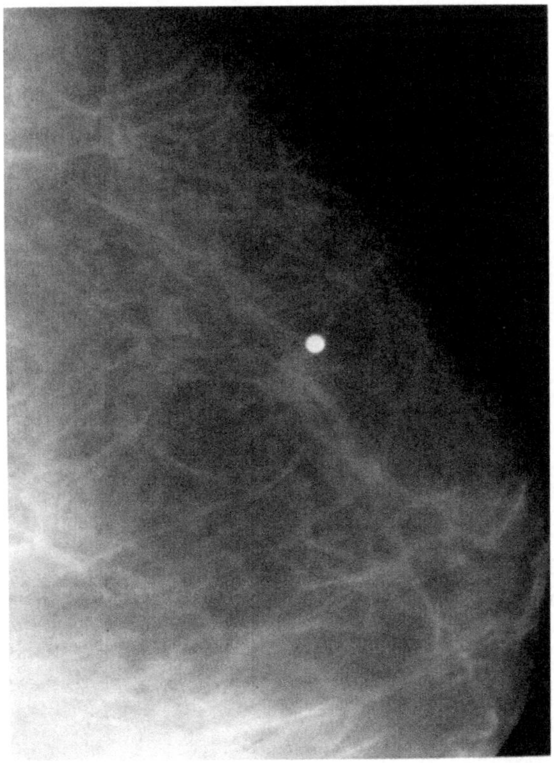

109

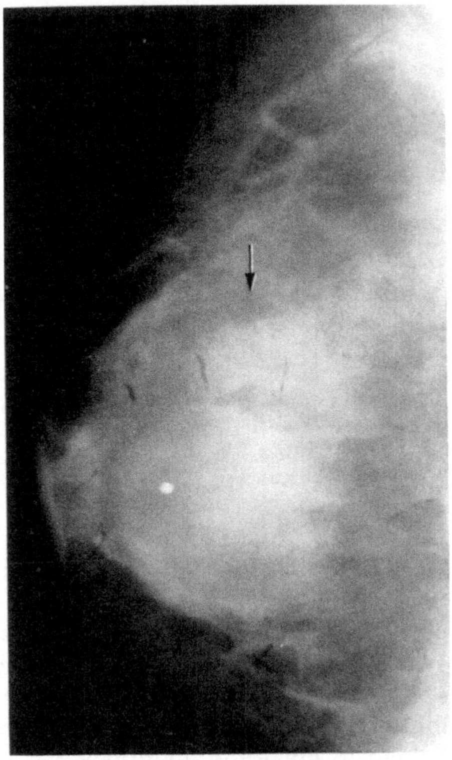

110

Fig. 111. Mastitis. Acute inflammation may easily be suspected clinically, but sometimes with difficulty on the X-ray film. The edema of the left breast blurs the structural details, and is best appreciated by comparing with the right

Fig. 112. Abscess (acute). An acute inflammatory process is present in the upper portion of the right breast. The edematous swelling, including the areolar skin, obscures the structural details as compared with the left breast. Increased skin temperature helped to make the diagnosis

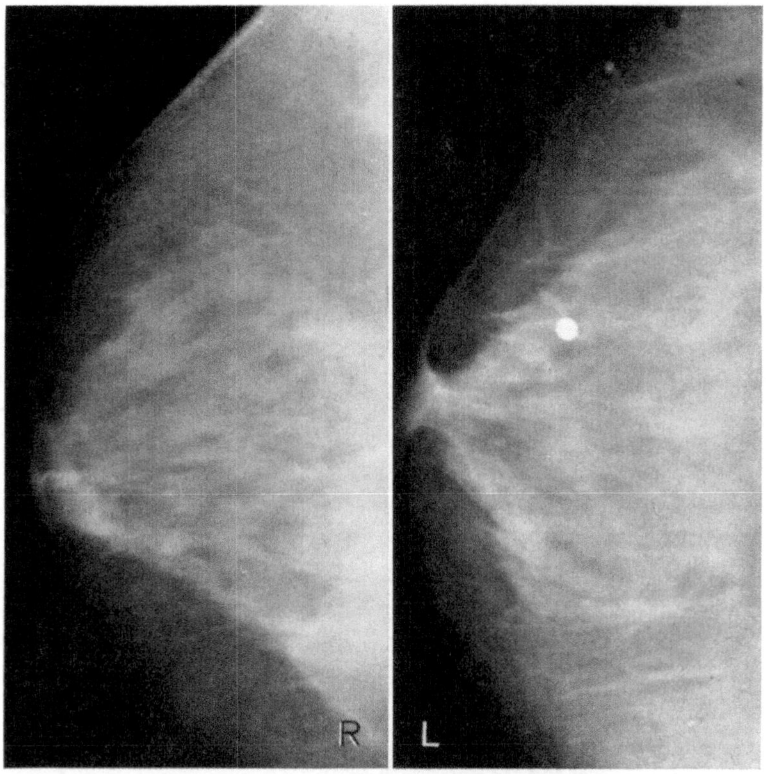

111

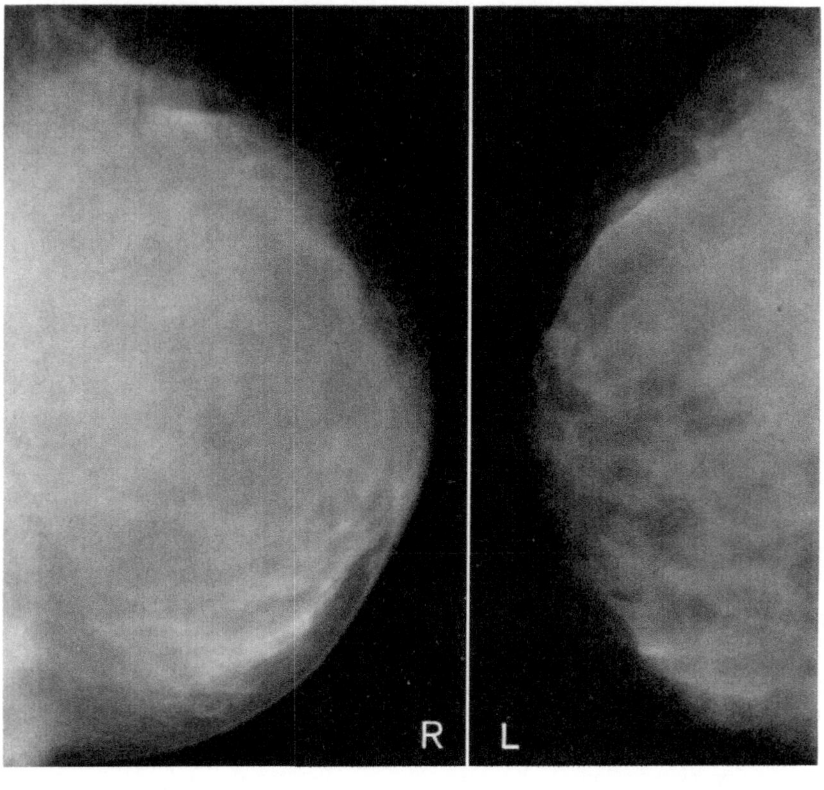

112

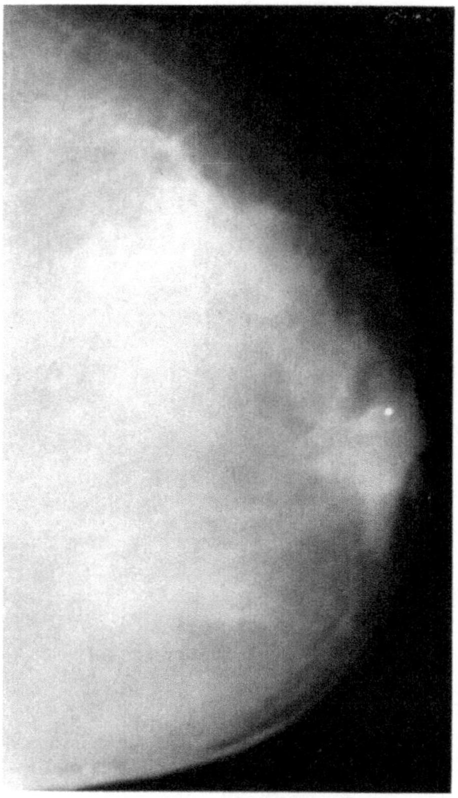

113

Fig. 113. Abscess (subacute). A mass of recent origin suggested cancer to both clinician and roentgenologist. An abscess can resemble cancer as it becomes localized and pseudospicules are formed due to edematous swelling of the perifocal trabeculae

Fig. 114. Chronic mastitis (localized). The edema and swelling of the skin and subcutaneous tissue in the areolar area of the right breast were present for 3 months before a draining mammillary fistula occurred and required resection

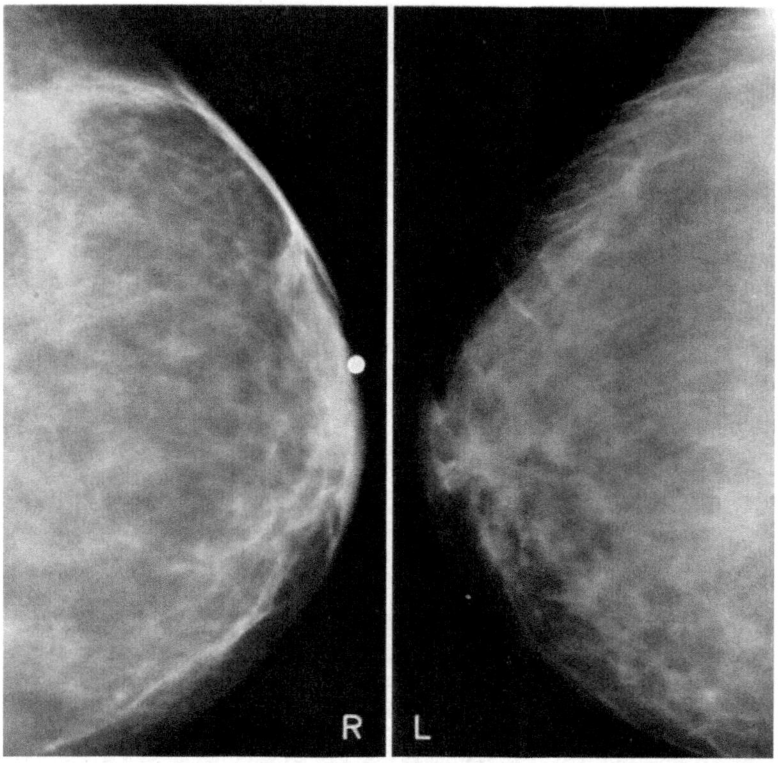

114

Fig. 115. Abscess (chronic). Abscesses are usually located in the areolar region near the nipple, and in the chronic phase their margins may be sharp and smooth, as in this case. Note edema of overlying skin

Fig. 116 A and B. Abscess (mammillary).
A
Lateral view of right breast reveals areolar and subareolar swelling, the limits of which are shown in
B
the cephalocaudad view. An abscess had been drained 4 months earlier, and a residual mammillary fistula is present. Note the pseudo-retraction of the nipple and the edema of the areolar skin

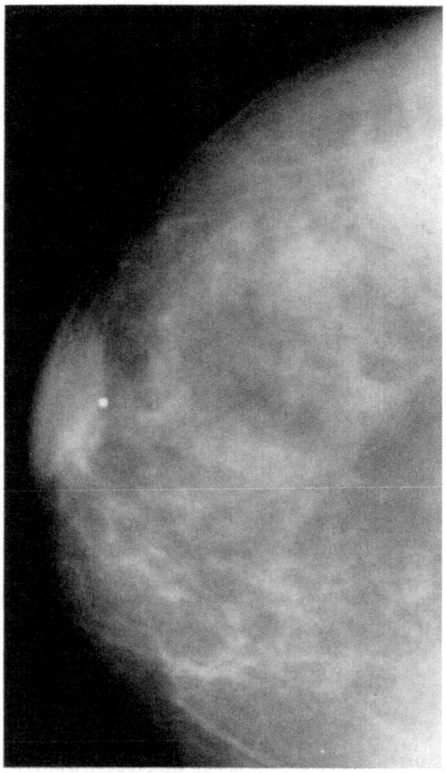

115

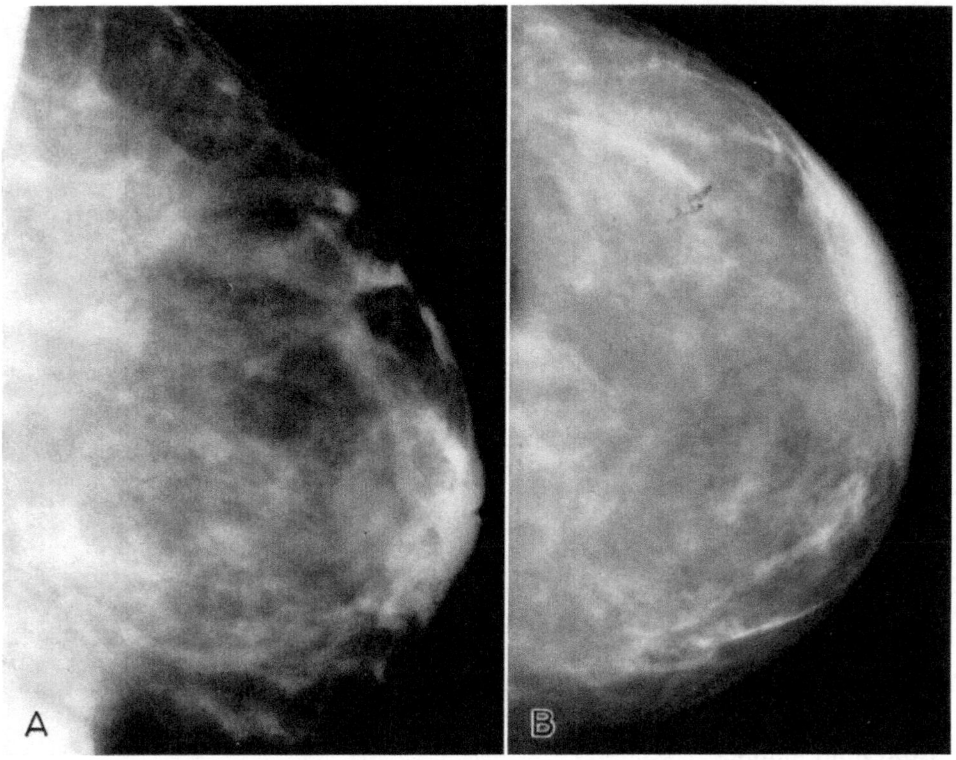

116

Fig. 117. Papilloma (arrow) in duct injected with contrast material (Renografin)

Fig. 118. Bilateral papillomatosis. The distorted duct in the right breast and the irregularly dilated duct in the left, encompassing a slightly calcified nodule, mark the location of papillomas associated with bleeding from both nipples

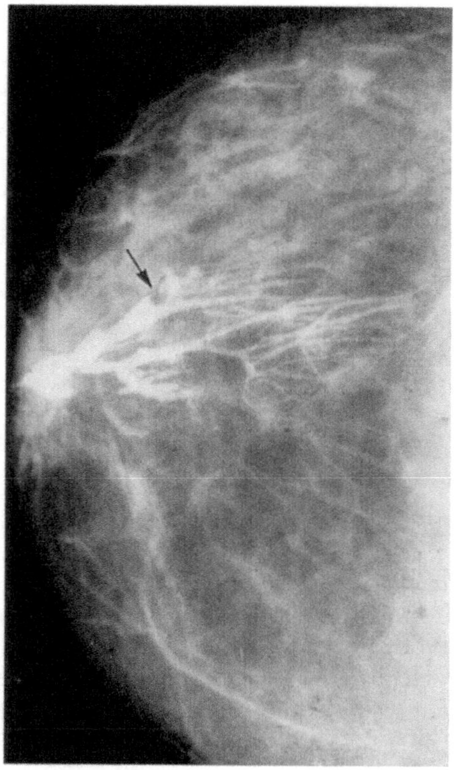
117

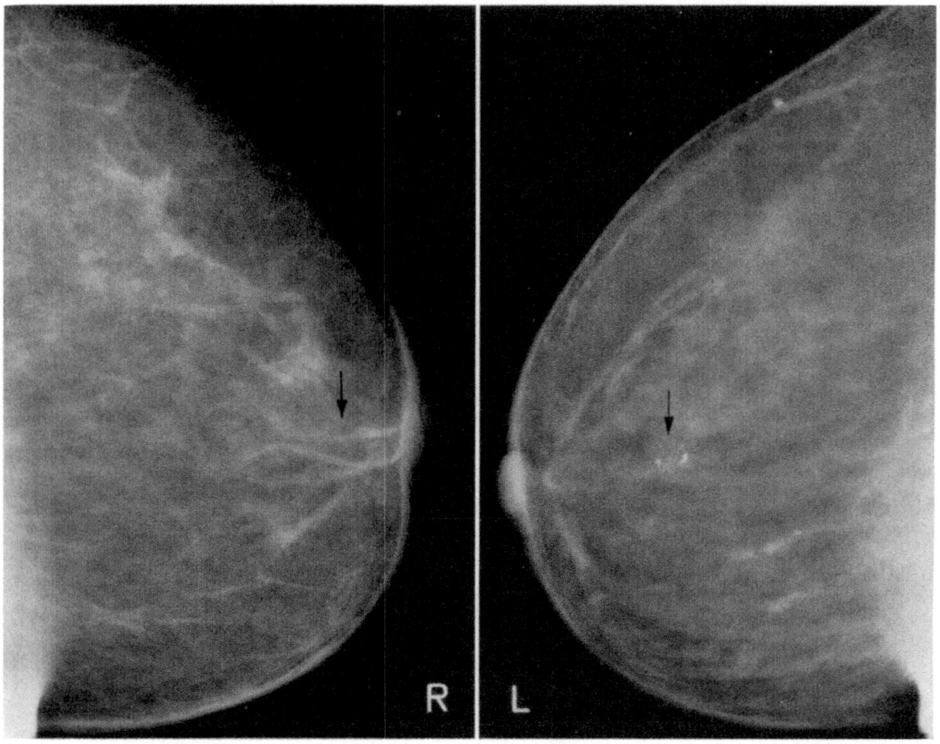

118

Fig. 119. Papilloma. Irregularly dilated, isolated duct segments (upper arrow) may mark site of intraductal papillomas, which must always be suspected in the presence of nipple discharge. A small fibroadenoma is present at the site of the lower arrow

Fig. 120. Papilloma. A short segment of a tortuous duct (arrow) is irregularly dilated. A papilloma may be suspected if there is a history of nipple discharge

Fig. 121 A and B. Papilloma. An isolated, irregularly dilated duct segment (arrows) may mark the location of a papilloma

A The lateral view

B The cephalocaudad view. A positive history of nipple discharge or bleeding is usually present

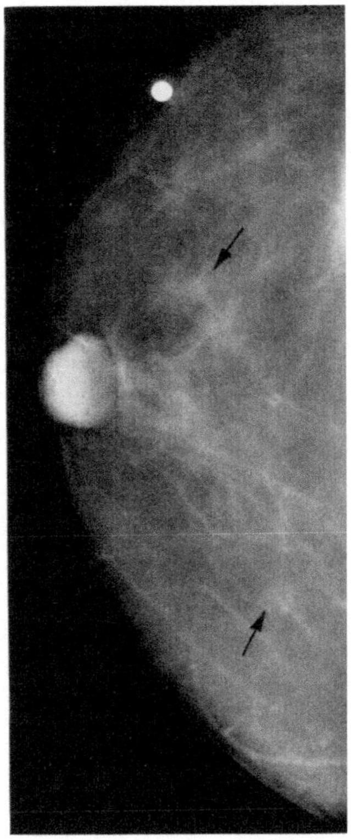

119

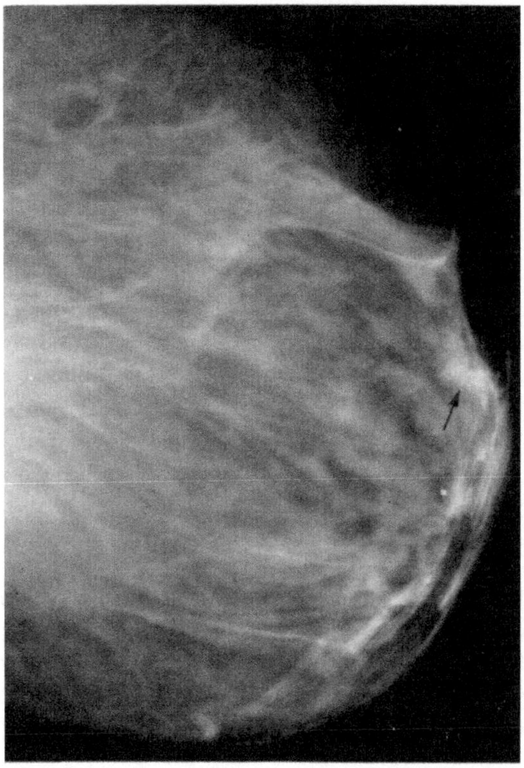

120

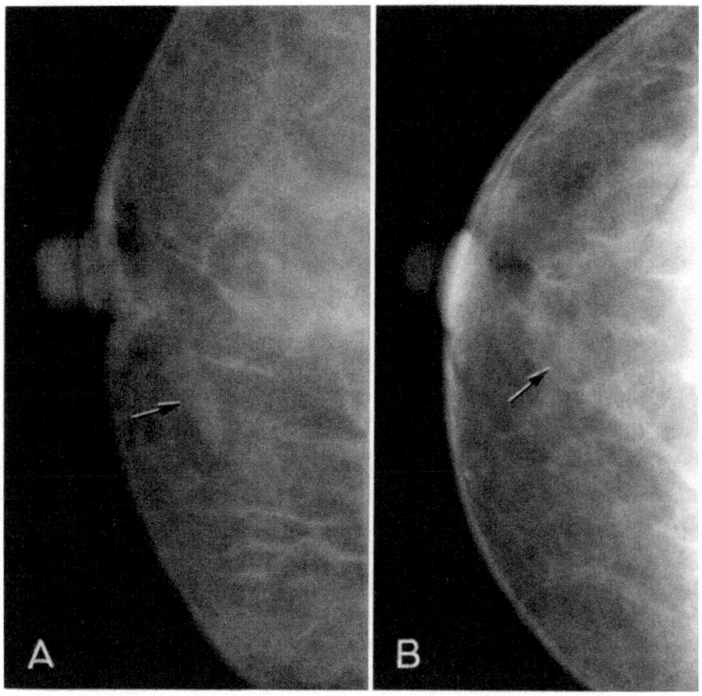

121

Fig. 122. Proliferative epithelial hyperplasia — papillomatosis (bilateral). The irregularly dilated ducts and numerous bulges are due to intraductal papillomas and fibroadenomas. Some are partially calcified

Fig. 123. Papilloma, intracystic. Intracystic papillomas may occur in the deeper recesses as well as in the larger superficial ducts. Distinguishing the smooth outlines of a papilloma or a fibroadenoma from those of a cyst is not usually possible on the X-ray film, although a papilloma within a cyst may be recognized by contrast if air is injected into the cyst after aspiration

Fig. 124. Papilloma (giant intracystic). Some cysts containing a papilloma can attain large dimensions and may resemble ordinary fibroadenomas or cysts

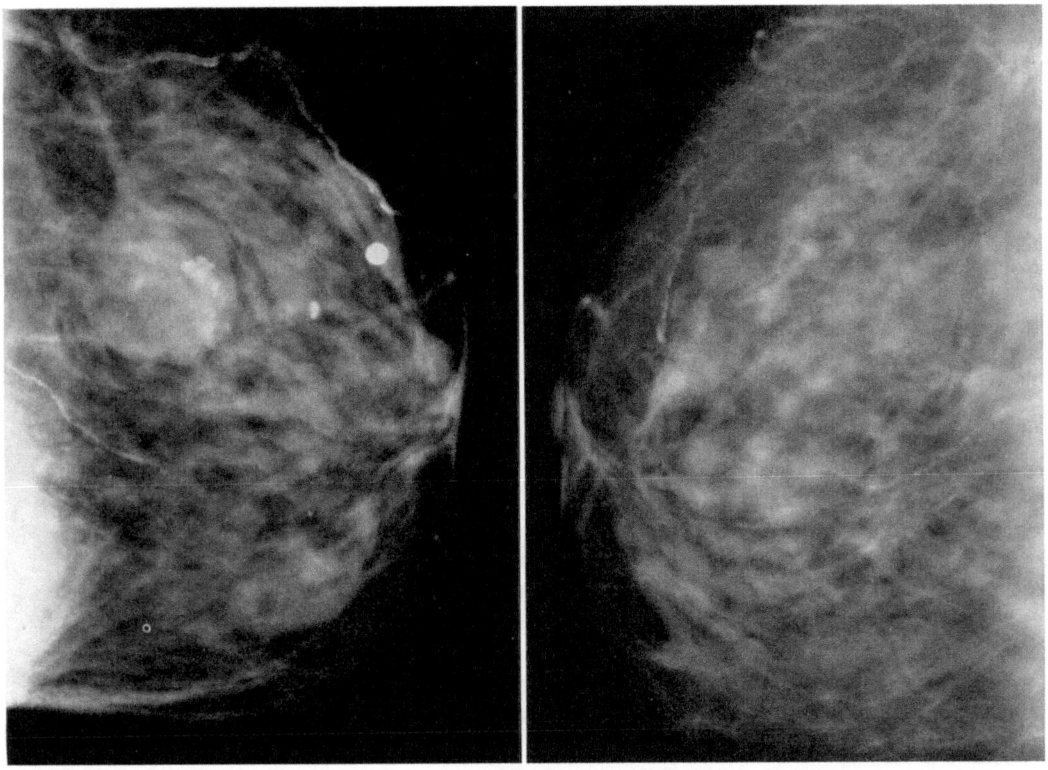

122

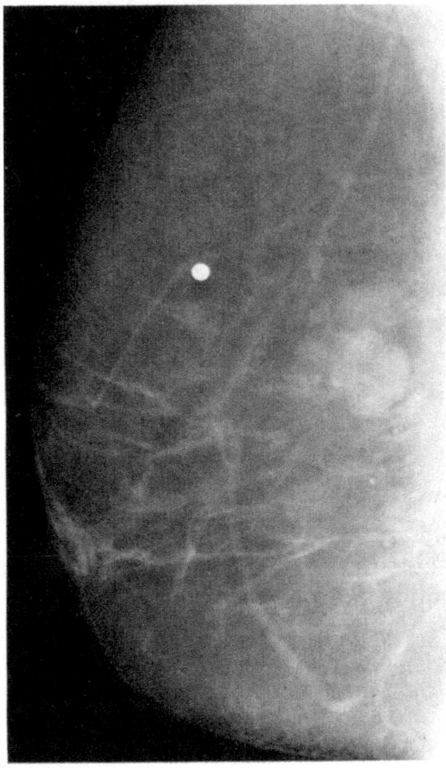

123

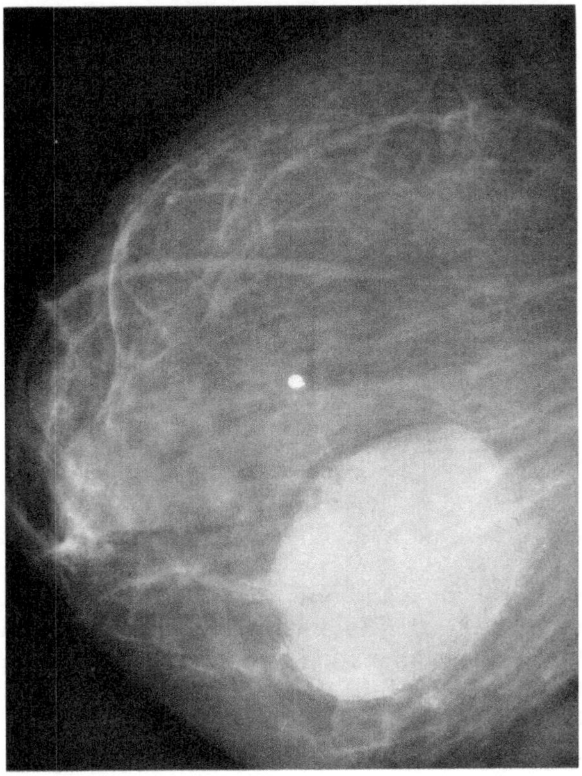

124

Fig. 125. Papilloma, intracystic. A circumscribed, smoothly contoured lesion suggests a fibroadenoma, a cyst, or a notched circumscribed carcinoma. An intracystic papilloma rarely may simulate these lesions. In women over 50 years of age, biopsy should be prompt

Fig. 126 A and B. Epithelial hyperplasia.
A
Microcalcifications are scattered throughout the breast. The small area indicated by the arrow when magnified 5 × better reveals the character of the particles
B
Most of them are minute and generally spheroid, but others are ring-shaped, unevenly calcified, and some of the rings of calcification are not complete. Such observations suggest epithelial excrescences, partially calcified in areas of epithelial hyperplasia and papillomatosis

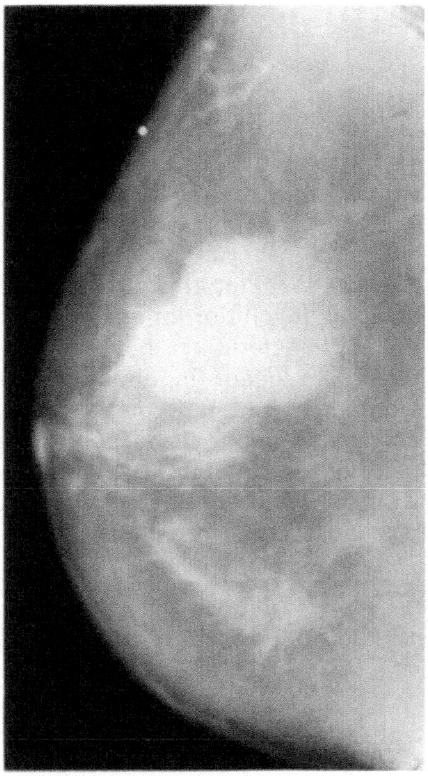

125

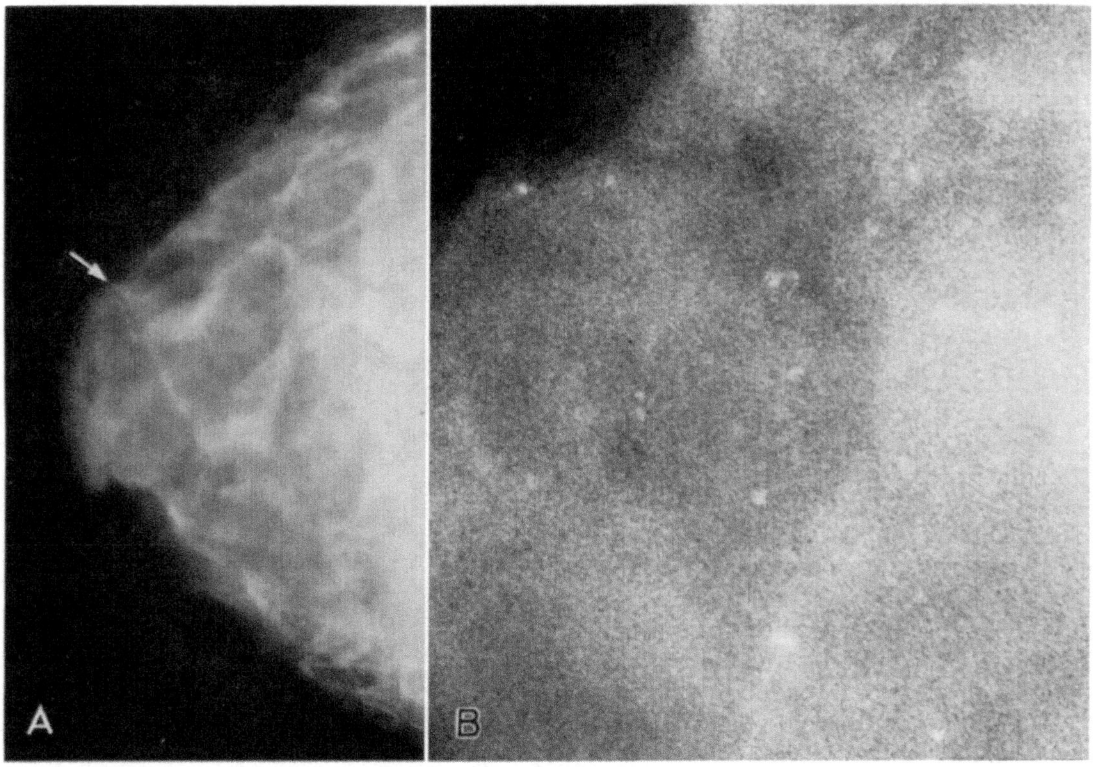

126

Fig. 127. Mastopathy. Instead of normal atrophic involution of active parenchyma at the climacterium, hyperplastic fibrosis seems to occur in about 40 per cent of women. The hyperplastic fibrosis and sclerosing adenosis in such breasts hamper cancer detection. In this 62 year old woman, a fibroadenoma was found in a field of hyperplastic fibrosis

Fig. 128. Mastopathy. When several dysplasias coexist without dominance of any one, the term "mastopathy" is found to be a convenient designation.
Tortuous dilated ducts due to epithelial hyperplasia may be present. Irregular zones of density due to adenosis in which epithelial pearls (arrows) are visible can occur. Sharply defined masses due to cysts and fibroadenomas, some of which exhibit the usual plaque-like calcifications, are commonly found. These combined dysplasias form the basis for this case of mastopathy. Cancer is far more prevalent in such breasts than in those mainly involved by a single type of dysplasia

Fig. 129. Mastopathy. When a combination of dysplasias is present with distorted fibrous ducts, irregular zones of homogeneous density due to fibrous and sclerotic adenosis (arrows), and scattered sharply outlined cysts and fibroadenomas, the term "mastopathy" is used for want of a better designation

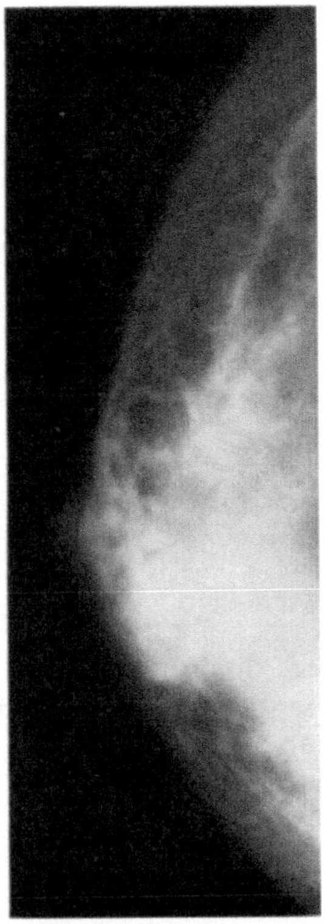

127

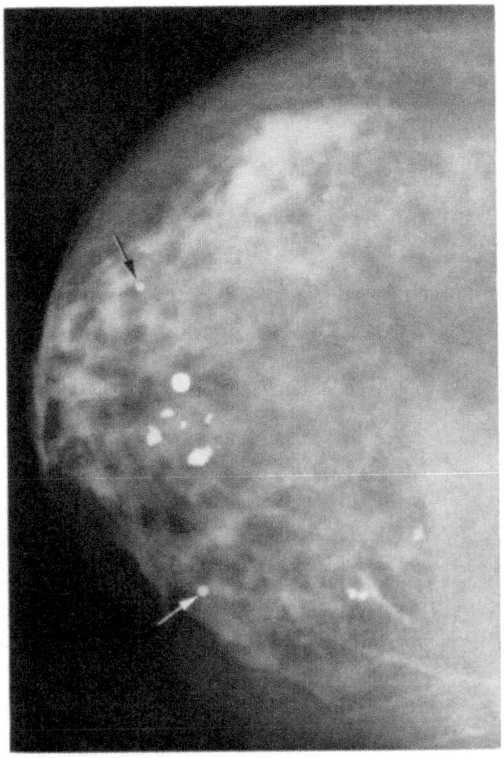

128

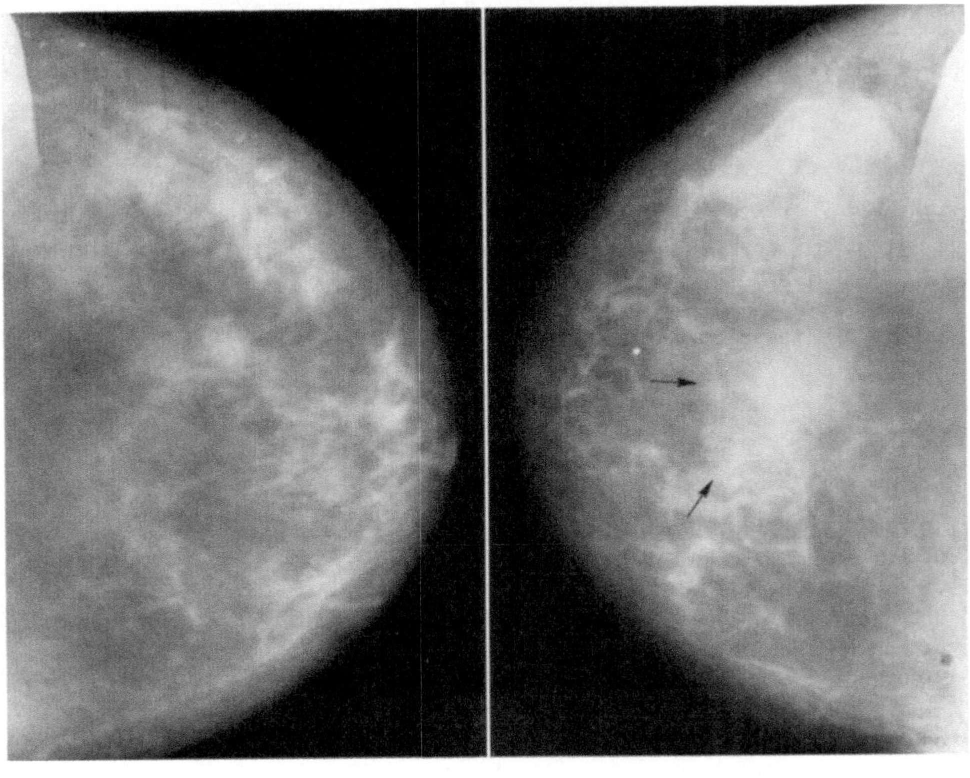

129

Fig. 130. Mastopathy. If both breasts are involved by irregularly dilated ducts due to epithelial hyperplasia (arrows), poorly defined areas of homogeneous density, due to adenosis, and several scattered cysts or fibroadenomas, these combined dysplasias are designated as "mastopathy." In the menopausal and postmenopausal periods, cancer is found more frequently associated with mastopathy than with any of the single dysplasias

Fig. 131. Mastopathy. When in the menopausal and postmenopausal periods residual dysplasias such as mazoplasia, adenosis, and epithelial hyperplasia persist, designated merely as "mastopathy," the higher incidence of cancer in such breasts must be kept in mind, and cancer in such breasts is often difficult to detect

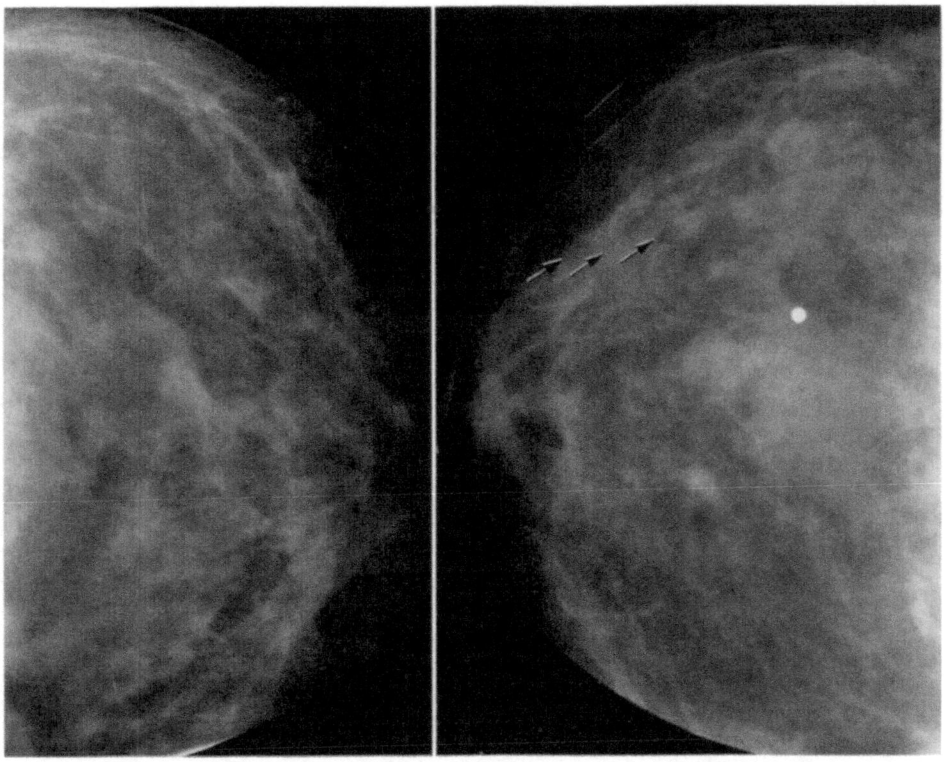

130

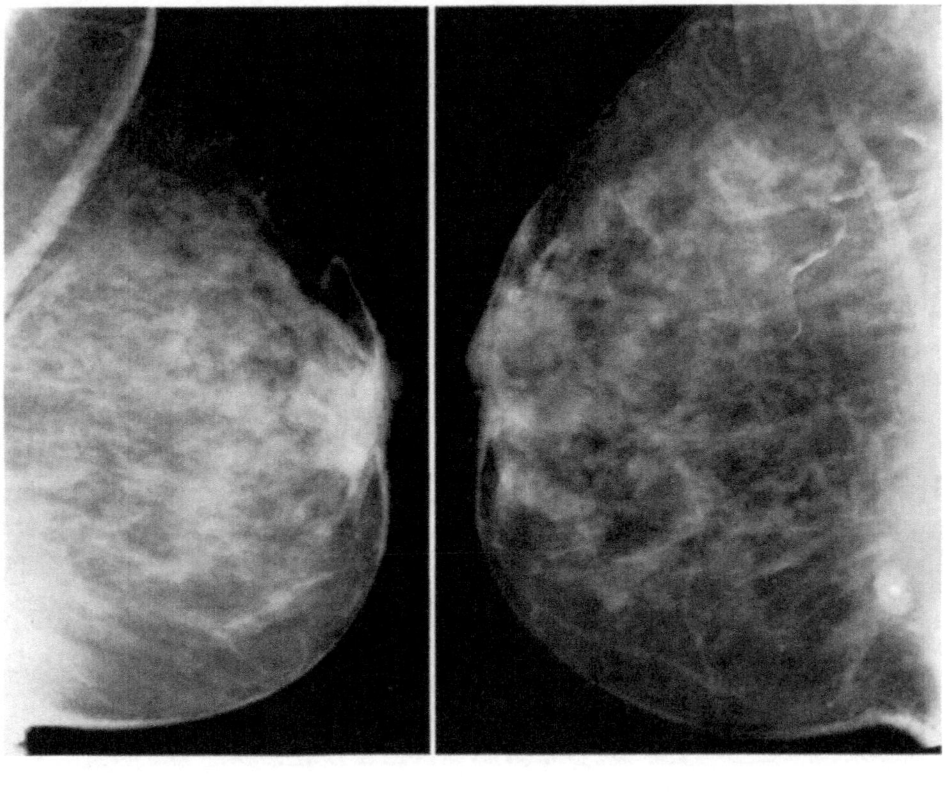

131

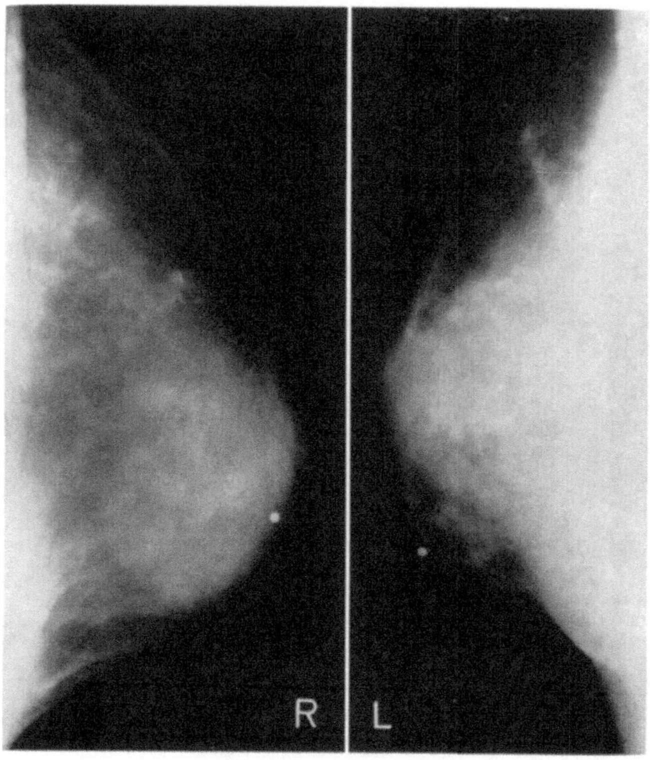

132

Fig. 132. Mastopathy. Postmenopausal hyperplastic fibrosis resulting from prolonged, excessive dysplasias is present in both breasts of a 59 year old woman. Palpable masses were present bilaterally under the skin markers. Biopsies were done to rule out cancer, which is hard to detect in such breasts

Fig. 133 A and B. Mastopathy with predominance of proliferative epithelial hyperplasia

A

Beaded, dilated, tortuous ducts due to epithelial hyperplasia dominate the fields of scattered areas of focal adenosis. An epithelial pearl is indicated by the arrow

B

An X-ray film of resected tissue enlarged 2 × reveals an epithelial pearl more distinctly

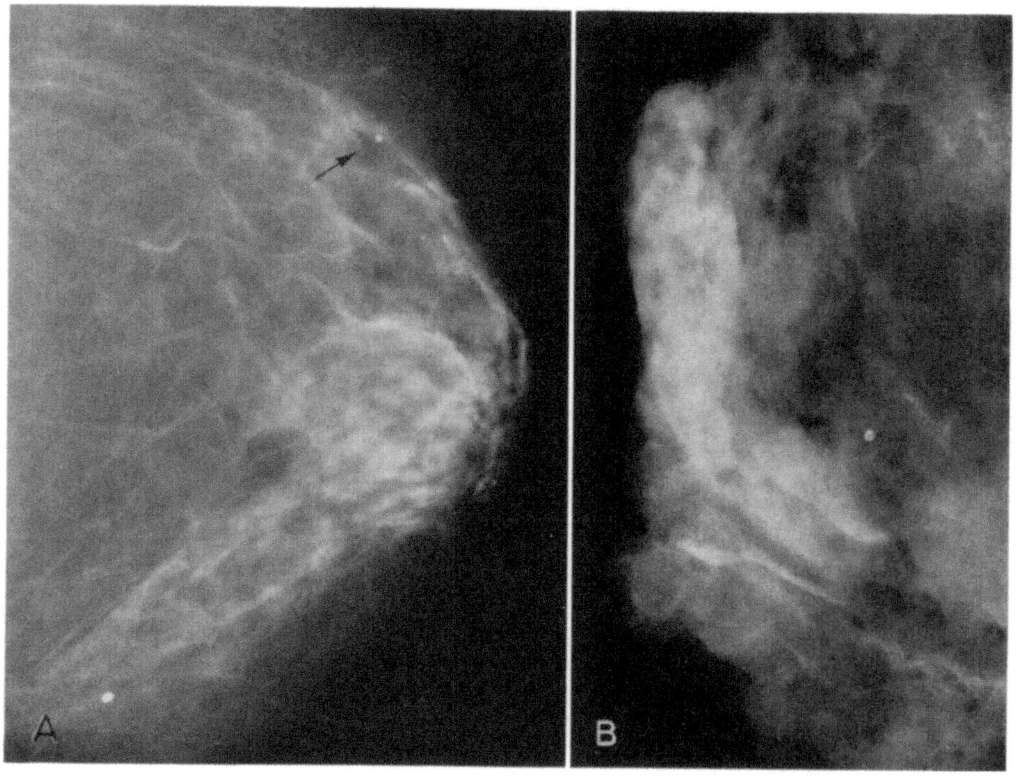

133

VI Differential X-ray Diagnosis of Benign Breast Lesions

For the reader's convenience, the principal sources of error in the X-ray diagnosis of benign lesions are summarized in the following paragraphs and in Table 1 (page 130).

1. *Adenosis*. Irregular lobular hyperplasia is extremely common. Minor grades of the disorder are often difficult to distinguish from normal breast tissue. For example, in the later stages of lactational involution, fluffy patches are seen which can only be interpreted correctly in light of a history of parturition some time previously.

In cases of doubt, the first consideration is comparison with the normal glandular type of breast. In generalized adenosis the homogeneous opacity at the base of the gland and the scattered fields about the trabeculae in the apical regions resemble the appearance of the normal breast. The coexistence of adenosis, cysts, and fibroadenomas must not be forgotten. Very careful search must be made for clusters of minute calcific particles which could betoken intraductal hyperplasia, carcinoma in situ, or duct cell carcinoma.

A spiculated opacity with perifocal edema should be examined with great care. At times the beginner will be confused by small stellate opacities which mimic early scirrhous carcinoma but are in reality distorted trabeculae or small fibrous scars. These must not be confused with the tentacles streaming from the body of a cancer. The presence of dilated ducts, especially clusters of small ducts, needs explanation. They are not part of adenosis but could be associated with intraductal hyperplasia.

Adenosis must be distinguished from early lobular carcinoma and from early cancers in which the tumor shows a lobular mode of spread. In both conditions the diagnosis is extremely difficult. On the X-ray film the carcinomatous areas resemble hyperplastic lobules.

2. *Mazoplasia Fibrosa*. Generalized mazoplasia fibrosa is uncommon in our experience. These breasts contain little fat and what has been said of immature breasts applies here. The chief difficulty is to visualize accompanying fibroadenomas.

Malignant tumors, fortunately, are rare; and they are extremely hard to recognize.

3. *Mazoplasia Cystica*. This condition is difficult to distinguish clinically from adenosis, but it is easy to diagnose on the X-ray film provided the cysts are seen. At times the cysts are masked by accompanying adenosis. The round, sharp margins of cysts are so distinctive that the diagnosis can usually be made if only a part of the cyst wall shows.

4. *Fibroadenoma*. Fibroadenoma occurs in young, dense breasts. The tumor is easy to feel but difficult to see. Sometimes it is necessary to push the tumor to the surface and take its X-ray picture in profile. Distinction from a cyst cannot as a rule be made on the X-ray film and should seldom be attempted. When a fibroadenoma is developing from adenosis, a sharp margin may be present on only one side of the mass. Coarse calcification is seen in long-standing fibroadenomas. It is a rather striking phenomenon and must not be allowed to distract the eye from more serious lesions such as carcinoma.

5. *Secretory Disease*. In making a diagnosis of secretory disease, the life history of the disorder should be borne in mind. In young women it often begins as an intermittent milky discharge following lactation. The lactiferous ducts will then be slightly dilated, but otherwise normal. In older women the chief changes are in the ducts. Two things to be looked for are: 1. thickening of the trabeculae; 2. dilatation, tortuosity, and sometimes beading of the ducts.

Besides dense fibrosis, long-standing cases of secretory disease show a variable amount of calcification along the line of the ducts. When dilatation and tortuosity are present the distinction from multiple intraductal papillomas is difficult, if not impossible. Nipple retraction occurs in older women with secretory disease but is very rare in papilloma. Of considerable assistance in diagnosis is the fact that secretory disease is nearly always bilateral. Nipple retraction, often present in long-standing cases, may be more marked in one breast but is to be expected in both, and is more easily seen on the film than in the patient.

6. *Plasma Cell Mastitis*. This complication of duct ectasia or secretory disease brings most patients to the doctor. It needs considerable care in diagnosis. On the X-ray film it appears as an irregular opacity or as multiple opacities. The lesion varies considerably in extent in different cases and may be bilateral. The margins are irregular, sometimes stellate, and

merge into the parenchyma. The area seen on the X-ray film is larger than that measured clinically, a very important point in differentiation from carcinoma. The presence of secretory disease in both breasts is of considerable assistance in the diagnosis and will distinguish plasma cell mastitis from adenosis.

Carcinoma and abscess are the two most important conditions to consider in differential diagnosis. With carcinoma, onset with pain is unusual although not as uncommon as is often thought. It is a notable feature in inflammatory carcinoma. In plasma cell mastitis onset with pain and swelling is the rule, but there are exceptions. A carcinomatous mass is usually denser and more sharply defined than the tumor of plasma cell mastitis. The presence of characteristic secretory disease in the contralateral breast may help to put the radiologist wise to the possibility of plasma cell mastitis, but it by no means excludes carcinoma.

7. *Abscess and chemical or plasma cell mastitis* have much in common. In fact, most intramammary abscesses originate in foci of plasma cell mastitis. The chief points in favor of abscess rather than chemical mastitis are thickening of the skin from edema and extreme vascular engorgement.

8. *Inflamed cysts*, either mazoplastic or secretory, often resemble circumscribed carcinomas. On the X-ray film the margins of the lesion may be blurred or even spiculated. The radiologist should report such cases as suspicious of carcinoma and let resection decide the issue.

9. *Mastopathy (Schimmelbusch's disease)* is diagnosed when a mixture of benign lesions is seen in the individual case. Separate dominant dysplasias cannot always be distinguished, but however complicated the appearances, exclusion of carcinoma in necessary and is nearly always possible. Even if a definite diagnosis cannot be made, the radiologist can play an extremely important part by insisting on biopsy of a suspicious area.

The busy radiologist is often tempted to shelve the differential diagnosis of dysplasia and be content merely to label a lesion benign or malignant. But if we are ever to learn how to recognize premalignant lesions, only by an accurate designation of the changes of gross pathology, as we roentgenologists see them, can we hope to exploit these opportunities for prevention of cancer.

Table 1. *X-ray Diagnoses of Benign Breast Lesions*

Adenosis	Mazoplasia fibrosa	Mazoplasia cystica	Fibroadenoma	Secretory disease	Mastopathy	Intraductal hyperplasia	Papilloma
Multiple bilateral, often circumscribed, opacities of glandular density	Compact, homogeneous dense breast; bosselated surface	Single or multiple rounded, sharply defined opacities	Bosselated or round, sharply defined opacity, often shows halo: difficult to visualize in dense breasts; occasionally, coarse calcification	Dilated lactiferous ducts; dense fibrosis in subareolar area, calcification in duct wall. Plasma cell mastitis: irregular, poorly outlined opacity with extensions in line of trabeculae	Mixture of any or all forms of dysplasia	Irregular dilatation of ducts, punctate calcifications, even when ducts are not seen	a) Intraductal: varicose distension of ducts. b) Intracystic: resembles solitary cyst but is more opaque
Differential Diagnosis							
Physiologic hyperplasia; lactational involution; plasma cell mastitis; early lobular carcinoma	Normal immature breast	Fibroadenoma (not always possible); other cystic lesions; circumscribed carcinoma	Cysts; sarcoma; circumscribed carcinoma	Carcinoma; papilloma; intraductal hyperplasia; other forms of mammary dysplasia; traumatic fat necrosis; abscess	Carcinoma	Carcinoma; benign papilloma; secretory disease	Occasionally secretory disease; mazoplastic or other cysts; fibroadenoma

VII Cancer

1. Classification

Classifications of mammary carcinoma based on gross and histologic features of the tumor are far from satisfactory. They are as varied as the pathologists who make them. The main groups are usually infiltrating duct cell cancer with and without scirrhus; medullary; lobular; adenocarcinoma; and Paget's disease of the nipple. Obviously, not all of these represent distinct types of carcinoma. Histological appearances are deceptive.

Variations in morphology may well be manifestations of the mode of spread rather than true differences in the type of cancer. Carcinoma cells grow along the line of least resistance. In soft, fatty tissue they spread in all directions. In firmer tissue they tend to travel along clefts between fibrous strands. They may use lymphatics or even blood vessels as paths. They are seen occupying and distending mammary ducts. When no ready-made channels present themselves the tumor will compress the parenchyma instead of infiltrating it. The result is a carcinoma which is almost encapsulated.

Besides growing by multiplication of tumor cells carcinomas also increase by malignant transformation of developing epithelium in their vicinity. The change may take place in lobules or in ducts.

Lobular spread is seen mainly in women in their early 30s who have adenosis. Here the carcinoma is often surrounded by an area of hyperplasia. The process may occur in a number of foci over a large area.

Malignant transformation of hyperplastic duct epithelium is characteristic of intraductal carcinoma. The tumor extends via ducts. It is preceded by intraductal hyperplasia and followed by carcinoma in situ before clinical carcinoma supervenes. Precancerous epithelial proliferation may be adjacent to the tumor or at a distance from it.

The above considerations suggest that the pattern of carcinomatous growth might be expected to change from one part of a tumor to another, depending on the texture of the mammary tissue in process of being infiltrated. While the appearance of a tumor is determined in part by other environmental factors, such as those concerned with differentiation and organization, wide differences in one and the same tumor are best explained by the nature of the adjacent tissue.

When we reviewed our films it soon became evident that the tumors fell into certain categories depending on their contour and on the presence and type of calcification seen in and around them. About 30 per cent had spiculated margins and corresponded pathologically to the so-called scirrhous carcinoma; another 20 per cent were more sharply outlined and circumscribed, more rarely of the medullary type. Some 35 per cent were ductal carcinomas, which in nearly all cases displayed punctate calcifications either in irregular clusters or spread linearly through the ducts. The other types of cancers fitted into such categories as lobular, mucoid, inflammatory, lymphomatous and sarcomatous types.

2. Growth Rate

A carcinoma may be termed "early" because it is small or because it is believed to have existed for only a short time. Both conceptions are extremely vague and serve no useful purpose. The only satisfactory definition of "early" carcinoma is a neoplasm which has not metastasized.

Metastatic growth is the lethal factor in most breast cancers. Collins and his associates in their study of secondary tumors in the lung showed that the neoplasms in various parts of the body from which the lung tumors were derived had nearly always metastasized before the primary lesion was discovered. We agree with Collins in a similar concept that "no palpable breast tumor is early."

The conclusion to be drawn from perusal of available literature is that not more than 20 per cent of *clinically diagnosable breast tumors are "early"* in the sense just defined. Evidently the ability to metastasize does not depend on size, and clinical duration seldom has any relation to the real state of affairs.

The first step in the resolution of these imponderables is to determine the average growth rate of specific tumors. The measurements of the tumor as seen on the X-ray film correspond closely to those of the actual specimen. Furthermore, experience has shown that it is possible to visualize a carcinoma on the X-ray film long before it becomes clinically palpable. If, following Collins' reasoning, a nodule 2 cm in diameter is a likely minimal size for clinical diagnosis, the tumor may have already run more than half its life cycle before being discovered. Knowledge of progress during the first half of the tumor's life is closed to us without X-rays. Not all early tumors are diagnosable at first and only persistent regular re-examinations will bring them to light on the X-ray film. The growth rate of such tumors can then be calculated by tracing and measuring their outlines from successive X-ray studies.

The determination of growth rate by this means is, however, open to certain criticisms. More data are definitely needed before actual duration can be determined. Constant rate of growth, hence a uniform increase in size, would be expected of tumors which grow in a relatively homogeneous organ such as the lung. But the mammary gland is not homogeneous and a uniform rate of growth cannot be postulated. The fact that breast tumors are seldom spherical is circumstantial evidence that growth is affected by the structure of the organ. The surroundings of a small tumor are apt to be more homogeneous than those of a large one, and a more uniform growth rate might be expected. Moreover, as tumors enlarge, the blood supply becomes uneven, so that the more centrally placed cells may undergo necrosis and thus modify growth characteristics.

Duct cell carcinomas differ from the other two common forms in that their spread occurs mainly via multicentric foci arising in duct epithelium. The primary tumor increases very slowly and may remain in the stage of carcinoma in situ for years. When the infiltrative stage is reached, the growth outside the ducts is apt to blend with the surrounding tissue. Grossly as well as radiologically no definite boundary may be seen. Clusters of calcified particles indicate the site of tumor nodules, but the growth itself cannot be measured.

Because of the difficulties of measuring the size of duct carcinomas, they pose a problem when it comes to estimating duration. While it is quite possible for the primary focus to remain stationary for long periods, secondary foci may be in a state of active proliferation. The possibility of multiple primary foci must also be thought of. A duct carcinoma which remains true to type may be localized to the breast for 10 years or more. The contralateral breast may be affected, but this could well be by a second primary. The prognosis becomes considerably graver when the duct carcinoma passes over into the scirrhous type. It then behaves like a scirrhus.

Foulds demonstrated multiple cancers in hyperplastic foci in mice which eventually coalesced to form a large tumor. The same thing happens in human breasts. On the X-ray film, it may be impossible to tell whether the tumor arose simultaneously at multiple points or whether a single primary cancer gave origin to others by a lobular mode of spread. In either case, a sudden increase in size might be due to coalescing of growths too small to have been detected on previous examinations.

The malignant progression in recurrent tumors described by Foulds (1949, 1954) in mammary glands of mice and by our own evidence would indicate that similar progression may occur in women. Murine tumors are hormone-responsive. They were found to grow during pregnancy. Some increased progressively; others regressed partially or completely after parturition. After a longer or shorter time, hormone responsiveness was lost but the tumors continued to grow. The time factor for loss of responsiveness was extremely variable. It might exceed the life-span of one animal and the change might be observed only after grafting the tumor into a second host.

The changes in Foulds' mouse plaques during regression following pregnancy are certainly akin to those of human adenosis. In some mice, minute foci of carcinoma were detected in the degenerating areas. A similar focus in humans would be far too small to be detected clinically, as a rule, and would have little chance of being included in a histologic section. Lobular hyperplasia initiated by pregnancy was preceded by tumor formation in the mice. Lobular hyperplasia (adenosis) can antedate carcinoma in women.

Although investigation of tumor duration is still in its infancy, two points are clear: 1. The average rate of growth of scirrhous carcinomas greatly exceeds that of circumscribed and duct varieties. The excess is well outside the margin of error and confirms previous observations that patients with scirrhus succumb to the disease earlier than do those with circumscribed or duct carcinomas. 2. Cancers have a much longer life-span and a greater variation in growth rate than clinicians usually realize. Animal experiments translated into human terms of life-span suggest that in man a carcinogenic agent takes 10 years or more to produce a tumor of clinical size. When all the data are taken into consideration, *it must be conceded that few palpable tumors may be thought of as "early."*

3. Diagnosis without Symptoms

Cancer of the breast in the late 1960s involved more than 65,000 women in the United States. Despite advances in surgical, chemotherapeutic, and radiotherapeutic techniques the survival statistics have not shown improvement. This fact suggests rather strongly that we are still not finding cancers when they are localized.

Possibly this is because in the United States we tend to place responsibility for detecting breast cancer chiefly on the woman herself. We urge women to examine their breasts periodically and report anything suspicious. The indoctrination has been highly successful; more than 95 per cent of women discover their own lesions. But statistics for these self-found cancers are very discouraging. Current data indicate that the lesion found in this manner averages more than 3.5 cm in diameter, is associated with metastasis in more than 65 per cent of cases, and has a mortality rate of 50 per cent within five years.

Some of the reasons for this sad state of affairs are these: 1. Fear often causes the patient to delay taking her findings to a physician. 2. When she does, often the advice she receives from her family doctor occasions further delay, for the physical findings when limited to inspection and palpation are often so doubtful that an unqualified decision to procure a biopsy seems unwarranted. Such unfortunate events probably contribute in large measure to the poor recovery rate for this tumor.

If we shifted the responsibility for the early detection of cancer from the patient to the physician skilled in breast examination, we should expect better results. Healthy women do not fear periodic physical examinations and X-ray studies. If they know in advance that no therapeutic decision will be made until both the physical and X-ray findings are reconciled, they are even more willing to subscribe to such a program.

In a survey project started by us in January 1956, using mammography among a group of 1,120 healthy volunteers over 35 years of age, periodic X-ray studies at 6-month intervals for 10 years resulted in the discovery of 36 cancers in 33 women, 3 of which were subsequently bilateral. Axillary metastasis was present in only 30 per cent, and the cancers averaged 1.1 cm in diameter.

In another group of 102 consecutive cases of breast cancer which we studied, 8 women had bilateral mastectomies over a period of 14 years. The initial operations were performed without benefit of mammography. Delays in seeking medical advice averaged 7 months and the lesions removed averaged 3.8 cm in diameter. All of the second operations were preceded by mammographic studies at 6-month intervals. All 8 cancers in the second breast were discovered by mammography alone.

No delays occurred before the removal of the second breast. The lesions averaged only 1.1 cm in diameter and only one of the 8 showed axillary spread.

A diagnostic resection is mandatory if the clinician, the surgeon, or the radiologist suspects the presence of cancer. The roentgenologist will suspect cancer in some 20 per cent of cases in which the clinician or the surgeon, or both, will be undecided. These will usually be multinodular breasts in which a dominant lesion cannot be pinpointed; lesions which feel benign by palpation but show malignant characteristics to mammography; palpable lesions which prove to be benign by X-ray but which are associated with a malignant lesion in another part of the breast or, rarely, an unsuspected malignancy in the opposite breast. If there were wider collaboration of the clinician, the surgeon, the pathologist, and the radiologist in such an effort, more biopsies would result and a greater number of localized and curable (Stage 1) cancers would be discovered.

4. Diagnosis with Symptoms

Since early, accurate diagnosis of breast cancer is so vital to prognosis, the radiologist must become familiar with both the clinical and the pathological manifestations of the disease. They are varied and insidious, yet classifications of mammary cancer are far from satisfactory. The categories are merely descriptive for the most part, or follow conventional arrangements as varied as the pathologists who formulated them.

The roentgenologist doing mammography will find the following categorization a good working plan based on X-ray findings: 1. spiculated masses; 2. circumscribed masses; 3. distorted structural patterns due to cancer; 4. microcalcifications with any of the above-mentioned patterns; 5. secondary signs due to lymphatic spread, edema, and inflammatory reactions. These radiologic terms must then be reconciled with those used by the pathologist.

Probably 90 per cent of all breast cancers are ductal in origin, and may be papillary, comedo, scirrhous, medullary, or colloid in type. Of these, the roentgenologist will identify most easily the infiltrating duct cell cancers with scirrhous formations. Medullary, lobular, and colloid cancers are more difficult to assess. Of the lobular carcinomas, only the infiltrating types are apt to be recognized on the X-ray film, by the presence of structural distortions, microcalcifications, or associated scirrhous involution.

Of the rare carcinomas, such as those arising from the so-called sweat glands or those which are intracystic, squamous, or spindle-celled, only by comparing the dissimilar architectural components of both breasts will the suspicion of malignancy arise in the mind of the roentgenologist. The same will hold true for the various forms of sarcoma which in essence cannot be differentiated on the roentgenogram from carcinomas.

Finally, Paget's disease will involve the nipple and ducts, and the minimal distortion it produces in the structures can easily fail to excite suspicion if the history of itching, scaling, and bleeding of the nipple is not properly appraised. The late stages, when secondary infiltrative lesions occur, may be obvious on the X-ray film.

When reporting these various pathologic conditions, the radiologist will use such terms as "increased localized density," "undue prominence of the ducts," "spiculated infiltration," "circumscribed but irregularly contoured lesion," "punctate calcifications," "architectural distortion as compared with the opposite breast," and the like. The secondary signs of malignancy, which are often easily discerned, will be described as "edema," "vascular engorgement," "thickening of the skin," "retraction of the nipple," etc. Some of these signs will also be obvious to the clinician at times, but at other times they are not, so the radiologist should report these findings because they may have extreme importance.

In the final analysis, the knowledge of gross anatomy and extent of the disease which the roentgenologist is particularly capable of furnishing may far outweigh the importance of microscopic classification. A combination of the two may yield even more information of significance.

a) Infiltrating Duct Cell Carcinoma with Productive Fibrosis (Scirrhus)

This is the most common form of breast cancer, comprising probably more than 70 per cent. The desmoplasia and productive fibrosis are what give the characteristic gross and roentgenographic appearance to these tumors. As these malignant proliferations break out of bounds of the ducts, scirrhous tumors form and the majority will not be rounded, but ovoid, ellipsoid, or discoid. Dendritic strands and striae radiate from the irregular margins of this fibrous tumor. It is the fibrous quality that accounts for the unyielding induration of these lesions to palpation. The pathologist easily recognizes the increased resistance of the cut surface and the striate, yellowish,

chalky streaks scattered over a generally grayish-yellow background. The histologist has little trouble confirming a diagnosis of malignancy, although much fibrosis may crowd the cancer cells into a limited field and make his diagnosis difficult.
On the X-ray film the radiating spicules, strands, threads, and burr-like formations of fibrosis in fatty breasts make accurate spotting of the lesions easy, and a firm diagnosis of malignancy can be made without benefit of a history or knowledge of the results of physical examination (Figs. 134—145).
At other times the reaction to the tumor is so limited to the periphery of the lesion that it will escape detection. Such lesions may appear to be circumscribed, resembling medullary cancers with undulating, notched margins. Often the reaction is not evident at all except for distortion of the perifocal trabecular architecture. A group of ducts or vessels may be stretched or tugged into unusual alignment, or there may be actual disruption of the adjacent glandular or ductal configuration. An edematous reaction in the surrounding tissue may blur the component structures and may be the first sign of an infiltrative process. By this time vascular engorgement, thickening of the skin, and displacement of the nipple may be obvious secondary signs, easily discerned on the roentgenogram. These reactive changes account for the common observation that the physical, external measurements of these tumors exceed those derived by measuring the lesion on the X-ray film (Figs. 146—157).
But when these scirrhous lesions develop in areas of dense mazoplasia, adenosis, or mastopathy, the tumor itself may be entirely obscured. What should be searched for are the radiating dendritic striae, which may extend into areas of fat between the trabeculae or in the subcutaneous zone. They then stand out as "sentinel strands" and should immediately arouse the suspicion of a hidden cancer (Figs. 158—165).
These reactive changes cause blurring of tissue due to edema or may result from extension of a malignant process into the lymphatics or to reactive cellular proliferation. As this process increases, the trabecular breast pattern fades and blurs, at first in localized areas around the initial lesions and later becoming more generalized to include the skin. Such edematous intramammary swelling may become familiar to the practiced eye, but to the uninitiated these changes will not be evident until the films of the opposite breast are compared.
In such circumstances, help from the history and physical findings can also serve in the balance. When such help fails, the

roentgenologist will be foresighted if he suggests a diagnostic resection, especially if the woman is past 40 years of age, has localized symptoms of recent origin, and the X-ray signs in the involved breast are different from those in the opposite breast (Figs. 166—178).

About 35 per cent of these tumors are associated with microcalcifications by the time they are discovered by X-ray. The curious punctate crystalline-like calcium deposits which are seen may be located within the tumor or about it. Finding these deposits on the roentgenogram requires proper exposure and meticulous searching. Preferably, the films should be slightly overexposed and viewed with brilliant illumination and a magnifying glass. The minuteness of these deposits may elude the unaided eye, and the film must be scrutinized carefully before the possibility of their presence is dismissed. Because a reliable diagnosis can be placed on the finding of these calcifications, no matter what other diagnostic ambiguities exist, a search for these patterns of calcareous change is exceedingly important.

A scirrhus may arrest attention because it contains punctate deposits, and further scrutiny may reveal similar deposits in surrounding ducts which have not yet been breached. The deposits have a crystalline quality, like grains of salt, and lie about helter-skelter in an unpolarized fashion. When confined to the ducts they are naturally strewn along the course of the ducts, usually very evident in some cases of comedo cancer and Paget's disease. The minuteness of these deposits results in only the faintest density contrast with surrounding tissues, so their discernment can be a difficult matter.

Coarser forms of amorphous calcification are also encountered in about 10 per cent of cancers, but they are nonspecific. They resemble the deposits seen in fibroadenomas and cysts. Mucoid carcinoma may occasionally contain lacy flakes of calcification. In proliferative epithelial hyperplasia, involutional changes may lead to deposits of minute calcification resembling those seen in cancer. These may pose diagnostic difficulties.

When only a few microcalcifications are discovered in small, localized areas in circumstances that raise no other reason to suspect malignancy, it is our habit to procure serial re-examination at intervals not exceeding 6 months. So long as the deposits do not increase in number and no other signs of malignancy supervene, we maintain a conservative approach to surgical intervention. But any increase in the amount of calcification or the appearance of other clinical or X-ray signs which could portend malignancy lead us to favor a surgical approach without further delay (Figs. 179—187).

b) Infiltrating Duct Cell Cancer without Scirrhus

Infiltrating duct cell cancer without scirrhus, while it is predominantly confined to the duct system, can be detected if the slight bulging and distortion of the trabeculae occur in fatty breasts (Figs. 188—192).

In dense, hyperplastic, fibrous breasts where a cancer might occur without the formation of a scirrhus or the development of microcalcifications, the skilled clinician may detect the cancer as a palpable "dominant mass" which eludes detection by the roentgenologist. In many of these cases, the secondary signs of edema and vascular turgescence may be evident to the practiced eye of an experienced roentgenologist, which will bolster his stand with the surgeon on his decision to operate (Figs. 193—199).

If such changes occur in the absence of a palpable "dominant mass," obtaining a biopsy may pose problems due to reluctance of the patient and/or the surgeon to proceed with an operation under such circumstances. Often the patient will have localized symptoms corresponding to the site of suggestive X-ray findings, in which case the roentgenologist can be more insistent on establishing a definitive diagnosis by advising a diagnostic resection. Otherwise, it is foresighted to arrange for periodic re-examinations at one- or two-month intervals. If local symptoms and X-ray signs persist, then biopsy should no longer be postponed, regardless of the absence of a palpable "dominant mass."

The main purpose of mammography is to obtain detection of small, *localized* cancers and the only way this can be effected is to get a biopsy whenever there is the slightest suspicion that a lesion might be a cancer, regardless of the physical findings. The reverse of this situation can also be valid, so that when the surgeon believes he can palpate a "dominant mass" even though it cannot be confirmed on the X-ray film, his conviction to operate should be supported.

When the malignant process is more advanced, even if the infiltration and permeation of the cancer itself cannot be recognized, the extensive edema with the resultant skin thickening will be obvious to both the clinician and roentgenologist alike (Figs. 200—204). Such cancers are not infrequently referred to as "inflammatory cancers, "which is a misnomer. These cancers have simply infiltrated widely to include the dermal lymphatics. While a moderate amount of desmoplasia accompanies the tumor cells, the X-ray appearance is not based on an inflammatory reaction, but is rather the result of an aggressive cancer infiltrating widely in all directions. The gross appearance can simulate lymphectasia due to mastitis and other causes as in Figure 205. Rarely, an unsuspected cancer may be found by the roentgenologist in such circumstances in the opposite breast (Fig. 206).

When microcalcifications are present, the roentgenologist may be the only consultant to suspect cancer, since a palpable "dominant mass" may not be present (Figs. 207—213).

c) Medullary Cancers

Medullary cancers with lymphoid infiltration are sufficiently distinctive to warrant a separate classification not only from the viewpoint of the pathologist but also from that of the roentgenologist. Because these tumors are circumscribed, the initial tendency is to confuse them with benign cysts and fibroadenomas on the X-ray film. But their nodular or globoid appearance is not the result of encapsulation, and careful scrutiny of the margins of these tumors will reveal a wavy, sinuous, undulating or notched contour which in one or more places will lead off into a comet-tail-like extension of fibrosis into the perifocal parenchyma. Many of these tumors when seen initially are 3 cm to 6 cm in diameter, and their clinical dimensions are usually greater than those measured on the X-ray film. Yet the prognosis of many of these cancers is better than most other varieties.

The tendency for the epithelial cells of these cancers to be large, oval, rounded, or polygonal with abundant basophilic cytoplasm and large vesicular nuclei is well known to pathologists. Another characteristic of these tumors is the abundant infiltration of small lymphoctyes. Hemorrhagic and anemic necrosis are common findings, especially in the larger tumors, which may even fungate and resemble inflammatory cysts.

All circumscribed tumors on roentgenograms must be carefully examined, and an *isolated*, circumscribed lesion more than 2 or 3 cm in diameter in a woman over 35 years of age should raise the question of malignancy. If the margins of such a mass are undulating or lack the sharp, smooth contour of a benign process; if a tongue-like projection of fibrosis leads away from any portion of the margin; and if blurring of the perifocal tissues due to edema is present, sometimes with other secondary changes such as vessel engorgement and thickening

of the skin, the suspicion of malignancy should be verified or ruled out by biopsy. The roentgenologist may not find it easy to convince the surgeon to operate, since many of these cases present misleading physical signs of a benign process.
On the X-ray film, most of these cancers are greater than 2 cm when first discovered, but some can be detected when they are less than 1 cm in diameter, especially if they occur in fatty breasts. The smooth contours may appear deceivingly benign, but close examination will disclose some undulation and signs of incomplete encapsulation which should raise a suspicion of cancer.
The margins around some tumors may be blurred due to perifocal edema. Rarely, tentacles or radiating striae may occur like those seen in ordinary scirrhus (Figs. 214—224). As these cancers grow larger, beyond 2 cm in diameter, edema of the surrounding tissues is apt to occur, blurring structural details, so that the peripheral fine or coarser tentacles and striae are more difficult to discern (Figs. 225—231). Finally, in the terminal stages, the tumors can become very large and the signs of secondary malignancy overshadow all other hallmarks. The tumors may then look cystic because of their bulging, smooth contours (Figs. 232, 233); or they may be partially obscured in areas of adenosis, clouded over by the extensive edema, so that it then becomes helpful to examine the other breast for comparison (Figs. 234, 235).

d) Lobular Carcinoma

Lobular carcinoma cannot be recognized clinically when it is still in situ. It is only when many localized lobules become involved in the process that the clinician may become aware of an ill-defined area of induration. All that the pathologist may see on gross sectioning are a few large lobules which stand out from the surrounding tissue by bulging because of their concentration. Under the microscope these large lobules may contain cells that are somewhat larger than the ordinary acinar cells, piled up in loose, compact fashion without orderly distribution or arrangement. The cells may have pale nuclei, sometimes resembling those seen in Paget's disease.
Localized lobular carcinomas are usually not found on roentgenograms. However, microcalcifications occur in probably 30 per cent of these tumors, and their presence will raise the question of malignancy for the roentgenologist.
Infiltrating lobular carcinomas are apt to resemble scirrhous types with their dendritic margins. The spicules are apt to be

very fine, and both the spicules and the tumor are apt to elude detection by the pathologist on gross section. This is one of the reasons pathologists at times have considerable difficulty in identifying these lesions from frozen sections. As a result, large sections of breast tissue must at times be inspected by the pathologist before he becomes aware of the infiltrating nature of these tumors.

When some of these lobular cancers occur in atrophic, fatty breasts the irregular and tentacled margins are easily discerned and properly labeled as cancer, although not necessarily lobular (Figs. 236, 237). If microcalcifications are also present, the diagnosis of cancer is further supported (Figs. 238—240). When these cancers occur in areas of dysplasia, however, only the secondary signs of malignancy may raise a suspicion of cancer (Figs. 241—246).

When lobular cancers spread beyond their original lobate confines, dendritic, spiculated, and tentacled scirrhous masses may supervene, and these are more easily recognized (Figs. 247 to 250). Many of these cancers are bilateral (Fig. 251).

e) Paget's Disease

A history of itching, crusting, or excoriations of the nipple should conjure the possible presence of Paget's disease.

If the process is confined, involving only the nipple portions of the ducts, nothing abnormal may be visualized roentgenographically. In instances where spread of the cancer has extended deeper into the breast, signs like those of infiltrating duct cell cancer with scirrhous formation may supervene (Figs. 252, 253).

f) Mammary Cancer in the Male

Carcinomas of the male breast can assume all the mammographic earmarks of those encountered in the female breast. The tendency to form a scirrhus seems greater in males, so the lesion which arouses attention is apt to be an isolated mass, irregular in outline, with blurred margins due to perifocal reaction and edema (Figs. 254—258).

Rarely, the lesions may be well circumscribed and smoothly contoured, but closer examination is apt to disclose the presence of surrounding edema including the skin (Figs. 259, 260).

In the more advanced stages, larger, infiltrating, tentacled masses may emerge with much attendant edema and thickening of the skin (Fig. 261). Intracystic papillary carcinomas may be exceptionally encountered (Fig. 262).

g) Unusual Malignancies

Unusual cancers, such as those designated sweat-gland carcinoma, mucinous carcinoma, adenocystic carcinoma, squamous cell carcinoma, spindle-cell carcinoma, intracystic carcinoma, intracystic papillary carcinoma, malignant cystosarcoma phyllodes, and sarcoma constitute a relatively small percentage of all breast malignancies.

a) Malignant Cystosarcoma Phyllodes. These tumors resemble fibroadenomas and can be suspected only if there are serial studies which indicate rapid growth of the tumor. Many times a resection of a fibroadenoma is followed by a recurrence, under which circumstances the possibility of a malignant cystosarcoma phyllodes should arise in the mind of the roentgenologist. (See discussion under fibroadenoma.)

b) Intracystic Papillary Carcinomas. As would be expected, these cancers resemble cysts on the roentgenogram. If it were a routine practice to inject air after the evacuation of fluid from all cysts and re-X-ray the suspect area, these tumors could easily be identified. Doctor Charles Gros of Strasbourg has reported finding several of these cancers by using this technique.

One would anticipate that these lesions would simulate cysts on the X-ray film, but curiously enough, they are rarely apt to resemble medullary cancers. Even an intracystic papilloma may be seen as a circumscribed tumor with sinuous, angulated, or notched margins (Fig. 263).

Intracystic papillary cancers usually are quite large when first seen, but, rarely, small lesions resembling a bossellated fibroadenoma or a multilocular cyst will be seen (Fig. 264). In general, the lesions are apt to be more than 2 cm in diameter, often with blurred outlines due to perifocal reaction and edema, but with smooth, angulated, or notched margins (Figs. 265 to 268). Lacy or granular calcifications occasionally occur in these lesions (Fig. 269).

c) Mucinous Carcinomas. Cancers designated "mucinous" conjure up a gelatinous, cystic type of tumor resembling intracystic papillary cancers or large, soft medullary cancers. The X-ray appearance is likely to be similar to that shown in Figs. 270—272. But the surprise occurs when the pathologist reports the lesion to be a mucinous cancer which resembles an infiltrating duct cell cancer (Fig. 273). The reason for this discrepancy may lie in the fact that the roentgenologist sees the whole picture, while the pathologist concentrates on the appearance of the microscopic section.

d) Sarcomas. Fibrosarcoma and lymphosarcoma are rarely encountered in the breast. They usually manifest themselves as isolated masses with smooth or irregular margins which might be sinuous or notched. Perifocal edema may blur the margins and the surrounding structural details (Figs. 274—278). Exceptionally, these lesions resemble those we associate with infiltrating duct cell cancer (Fig. 279). Thus, these tumors resemble the nodular scirrhous aspects of more common cancers, and the final diagnosis rests with the pathologist.

h) Cancers Rarely Discerned Roentgenographically

a) Non-infiltrative Duct Cell Cancers. All breast cancers are derived from epithelium, so that variations in morphology may actually be manifestations of the mode of spread rather than true differences in type. Carcinoma cells grow along the line of least resistance. When they occupy, extend along, and distend ducts their presence can readily be overlooked by the roentgenologist, and non-infiltrative duct carcinoma is one of the most difficult forms of cancer for the roentgenologist to recognize (Fig. 280).

b) The Comedo Form of Duct Carcinoma. In this type, the growth is confined within the ducts in more solid columns which tend to undergo central necrosis. This type of cancer is also quite rare, comprising probably no more than 1 per cent.

On gross sectioning, the cords and nodules of cancer tissue within the ducts can be expressed as soft or semi-solid greasy material. These lesions may involve the smaller as well as the larger duct radicles. The microscopic character of the cancer cells is much easier to identify than in the papillary type.

On the roentgenogram this rare form of malignancy will be evident usually after infiltration locally with distortion of one or more ducts. The diagnosis is seldom made outright, but these findings in a woman over 45 years of age with a recent discovery of a palpable lesion should arouse suspicion and lead at least to a diagnostic resection, especially if microcalcifications are present (Figs. 281—283).

c) Papillary Duct Cell Cancers. These cancers usually incite little reactive fibrosis, so that they grow as circumscribed but not truly encapsulated masses. When the lesion is confined to ducts as in Fig. 284, local density may be greater than in the neighboring tissue, following the pattern of the ductal trabeculae. When the process is infiltrative, the margins may be angular, notched, or partially dendritic, as in Figs. 285—289.

These tumors are rare and comprise probably no more than 2 per cent of breast cancers.

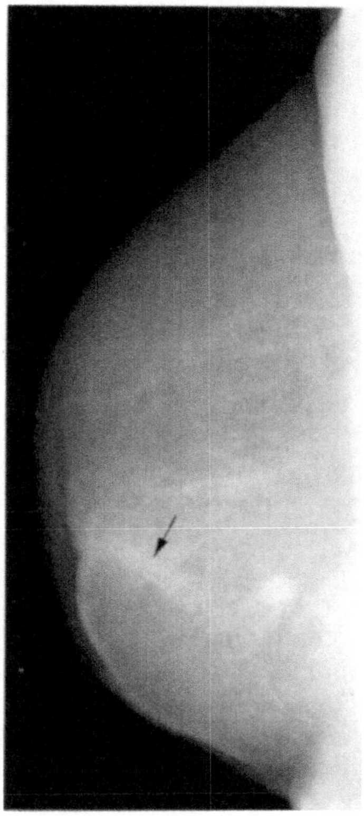

134

Fig. 134. Infiltrating duct cell carcinoma with scirrhus. The infiltrating cancer distends and distorts a duct complex (arrow). A small secondary nodular scirrhus, which first strikes the eye, is visible deeper in the breast. Perifocal edema and lymphatic involvement include the skin, which is thickened

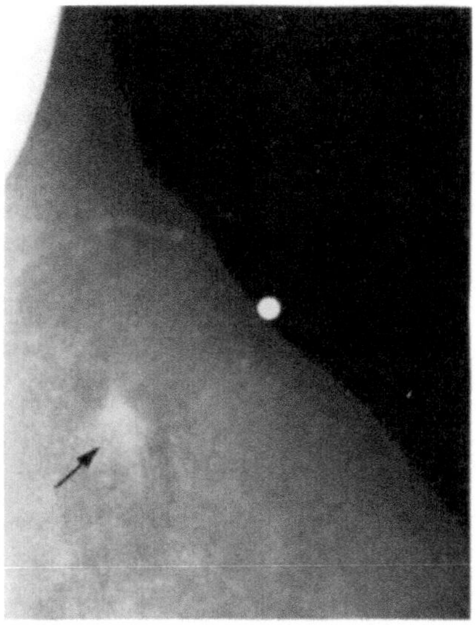

135

Fig. 135. Infiltrating duct cell cancer with scirrhus. The tentacled lesion was only 8 mm in diameter. No axillary node metastasis was present. The patient, 65 years old, felt a lump two months earlier, and the mass was thought to be 1.5 cm in diameter clinically

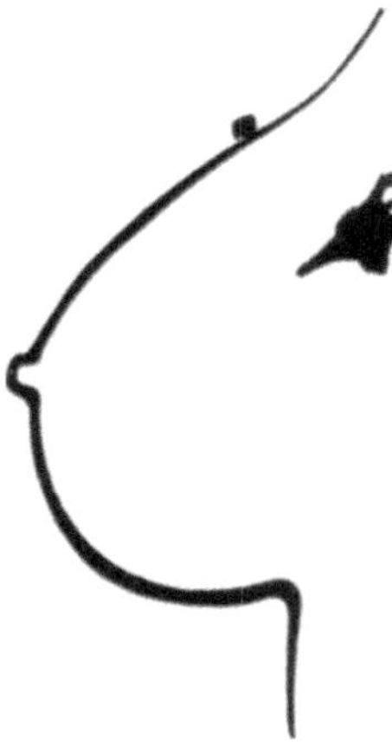

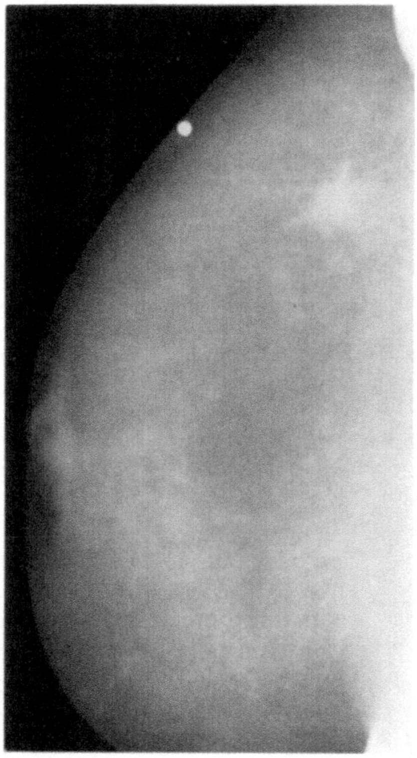

136

Fig. 136. Infiltrating duct cell cancer with scirrhus. A faintly visible tentacled mass was palpable under the skin marker in a 64 year old patient. It measured 2 cm in diameter clinically and 1 cm in diameter on the X-ray film

Fig. 137. Infiltrating duct cell carcinoma with scirrhus. Scirrhous carcinoma with long radiating fibrous strands, associated with thickening of the skin and retraction of the nipple, around which there is localized edema

Fig. 138. Infiltrating duct cell cancer with scirrhus. Radiating fibrous strands with thickening and retraction of the overlying skin are present

Fig. 139. Infiltrating duct cell carcinoma with scirrhus. The radiating strands issuing from the periphery of the scirrhous mass may be seen as "sentinel strands" (arrows), often pointing to a cancer hidden in a mass of adenosis

Fig. 140. Infiltrating duct cell cancer with scirrhus. The infiltrating margins and perifocal edema identify the lesion. Note the "sentinel strand" (arrow)

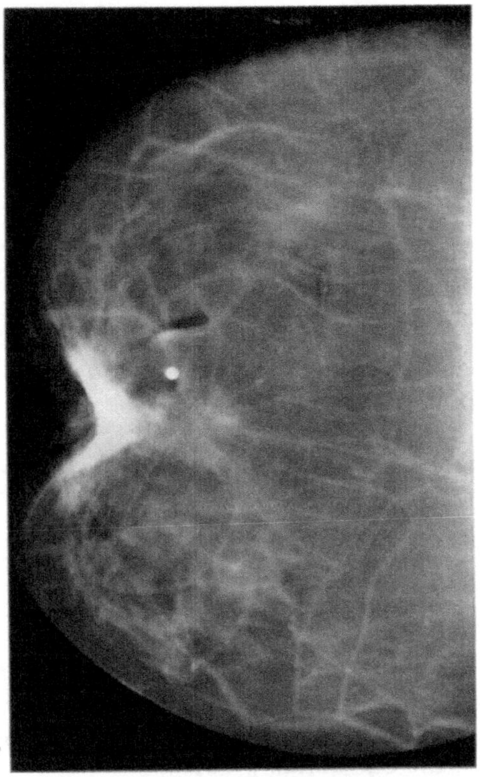
137

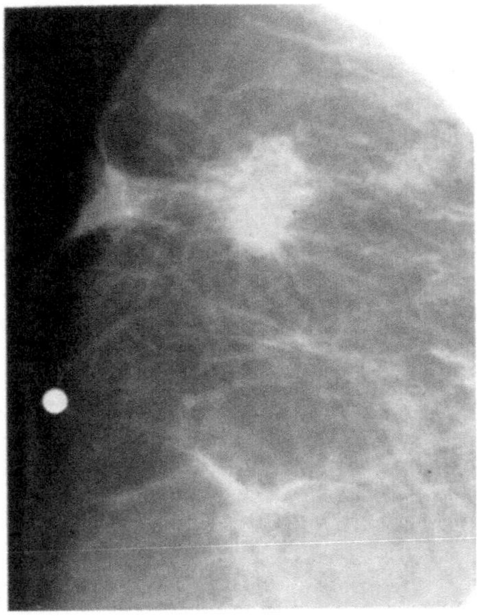
138

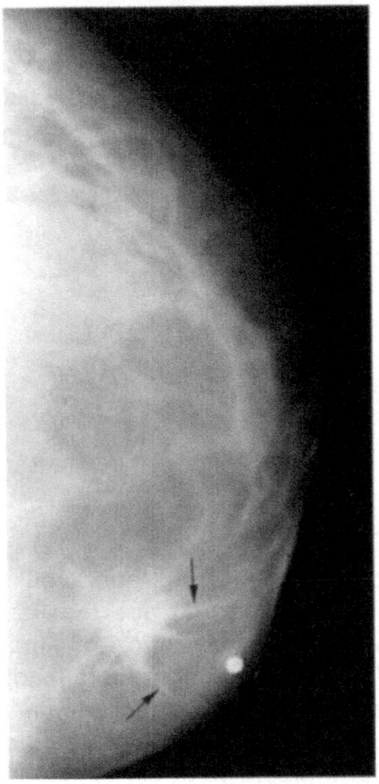
139

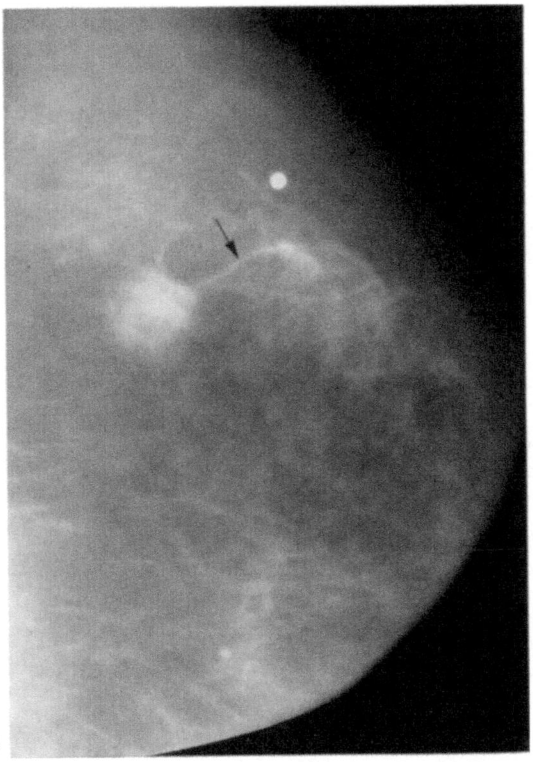
140

Fig. 141. Infiltrating duct cell cancer with scirrhus. The increased density and tentacles of the scirrhus are easily identified. The fibrous ducts leading from the nipple are distorted and stretched

Fig. 142. Infiltrating duct cell carcinoma with scirrhus. The tumor has spiculated margins and there is skin thickening due to the surrounding edema

Fig. 143. Infiltrating duct cell carcinoma with scirrhus. A dense tentacled mass is easily recognized as a cancer

Fig. 144. Infiltrating duct cell cancer with scirrhus. One can see the usual marginal spiculations, retraction of nipple, perifocal edema, and swollen ducts leading from the nipple. The skin is thickened and the superficial veins are turgid. Calcification in an arterio sclerotic artery is visible

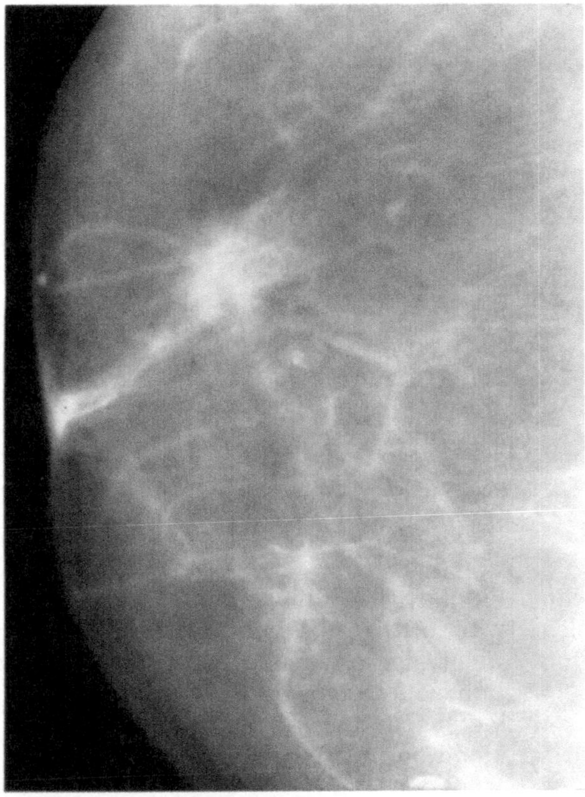
141

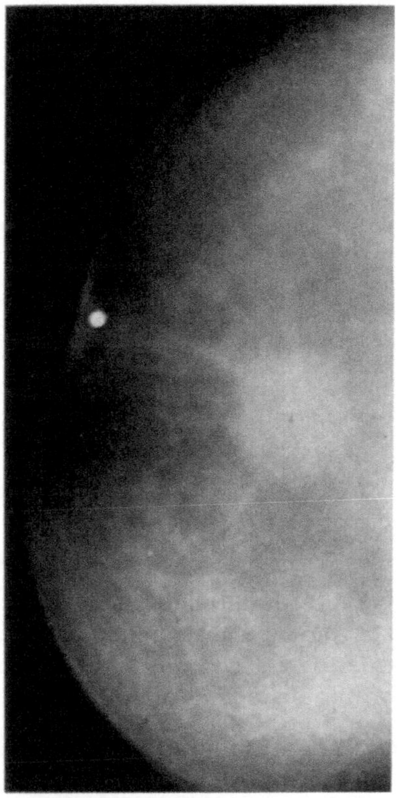
142

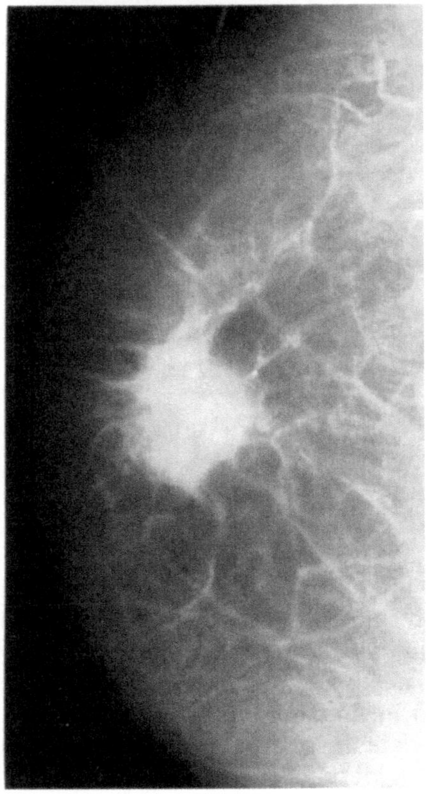
143

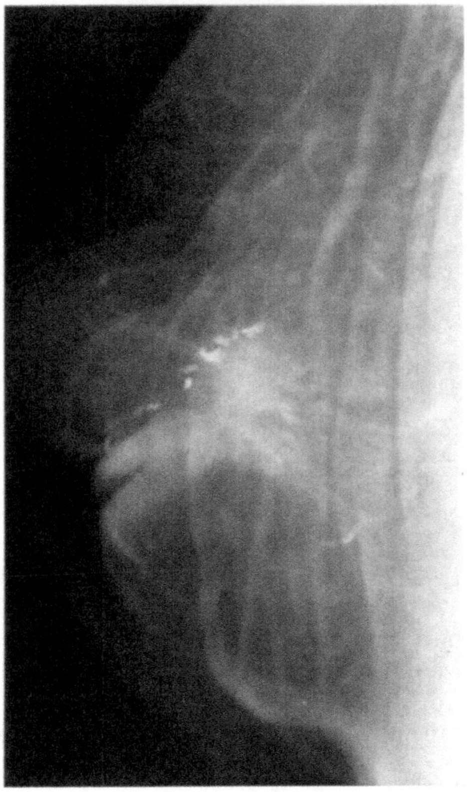
144

Fig. 145. Infiltrating duct cell cancer with scirrhus. Long radiating fibrous tentacles extend widely from the scirrhus and tug on the distended ducts

Fig. 146. Infiltrating duct cell carcinoma with scirrhus. Tumor under skin marker was 8 mm in diameter with short tentacles. It measured 2 cm in diameter clinically. The increased density of the tumor makes it stand out in an area of adenosis

Fig. 147. Infiltrating duct cell carcinoma with scirrhus. Invasion has extended beyond the ducts with the formation of a circumscribed scirrhus which resembles a nodular medullary type. The margins of the scirrhus are blurred due to perifocal edema

Fig. 148. Infiltrating duct cell cancer with scirrhus. Thin strands which radiate from the irregularly contoured mass are hardly visible. The five prominent tortuous ducts leading from the nipple suggest the presence of ectasia or secretory disease and epithelial hyperplasia

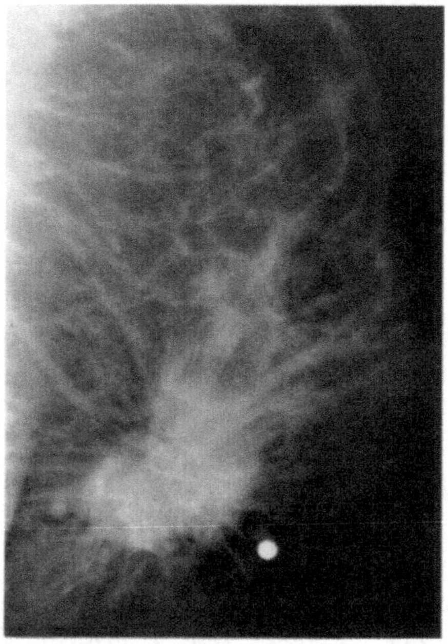

145

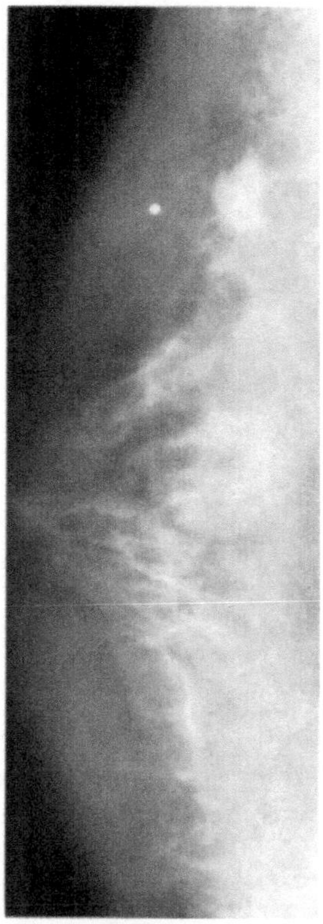

146

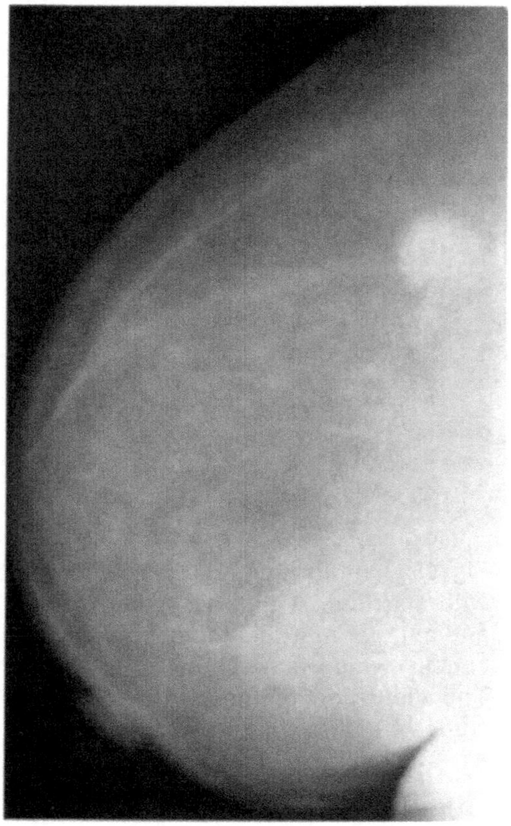

147

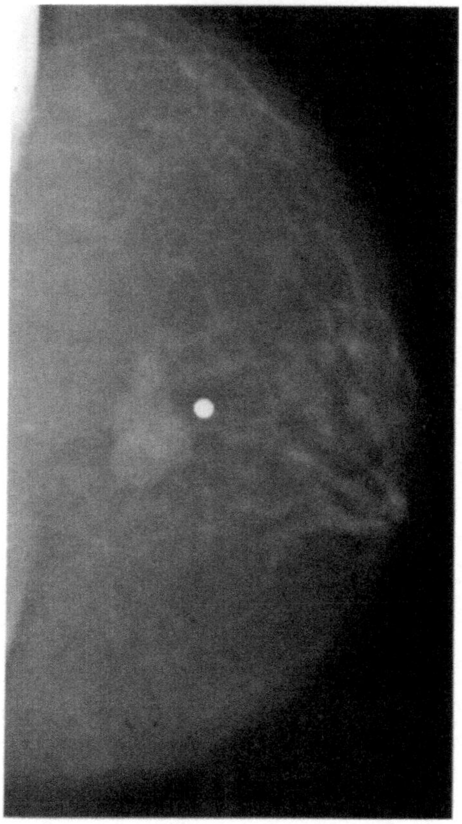

148

Fig. 149. Infiltrating duct cell carcinoma with scirrhus. Delicate fibrous strands which are hardly visible radiate from the periphery

Fig. 150. Infiltrating duct cell carcinoma. Cancer involves the ducts near the nipple and extends upward into smaller branches. Under the skin marker a scirrhus has formed, and its globoid contours resemble those of a medullary cancer

Fig. 151. Infiltrating duct cell carcinoma with scirrhus. A mass in the breast was known to this patient for 5 years. Its circumscribed contours resemble those of a medullary cancer. Because of extensive metastasis, no operation except biopsy was done. This confirmed the presence of a duct cell carcinoma

Fig. 152. Infiltrating duct cell carcinoma with scirrhus. A globoid mass with sinous and angular margins resembles a medullary cancer, which may characterize a scirrhus. The distortion of the perifocal tissues includes traction on the vessels

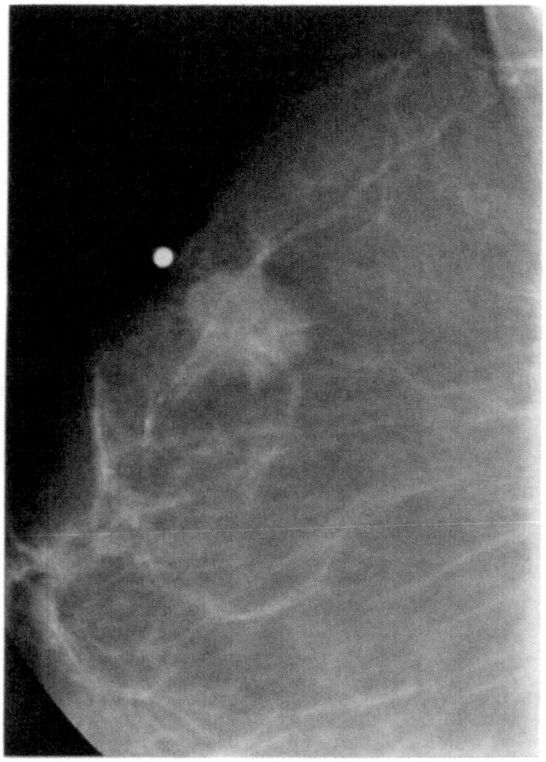
149

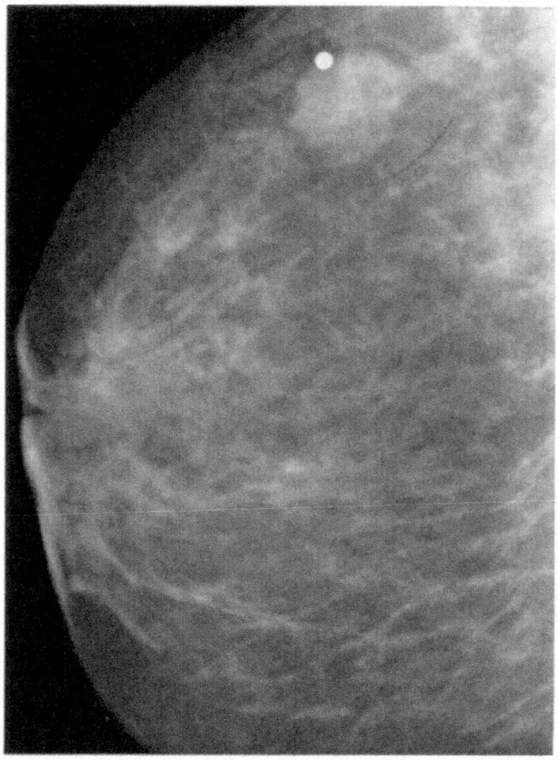
150

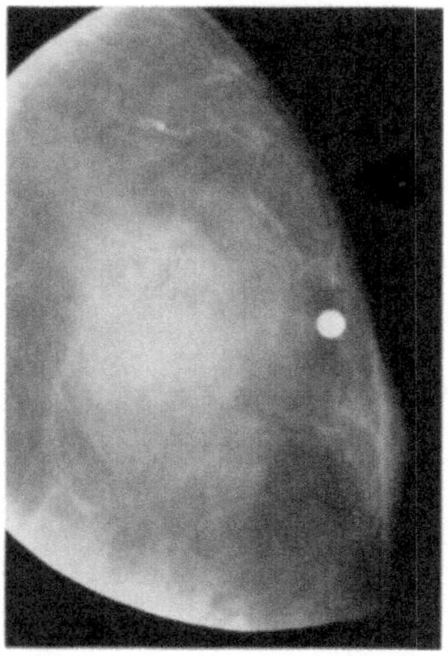
151

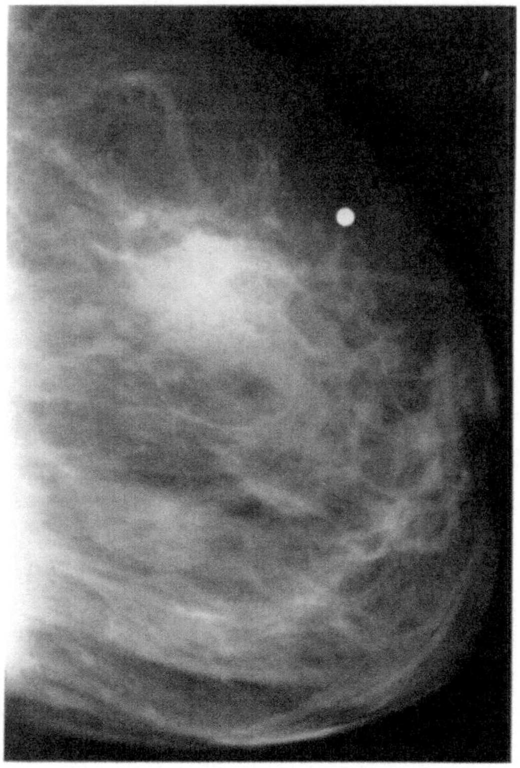
152

Fig. 153. Infiltrating duct cell carcinoma with scirrhus. The perifocal striate fibrosis is prominent. These striae or strands may be the only evidence of a cancer when it is obscured by a zone of adenosis

Fig. 154 A and B. Infiltrating duct cell cancer with scirrhus.

A

Lateral view.

B

Cephalocaudad view. The carcinoma resembles the medullary type. In a 60 year old woman, an isolated nodular mass with irregular, notched margins is apt to be a carcinoma. The distinction between a scirrhus and a medullary cancer under these circumstances can sometimes be almost impossible

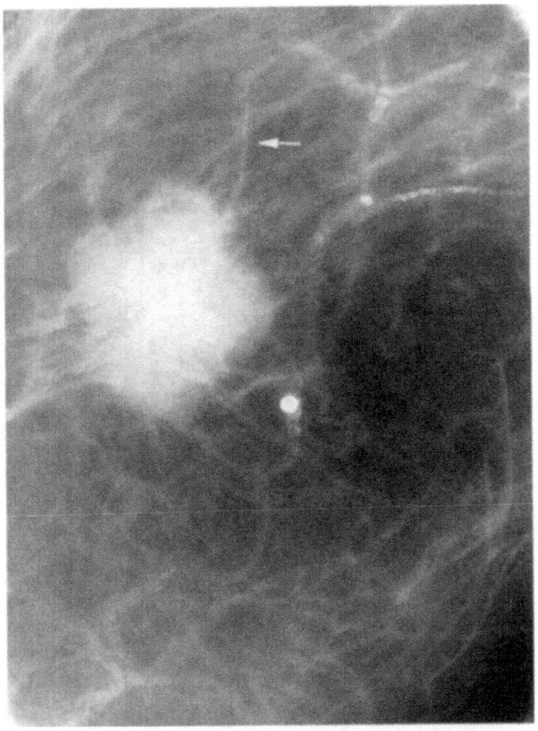

153

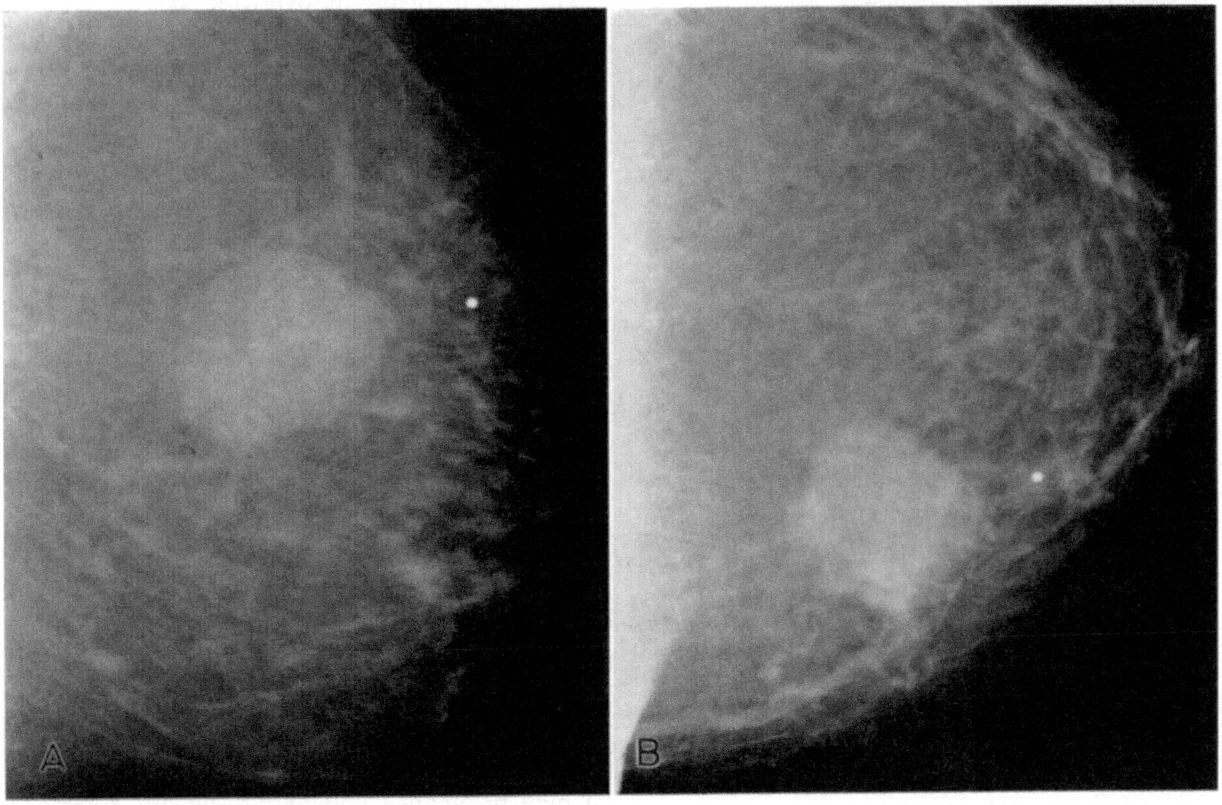

154

Fig. 155. Infiltrating duct cell carcinoma with scirrhus. A dense, irregular scirrhous mass has formed among medium-sized ducts with minimal distortion of the surrounding tissues. The circumscribed character of the tumor begins to resemble a medullary type of cancer

Fig. 156. Infiltrating duct cell cancer with scirrhus. The nodular appearance of some of these cancers may rarely resemble a medullary cancer with its associated comet-tail extension (arrow). Blurring of detail stems from the surrounding edema, which here also involves the overlying skin

Fig. 157. Infiltrating duct cell carcinoma with scirrhus. This cancer was of more than 5 years' duration. Only the irregular margins differentiate it from a circumscribed medullary cancer which it resembles

Fig. 158. Infiltrating duct cell carcinoma with scirrhus. In a breast with extensive adenosis and mazoplasia cystica, these cancers may be obscured. A dominant mass was palpable, localized by the skin marker. Under it may be seen a spiculated scirrhus near a smoothly outlined cyst

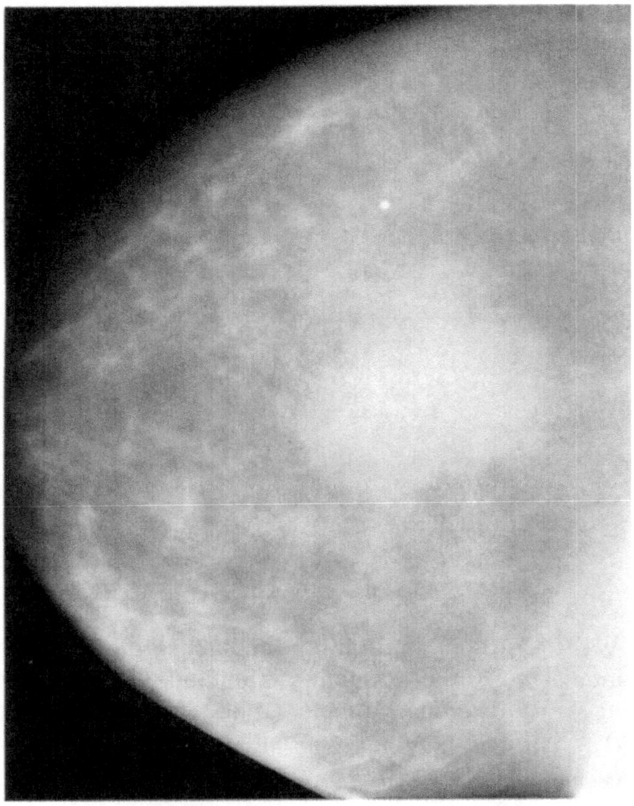

155

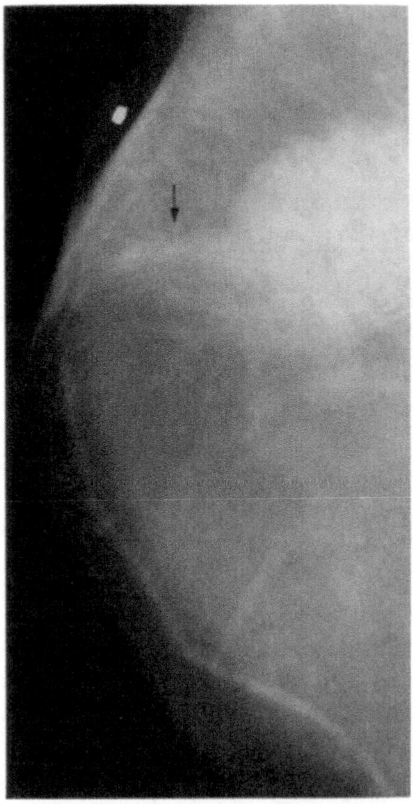

156

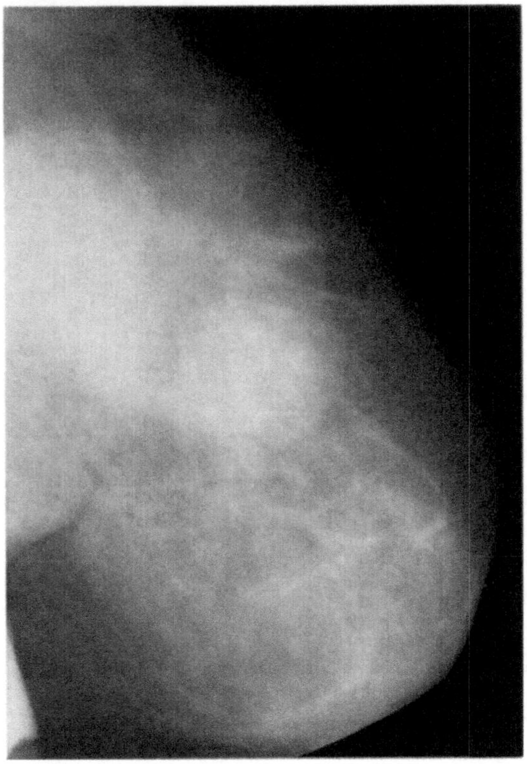

157

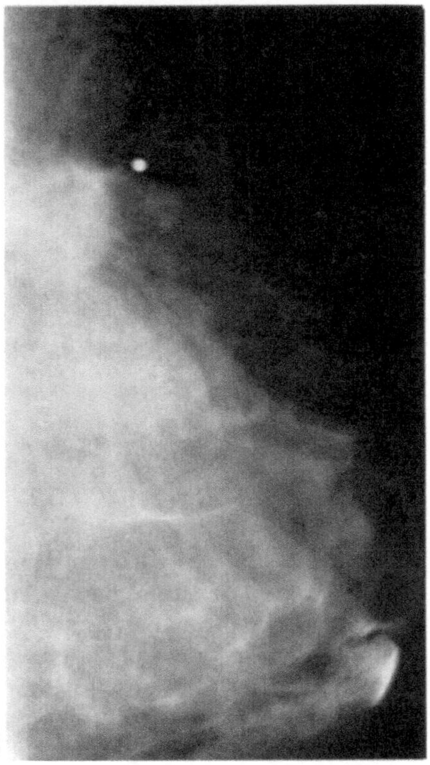

158

Fig. 159. Infiltrating duct cell cancer with scirrhus. Duct ectasia, or secretory disease, with calcifications and epithelial pearls. A supervening scirrhus is present (arrow)

Fig. 160. Infiltrating duct cell carcinoma with scirrhus. Radiating spicules, edema, and thickened skin mark site of scirrhus. The linear calcific deposits are in an area of healed secretory disease

Fig. 161. Infiltrating duct cell cancer with scirrhus. The skin marker on the right localizes site of a palpable tumor which is mostly obscured by the hyperplastic fibrosis. Only the "sentinel strands" (arrows) suggest the malignant character of the mass. The left breast is relatively normal in appearance for a woman of this age (52 years)

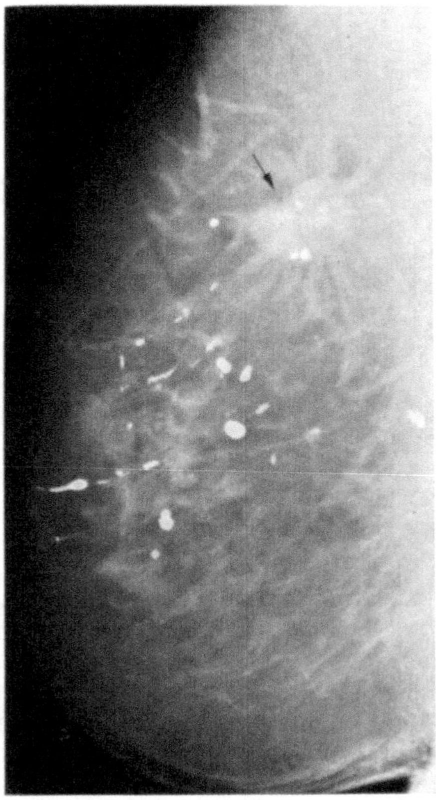

159

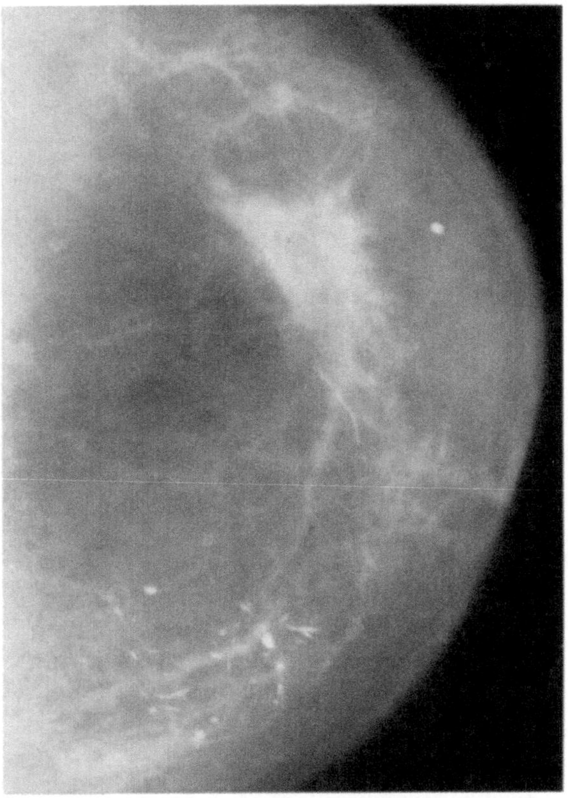

160

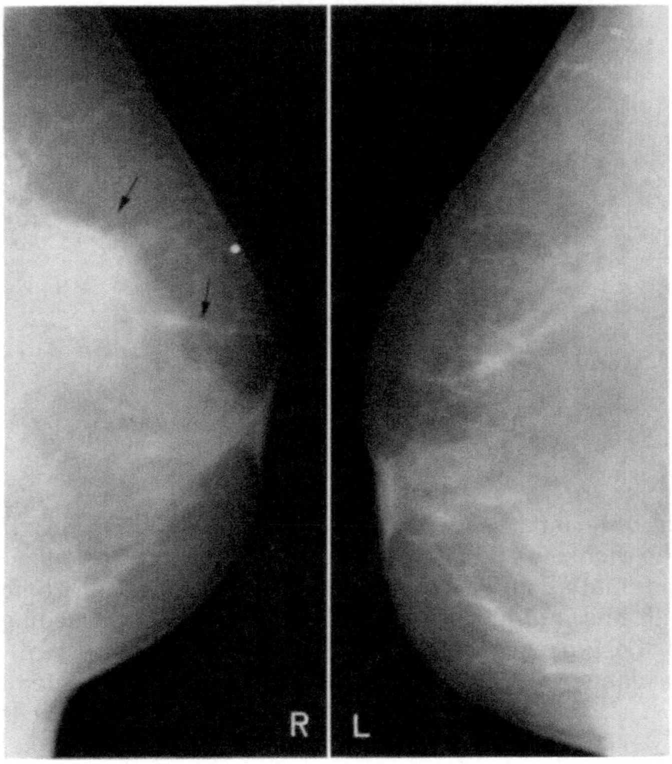

161

Fig. 162. Infiltrating duct cell carcinoma with scirrhus. Broad fibrous strands radiating from the dense mass identify the scirrhus in an area of trabecular distortion

Fig. 163. Infiltrating duct cell carcinoma with scirrhus. Edema of skin and of surrounding tissues blurs details. Only the dendritic "sentinel strands" are visible of the discoid tumor, which is partially obscured by a field of adenosis

Fig. 164. Infiltrating duct cell carcinoma. The increased density, spiculated margins, and distortion of the breast architecture with blurring due to perifocal edema point to the presence of a cancer in a zone of adenosis

Fig. 165. Infiltrating duct cell carcinoma with scirrhus. A fusiform scirrhus is present with thin radiating fibrous strands and thickening of the skin. Traction and straightening of the trabeculae leading from the retracted nipple are evident. The long intraductal casts of calcification are due to old healed secretory disease

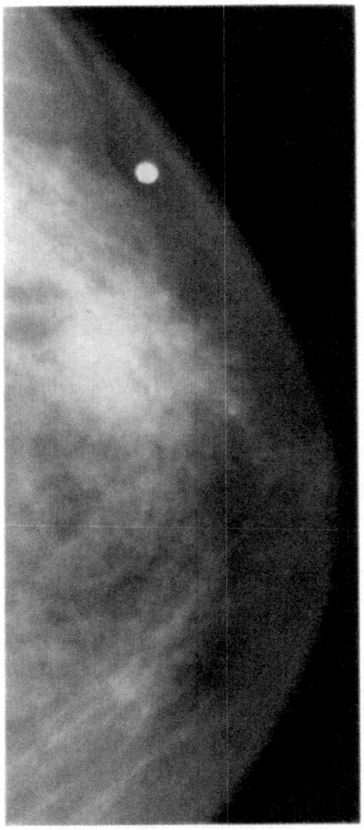
162

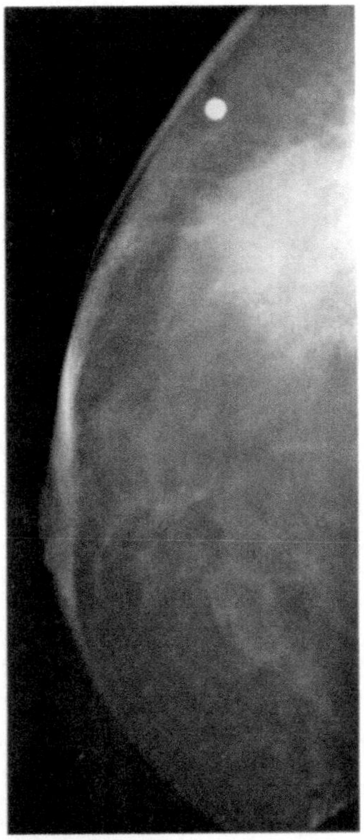
163

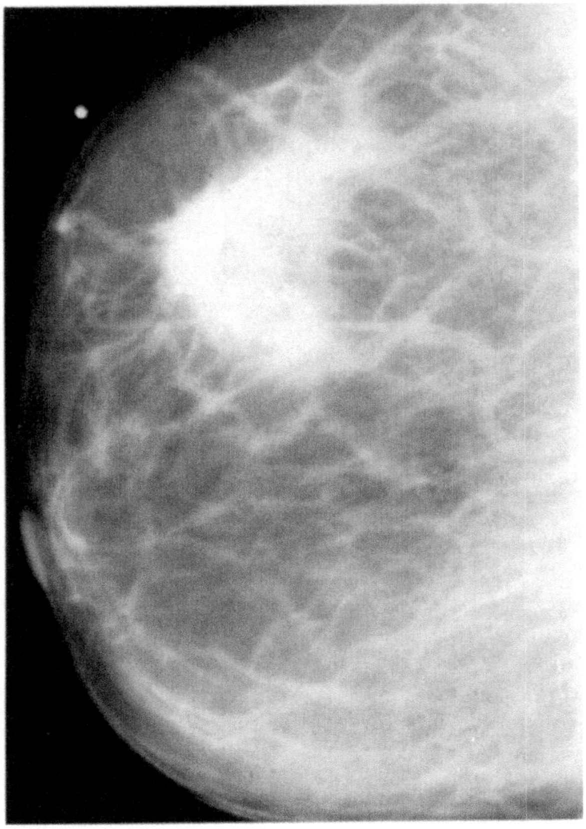
164

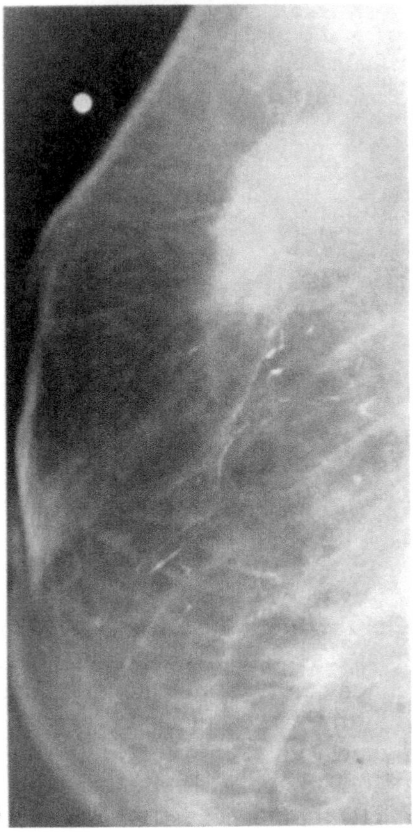
165

Fig. 166. Infiltrating duct cell carcinoma with scirrhus. A group of ducts near the nipple is involved with a secondary scirrhus which was palpable. Distortion of the duct complex is present behind the nipple

Fig. 167. Infiltrating duct cell carcinoma with healed secretory disease. A small spiculated cancer, not palpable (arrow), may be difficult to recognize in the presence of fibrous tissue. The fibrous ducts bunched together behind the nipple are due to healed secretory disease

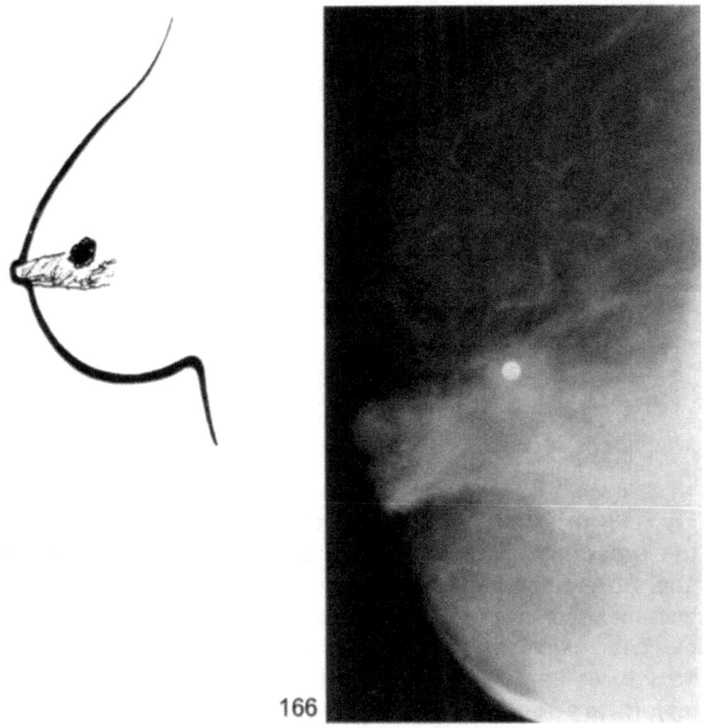

166

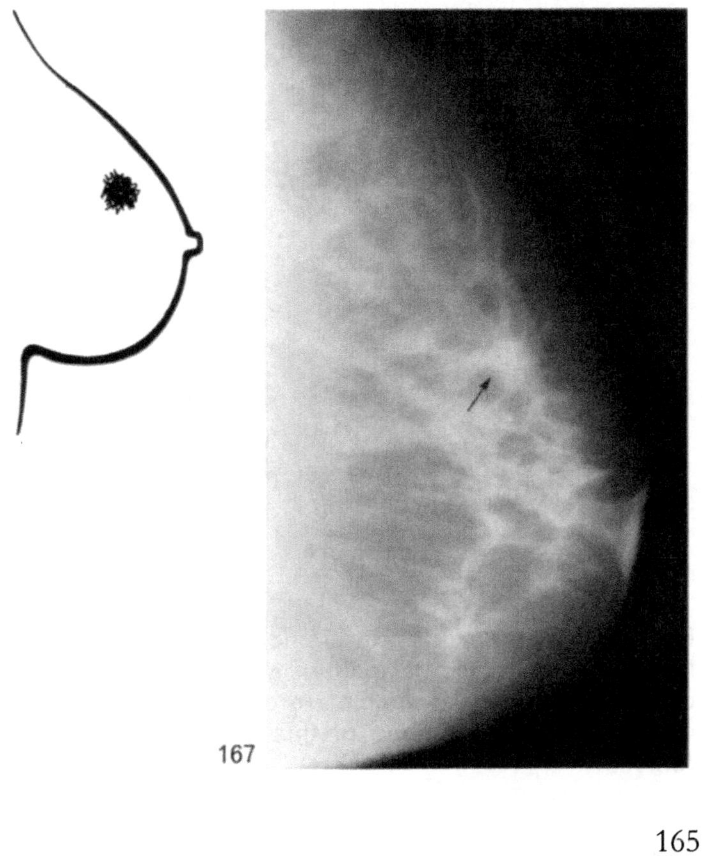

167

Fig. 168. Infiltrating duct cell carcinoma. In the presence of mastopathy due to healed secretory disease and sclerosing adenosis, two masked palpable tumors are localized by the skin markers. The surrounding structures are distorted; otherwise the lesions are obscured by the perifocal edema. The tubular calcifications are those seen in the late healing stages of secretory disease or duct ectasia

Fig. 169. Infiltrating duct cell carcinoma. Cancer was suspected by the clinician at the site of the skin marker. He may have palpated the more superficial area of sclerosing adenosis rather than the more deeply placed cancer, whose margins are irregular and blurred due to edema (arrows)

Fig. 170. Infiltrating duct cell carcinoma. Distortion of the structural pattern and blurring of detail due to edema are often the only X-ray manifestations of this type of tumor

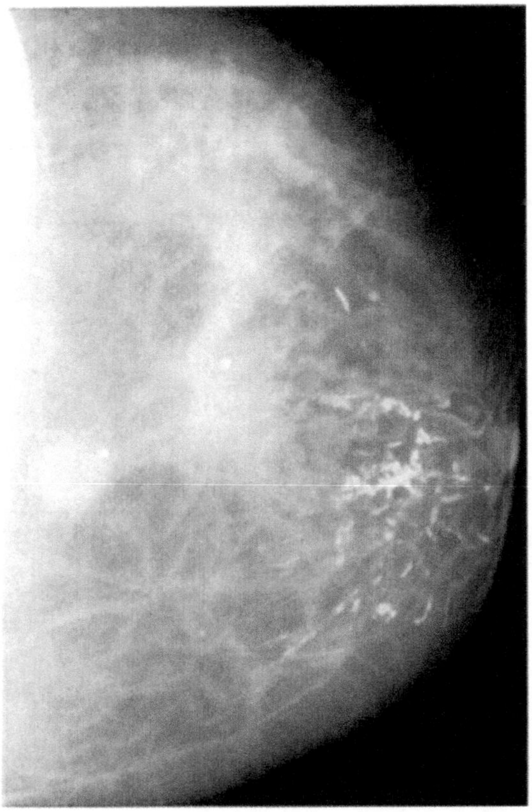

168

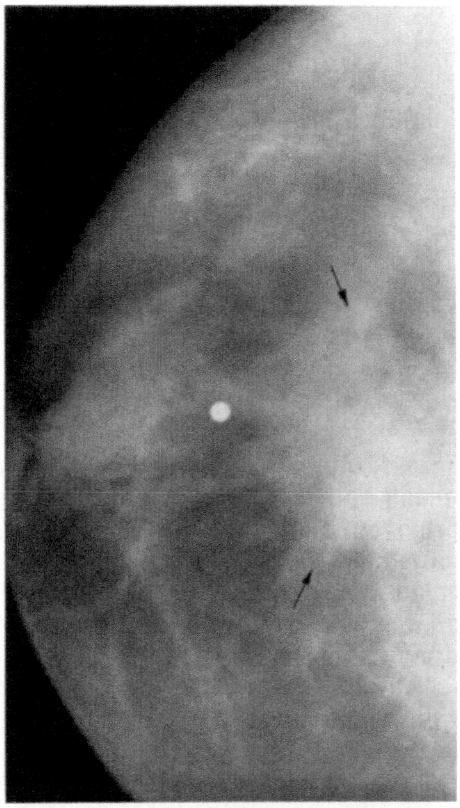

169

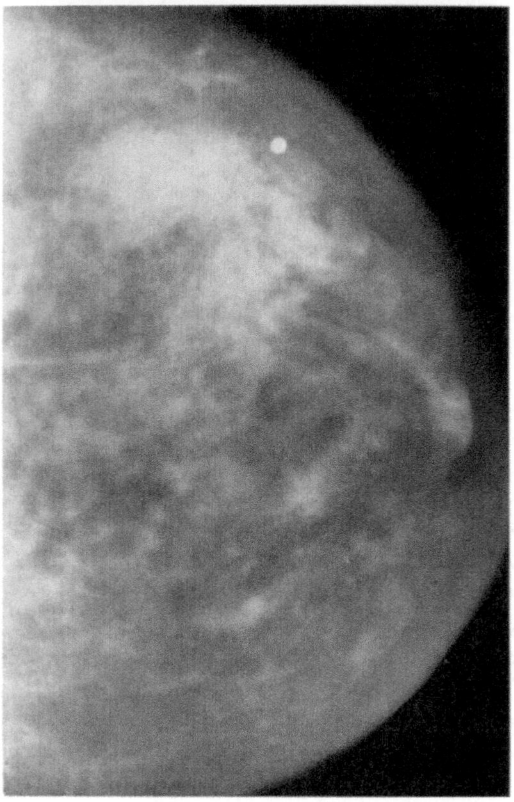

170

Fig. 171. Infiltrating duct cell carcinoma, left breast, with extensive adenosis. The distorted structural patterns and venous engorgement (arrow heads) are best appreciated when similar areas of the right breast are compared. They suggest the possibility of cancer and need for prompt biopsy, especially in a woman over 40 years of age with symptoms of a "drawing sensation" localized to this area

Fig. 172 A and B. Infiltrating duct cell cancer.

A

A sharply outlined lesion resembling a cyst or fibroadenoma (arrow) is partially obscured in a field of sclerosing adenosis. The lesion was not recognized as a cancer until the next examination.

B

Twenty-two months later, extensive invasion and blurring of detail due to edema indicated presence of a cancer

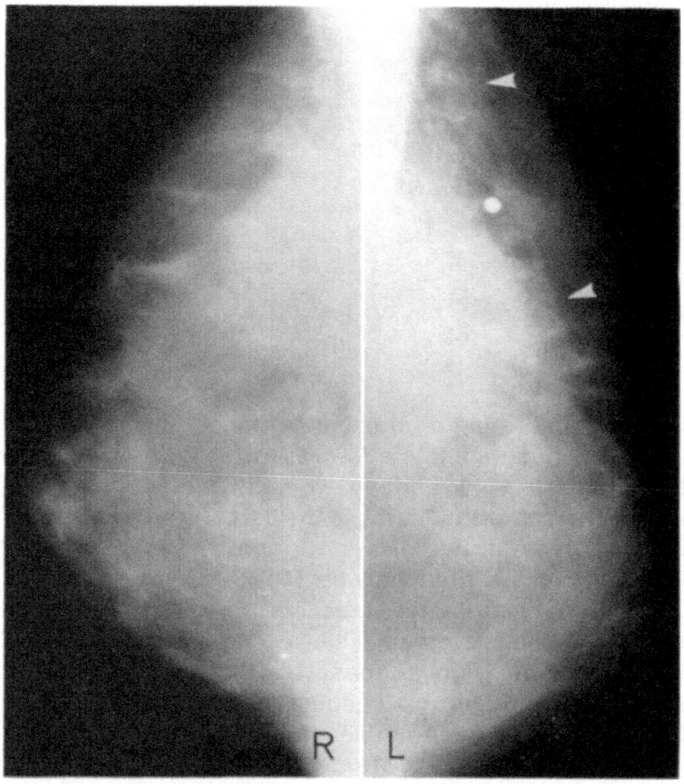

171

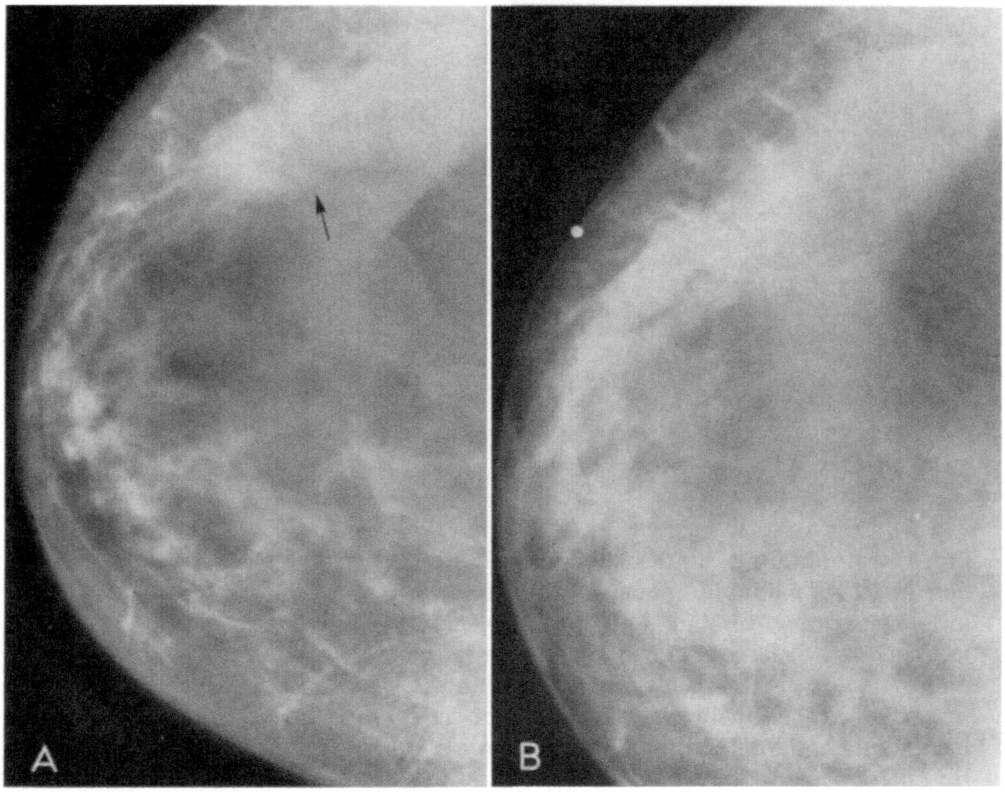

172

Fig. 173. Infiltrating duct cell carcinoma, left breast. Diffuse adenosis is present in both breasts of this 40 year old woman, and is much more pronounced on the left. Intermittent pain of two years' duration was localized to the area between the arrows. The poorly marginated area of increased density in the left breast, due to edema, is the only X-ray sign suggestive of cancer. It is very difficult to suspect cancer in breasts of this type unless the mammograms of both breasts are compared

Fig. 174. Infiltrating duct cell cancer with scirrhus. A palpable mass in the upper inner quadrant of the left breast (skin marker) is totally obscured by the dense adenosis and mazoplasia cystica. The diagnosis of cancer in breasts of this type is hazardous and often impossible, and should be so reported

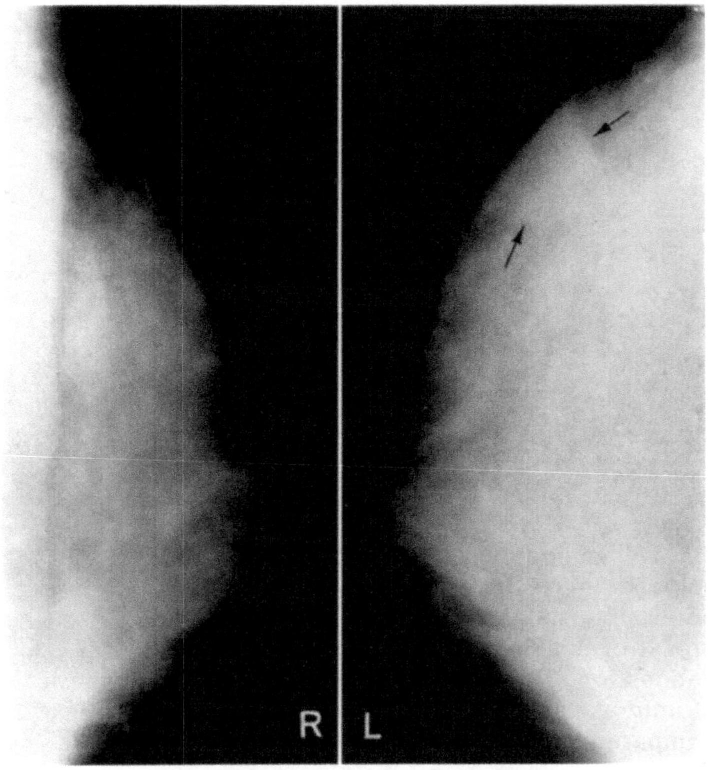

173

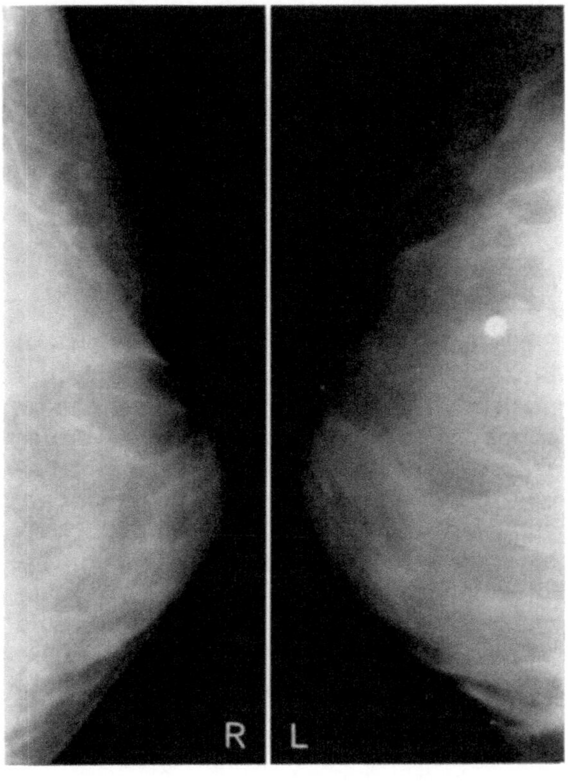

174

Fig. 175. Infiltrating duct cell carcinoma. A palpable mass at site of skin marker is not visible on the X-ray film of the right breast of this 69 year old women. The only suggestion of cancer is the blurring of structural details of the involved breast as compared with those of the opposite (left) side

Fig. 176. Infiltrating duct cell carcinoma, left breast, with widespread sclerosing adenosis. An X-ray diagnosis of cancer can be almost impossible in such cases. The increased density in the area of symptomatology of the left breast, with such secondary signs as generalized edema and thickening of the skin in a 69 year old patient, excites suspicion of malignancy. The clinician suspected cancer because he could palpate a hard, fixed mass 5 cm in diameter. What he was actually palpating was probably an area of sclerosing adenosis. No axillary lymph node metastasis was found

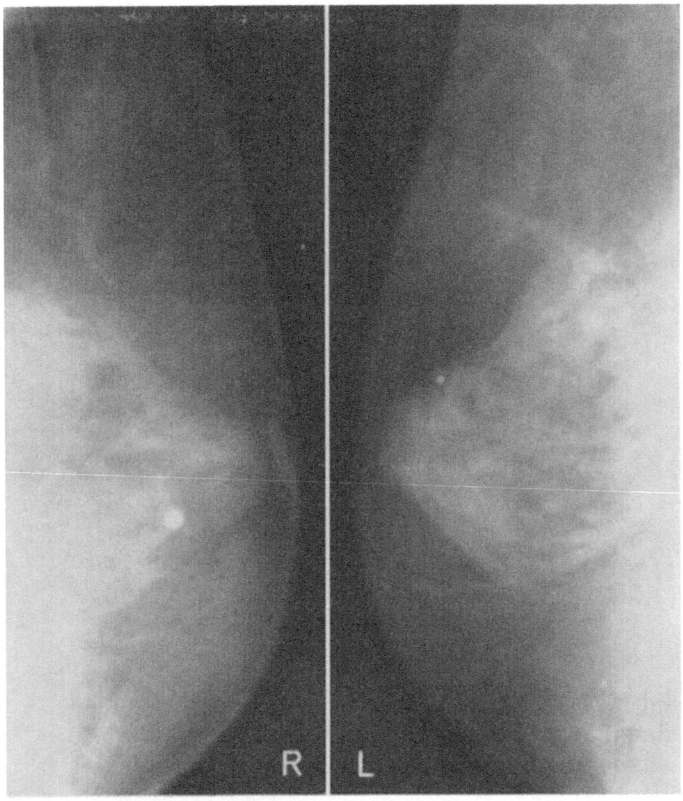

175

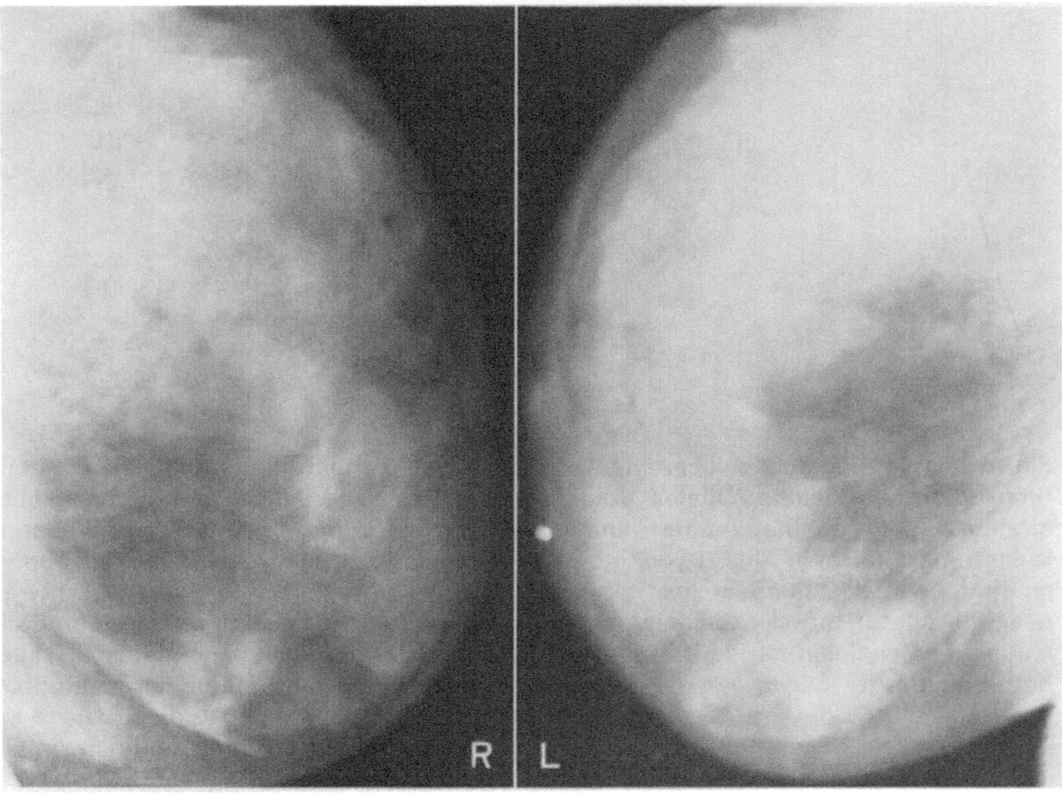

176

Fig. 177. Bilateral cancers. Advanced inflammatory cancer of left breast, and unsuspected scirrhous cancer (arrow) of right breast

Fig. 178. Infiltrating duct cell carcinoma with three scirrhous lesions. Dilated ducts are stretched between the anterior and posterior tumors (arrow). This 76 year old woman first noticed a lump in her left breast near the site of the skin marker one week earlier. The clinician felt several masses in both breasts

Fig. 179. Infiltrating duct cell cancer. The limited aggregate of microcalcifications (arrow) in the presence of epithelial hyperplasia in so many ducts led the roentgenologist to suggest biopsy. The X-ray examination of the specimen after operation confirmed removal of the tissue in question and helped the pathologist to pinpoint the area for histologic studies. These procedures should be done routinely in similar circumstances

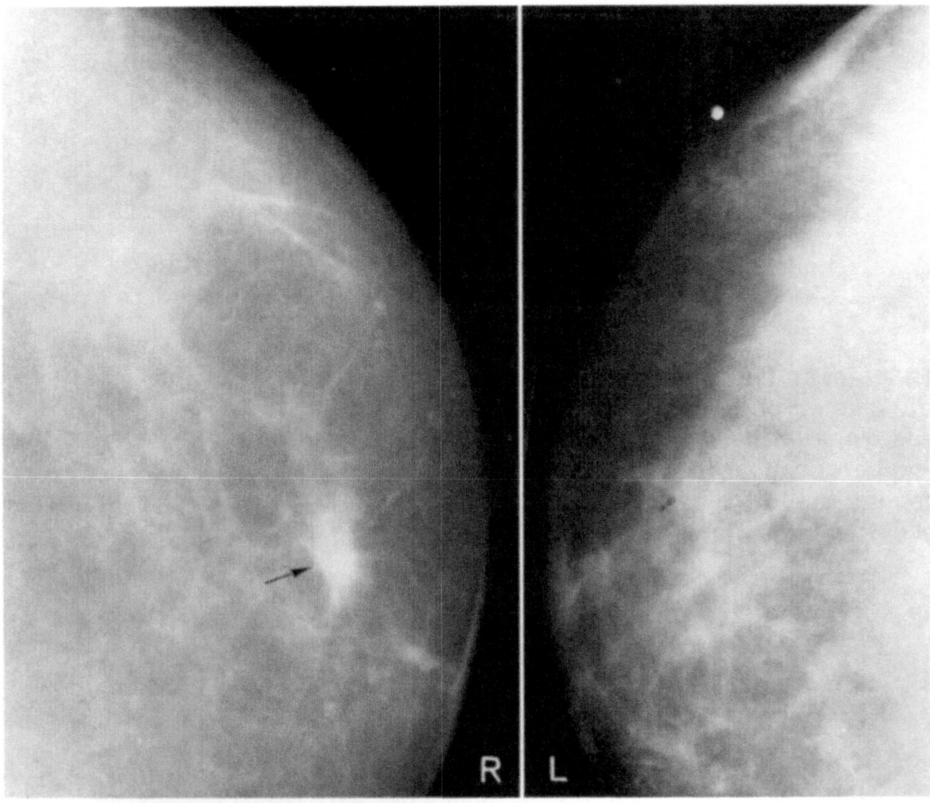

177

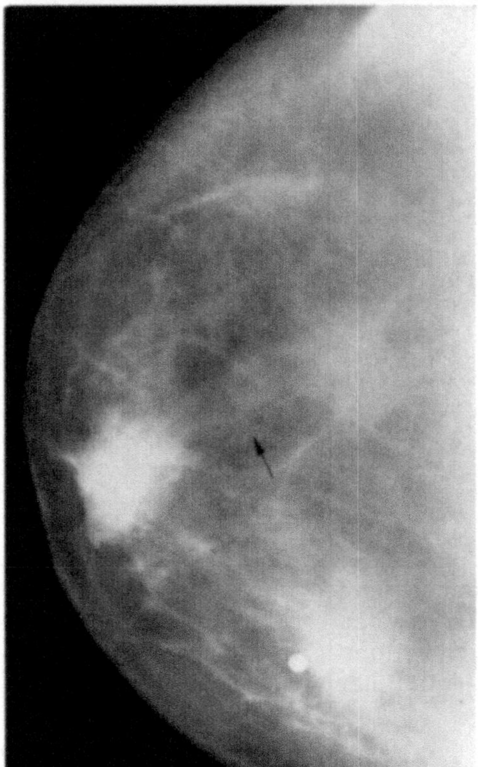

178

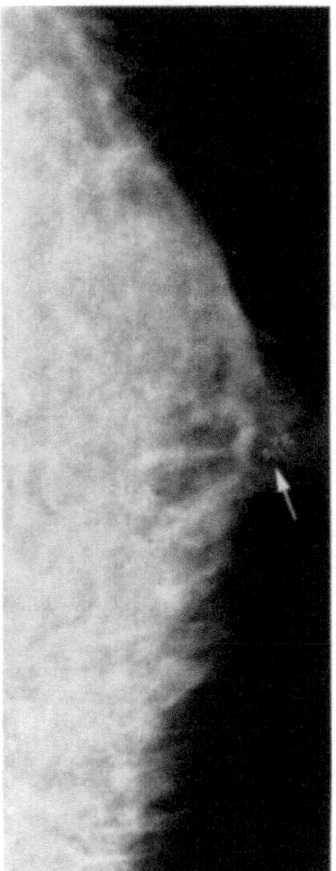

179

Fig. 180. Infiltrating duct cell carcinoma. A small cluster of unpolarized calcium deposits close to the skin marker reveals the presence of cancer in an area of "burning sensation" reported by the patient. No palpable tumor was present

Fig. 181. Infiltrating duct cell cancer. The tumor is revealed merely by the presence of a small cluster of punctate calcifications (arrow) in a dense area of multinodular adenosis

Fig. 182. Infiltrating duct cell cancer. Cluster of punctate calcium deposits (arrow) is visible in region of smaller terminal ducts where the cancer was present. Close by are two small cysts which were palpable and thought to be benign, while the cancer itself was not clinically suspected.

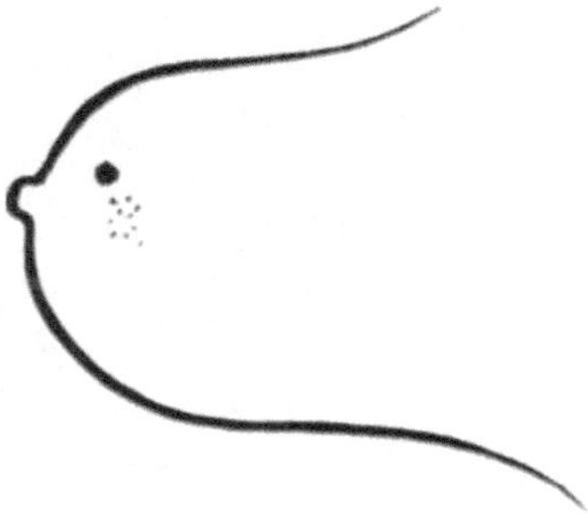

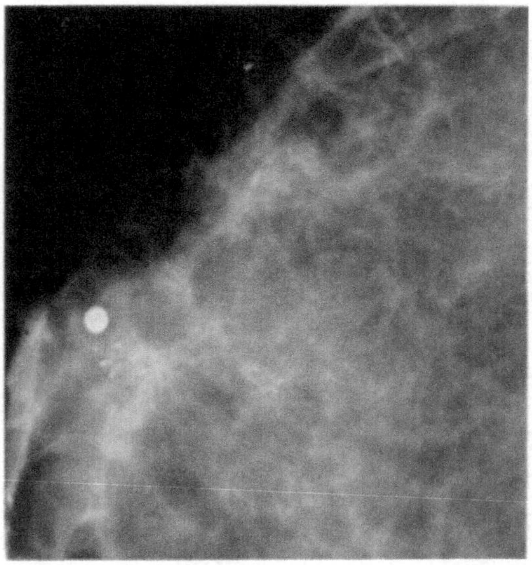

180

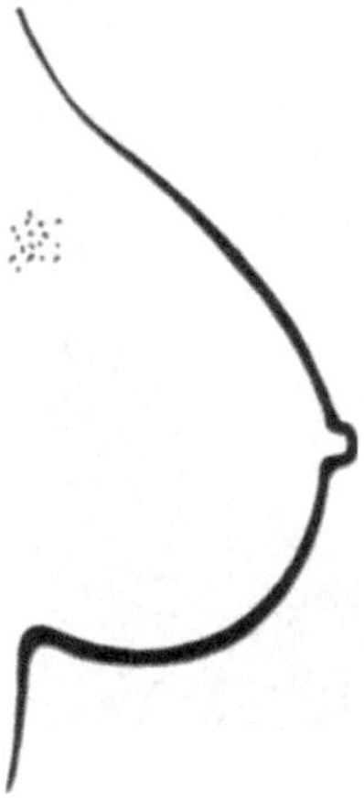

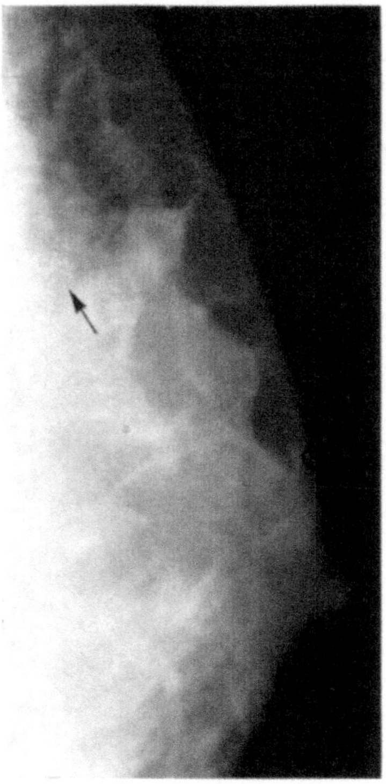

181

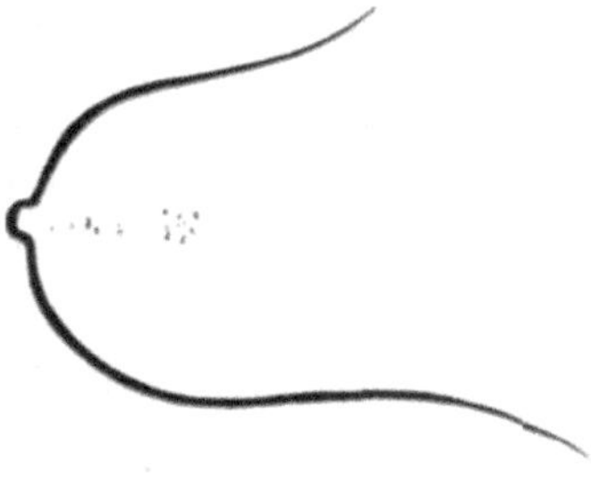

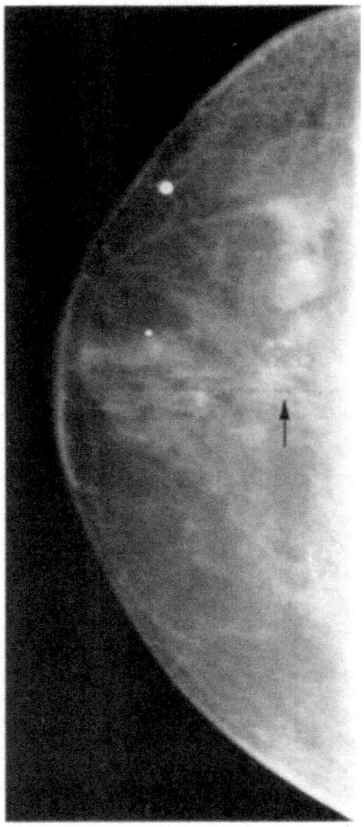

182

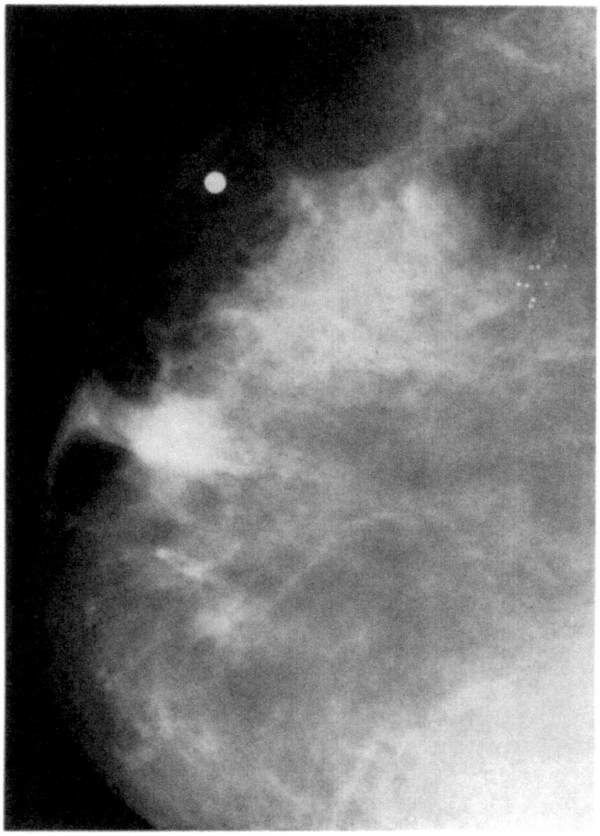

Fig. 183. Infiltrating duct cell cancer. The diagnosis is based on the presence of a distorted structural pattern, blurred detail due to edema, retraction of the nipple, and microcalcifications

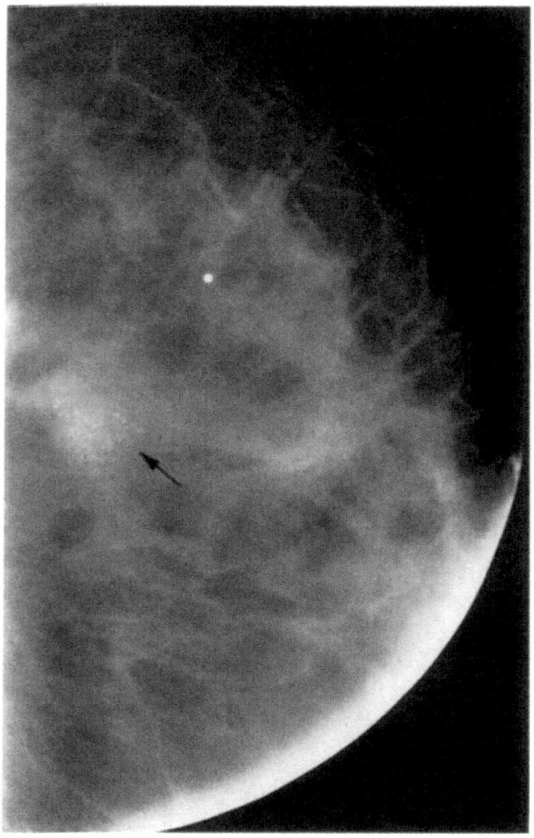

Fig. 184. Infiltrating duct cell cancer. Microcalcifications in clustered arborization appear in the tumor, which is almost obscured by an area of sclerosing adenosis. No mass was palpable. The patient requested X-ray examination because a sister had died of breast cancer

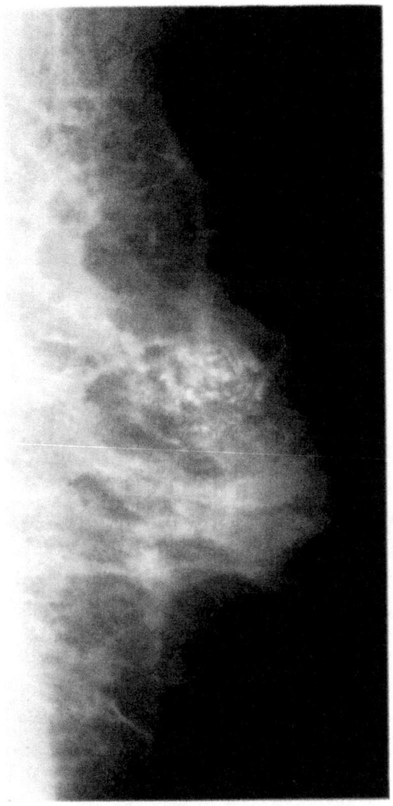

Fig. 185. Infiltrating duct cell cancer. Arborized cluster of irregularly-shaped microcalcifications in an area of sclerosing adenosis suggested cancer to the radiologist. This was not suspected clinically

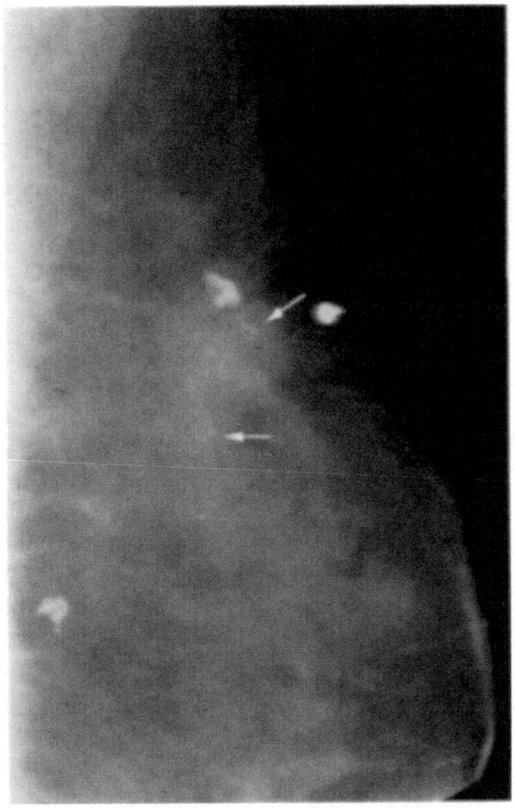

Fig. 186. Infiltrating duct cell carcinoma with scirrhus. Dendritic margins with punctate calcifications scattered in the tumor and among nearby ducts (arrows) identify the cancer. The larger calcific flakes were found in small adenomata. The perifocal edema blurs detail and has caused thickening of the skin

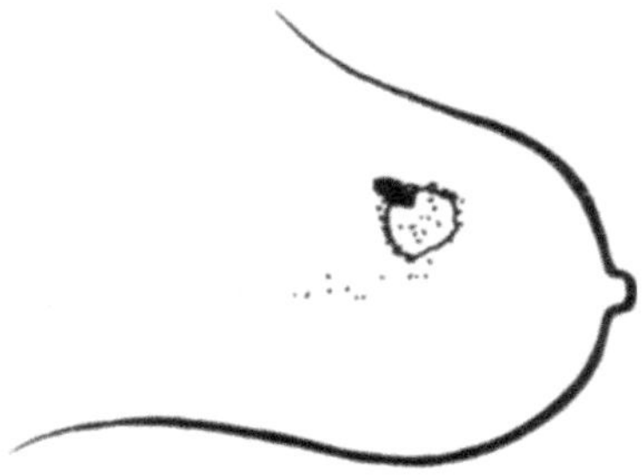

Fig. 187 A—D. Infiltrating duct cell carcinoma with microcalcifications.

A

8. 5. 59. A biopsy of this breast had been suggested because punctate calcifications suggested the presence of cancer. The pathologist reported only "cystic mastitis." This postoperative roentgenogram reveals that the aggregate of punctate calcifications had not been removed by the surgeon

B

3. 25. 60. Re-examination reveals spread of calcifications, but no tumor was palpable, so biopsy was refused by the surgeon.

C

4.21.61. More calcifications and still no tumor was palpable

D

6.1.62. Re-examination was requested by the roentgenologist, who prevailed upon the surgeon to operate despite absence of palpable tumor. A widespread infiltrative duct cell carcinoma was found, curiously not associated with metastasis to 12 axillary nodes

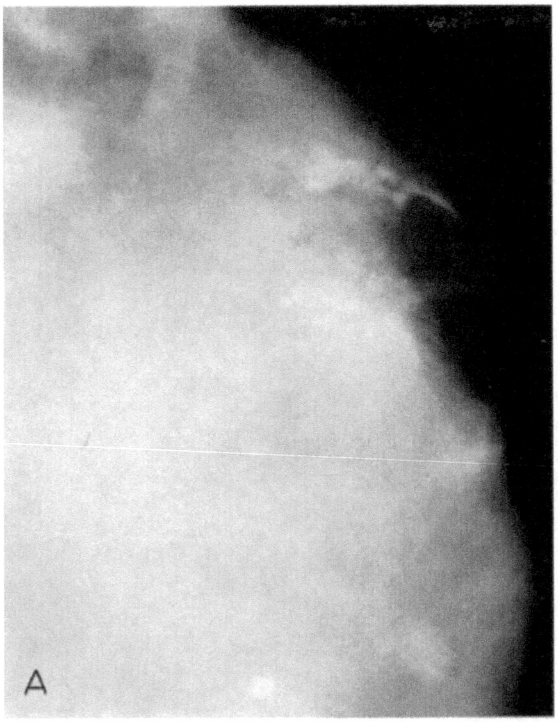

187

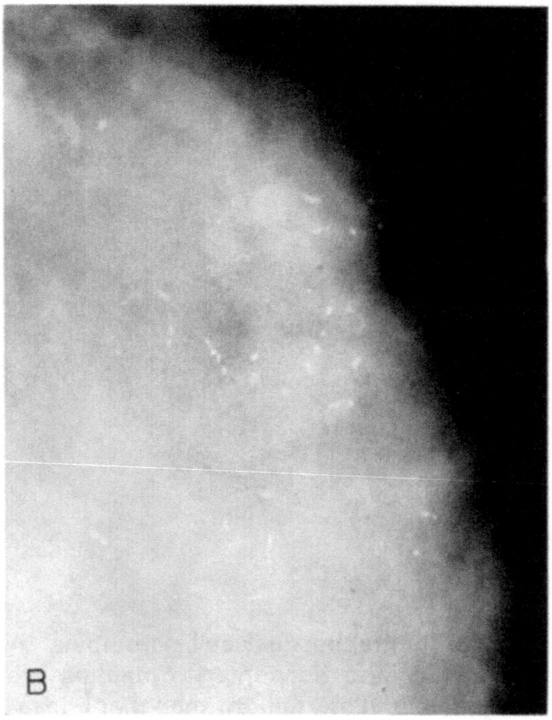

187

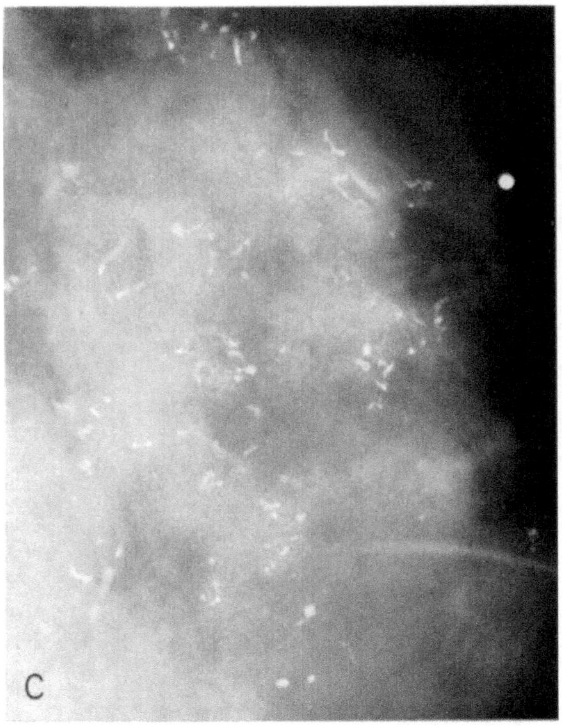

187

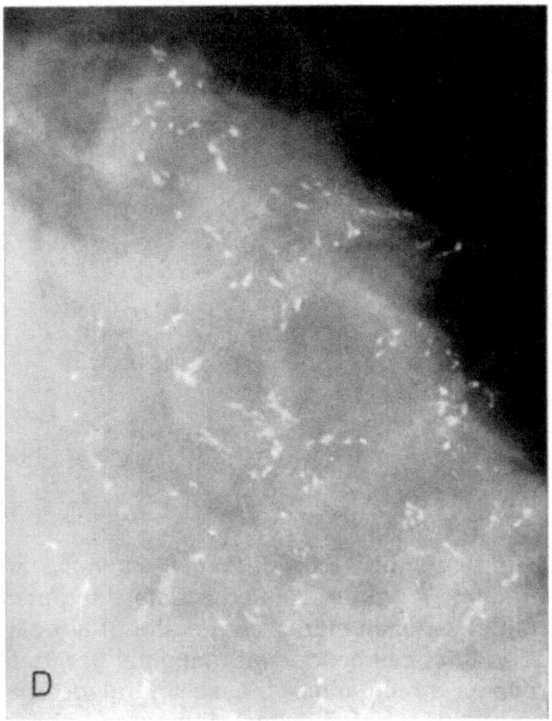

187

Fig. 188. Infiltrating duct cell carcinoma. A single duct and its primary branches are swollen and distorted by malignant invasion. Growth has breached the duct confines in the region where a dendritic scirrhus is forming (arrow)

Fig. 189. Infiltrating duct cell cancer, left breast. A short dilated ductal segment under the skin marker is the site of a localized duct cell cancer with minimal perifocal edema which blurs the structural details, best appreciated when compared with a similar area of the opposite (right) breast

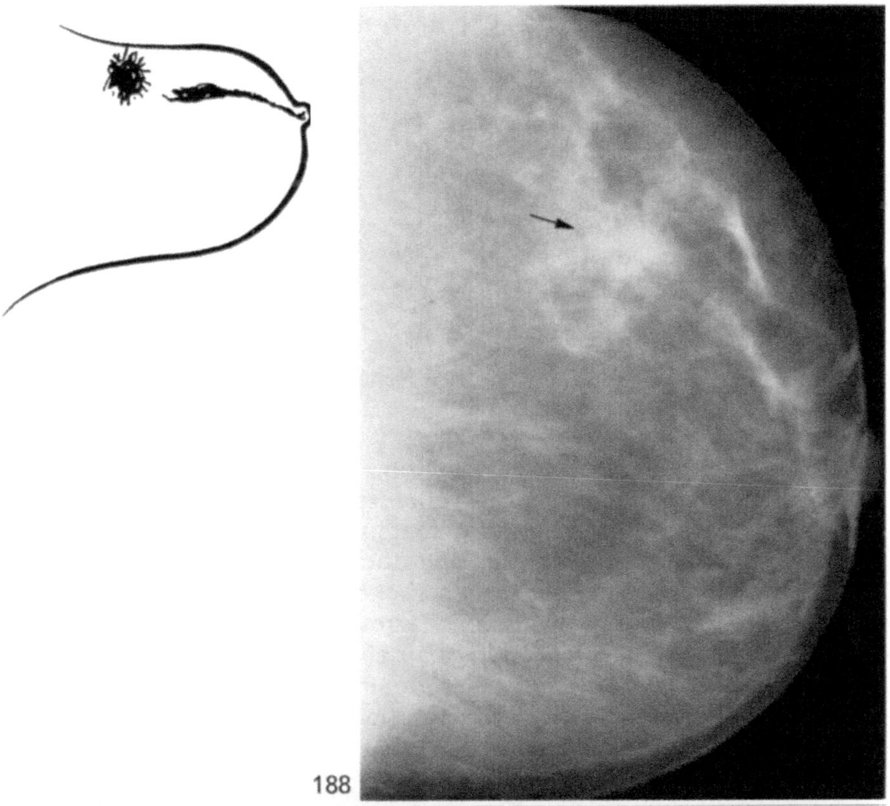

188

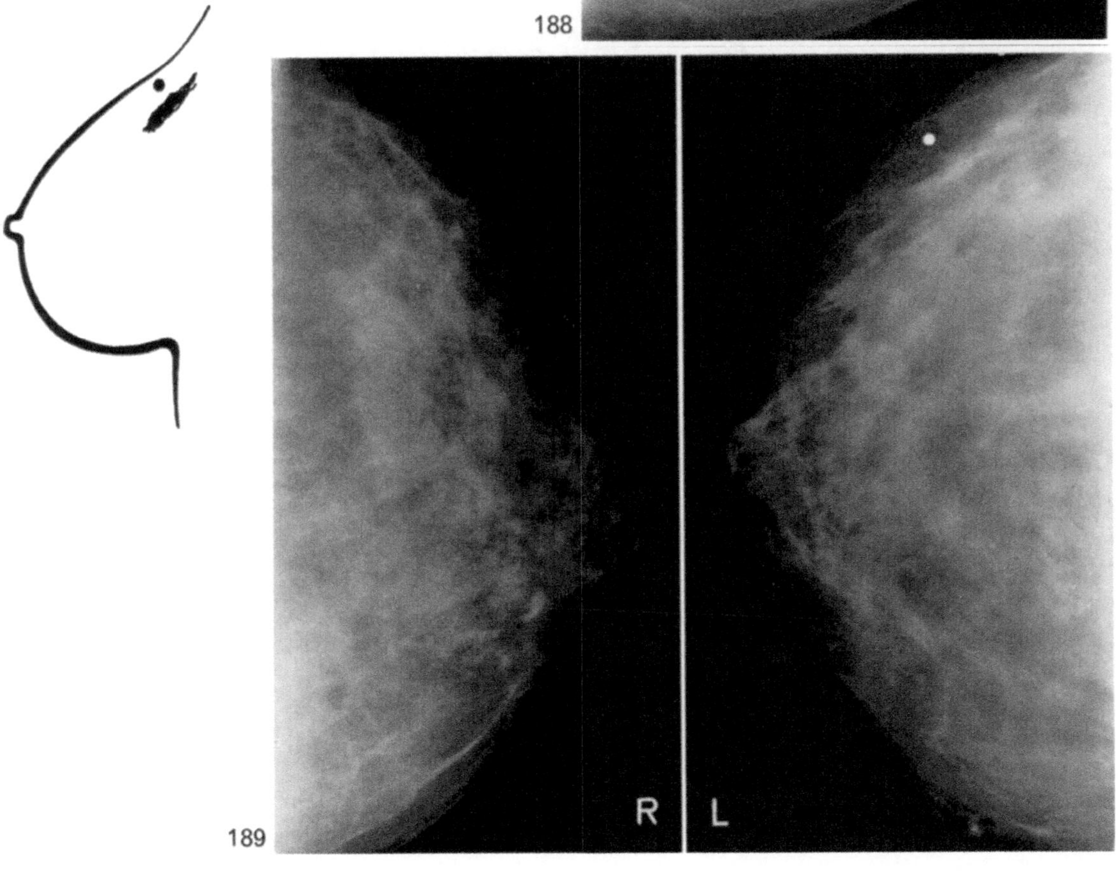

189

Fig. 190. Infiltrating duct cell carcinoma, right breast. The right nipple is retracted and the surrounding tissue is edematous, including the skin of the areola. The ducts are distorted, and extension has reached an area of scirrhous involution (arrow) which comprised the clinically palpable mass, suspected to be cancer. Sclerosing adenosis was found in the opposite (left) breast, where cancer was also suspected

Fig. 191. Infiltrating duct cell carcinoma, right breast. Localized edema and vessel prominence are present. The ducts are prominent in both breasts, but in the upper right breast they are locally distended, distorted, and ballooned corresponding to a mass palpated by both the patient and her physician, who thought he was confronted with "swollen milk ducts." These roentgen findings in a 41 year old woman correctly raised the suspicion of malignancy, which was confirmed by the pathologist. No axillary lymph node metastasis was present

190
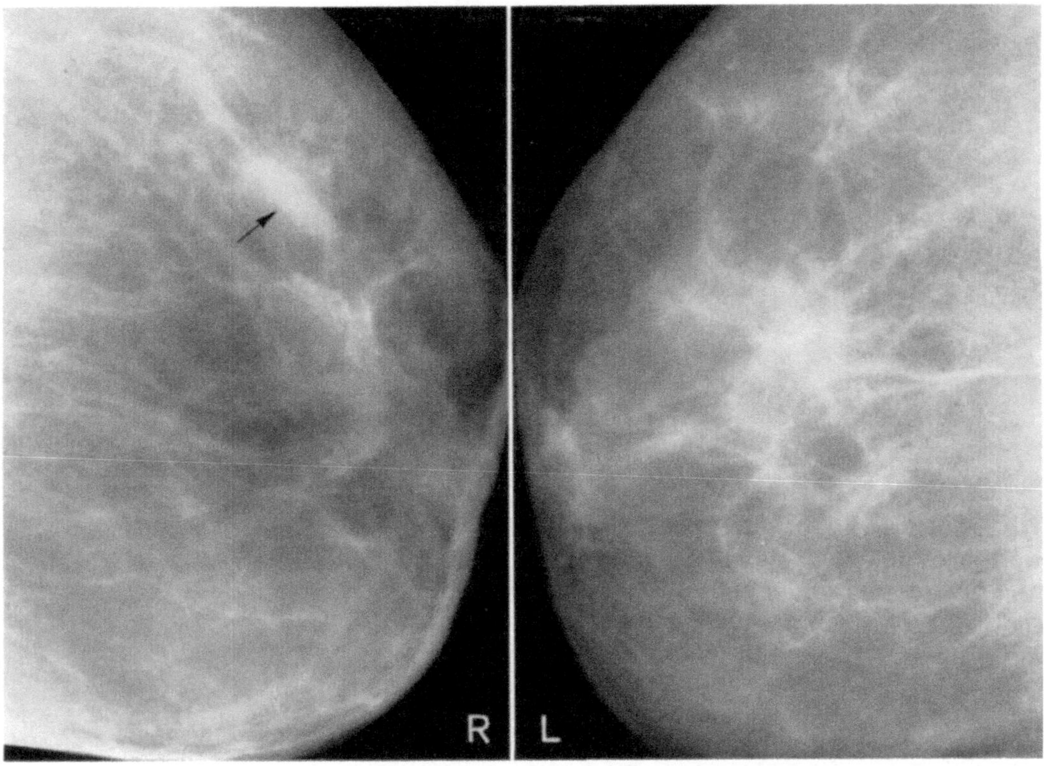

191
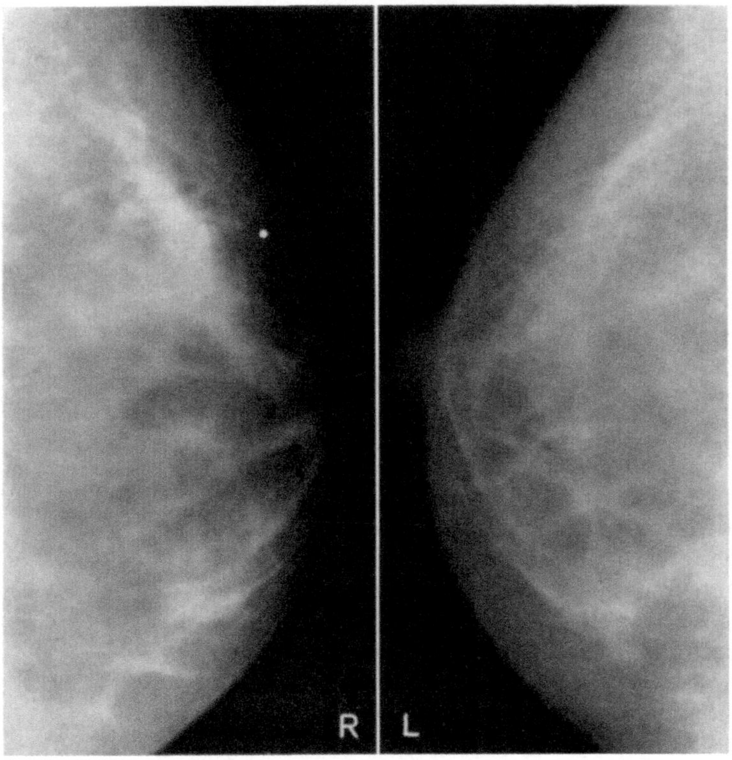

Fig. 192. Infiltrating duct cell carcinoma, right breast. A complex of ducts is dilated and distorted in the upper right breast, and there is also much perifocal edema, vascular turgescence, and thickening of the skin. This 43 year old patient noted the presence of a lump for five weeks. An ill-defined nodular mass was palpated by the clinician, which both he and the roentgenologist suspected might be malignant

Fig. 193. Infiltrating duct cell carcinoma. In an area of the right breast where the patient localized pain (arrow heads), the structural pattern is blurred due to edema. Comparison with the opposite (left) breast helps one to appreciate the differences in trabecular patterns. The homogeneous densities in both breasts, with curvilinear margins outlining areas of adenosis, pose diagnostic difficulties

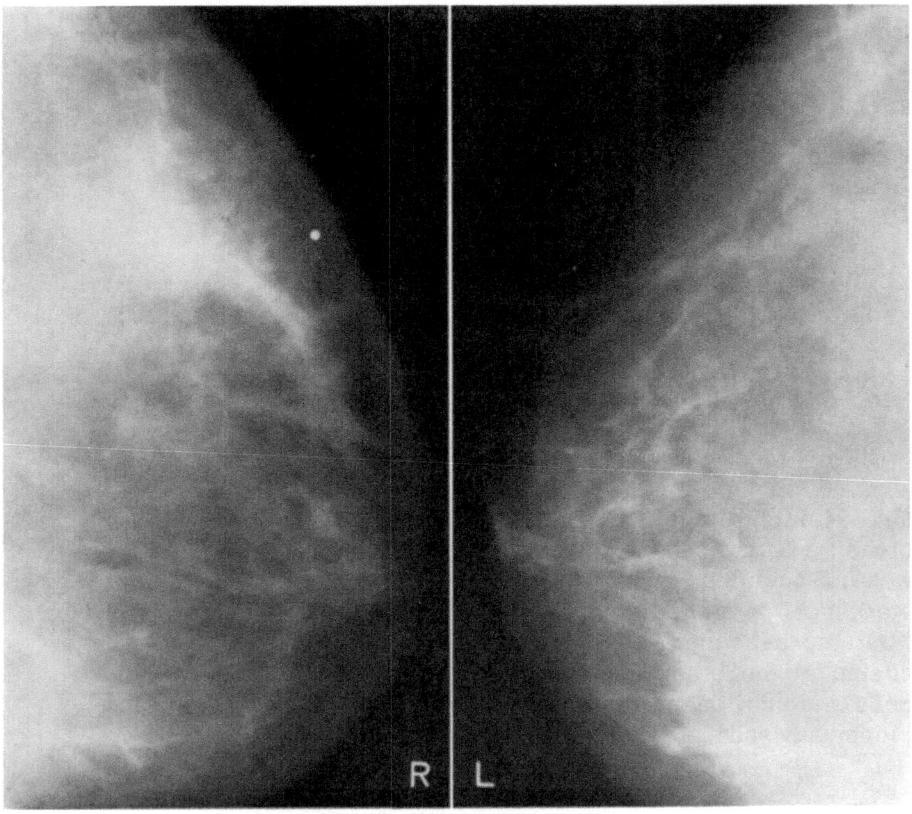

192

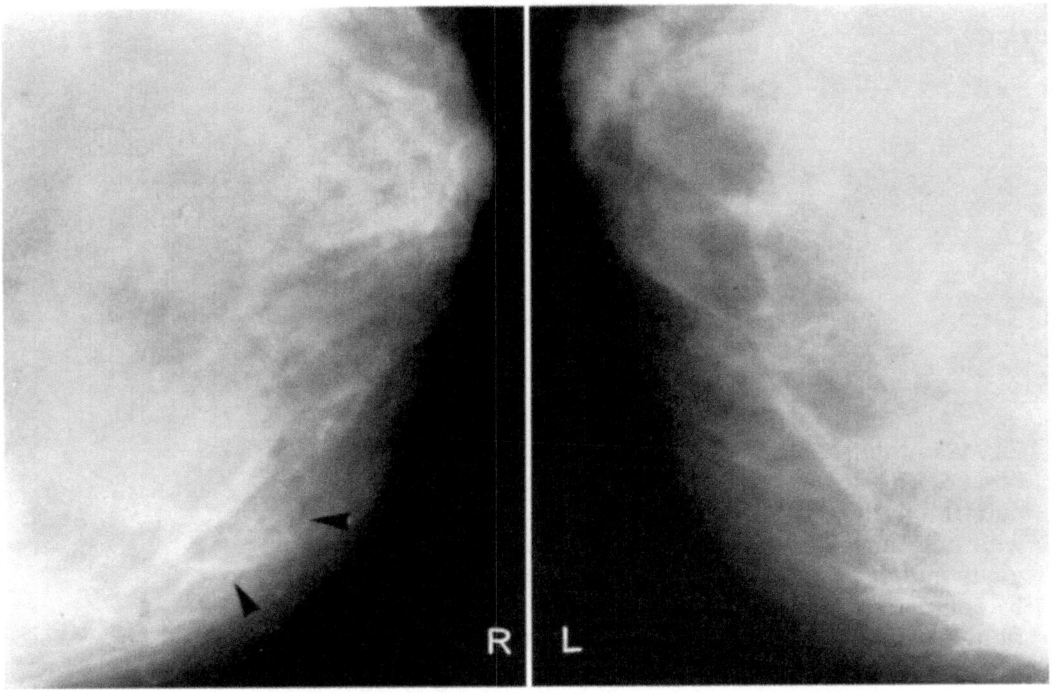

193

Fig. 194. Infiltrating duct cell carcinoma, left breast. The cancer under the skin marker was not palpable (it was only 9 mm in diameter), but the patient was conscious of a "burning sensation." Only because of the edema of the breast, best appreciated by comparison with the opposite breast, was biopsy advised

Fig. 195. Infiltrating duct cell cancer, left breast. The localized distorted trabecular pattern in the left breast (arrow heads), with blurring of details due to edema, suggests a duct cell cancer, better appreciated by comparison with structural details of the right breast. Patient complained of a "drawing sensation." No mass was palpable

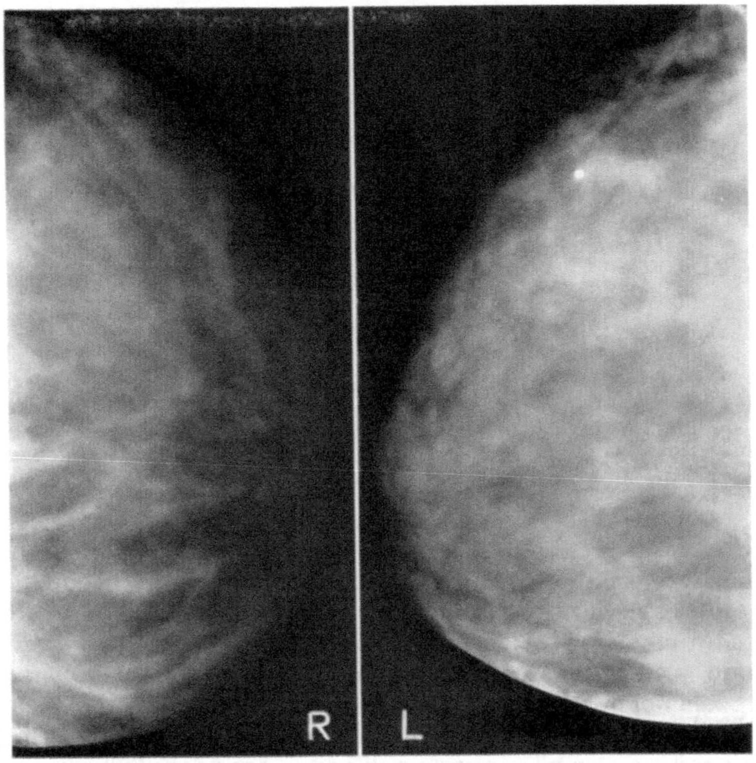

194

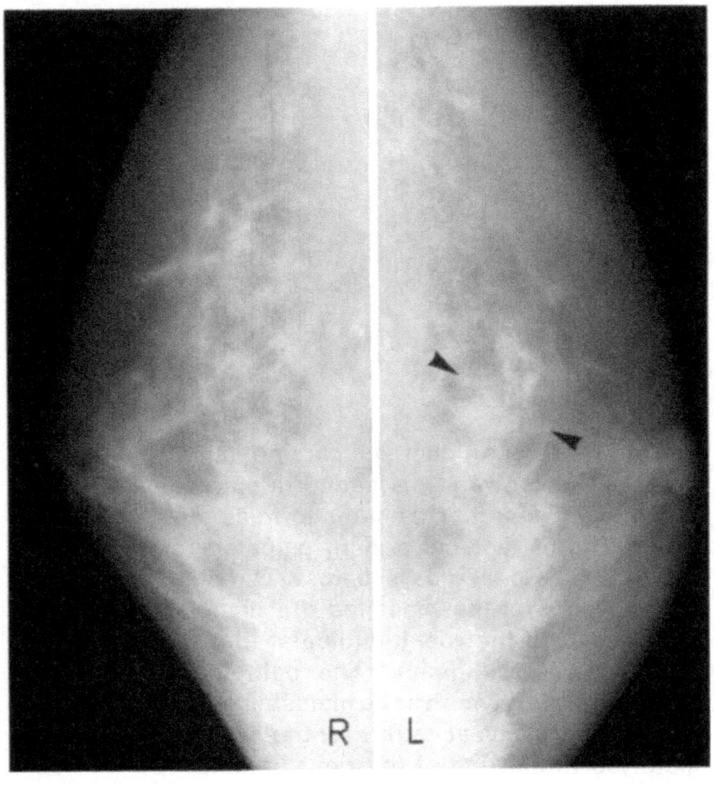

195

Fig. 196. Infiltrating duct cell carcinoma, left breast. For two months this patient had felt a mass in the left breast. On examination, a discrete, flat induration about 2.5 cm in diameter was palpable and thought to be benign. The lateral roentgenograms disclosed a small, poorly-outlined mass (arrow), slightly denser than the surrounding involuted fibrous tissue. The tissues of the breast are blurred due to edema, *better appreciated by comparison with roentgenogram of right breast*. Remarkable in this case was the fact that the pathologist found a cancer which was only 8 mm in diameter but which was associated with considerable small round-cell infiltration

Fig. 197. Infiltrating duct cell carcinoma, left breast. The crowded distended ducts with much reactive perifocal edema form a mass which this 65 year old patient palpated for the first time only 8 days before. Dimpling of the skin over the mass led the clinician to agree with the roentgenologist that the process was malignant. The pathologist found no axillary lymph node metastasis. Epithelial hyperplasia accounts for the swollen, distorted trabeculae of the right breast

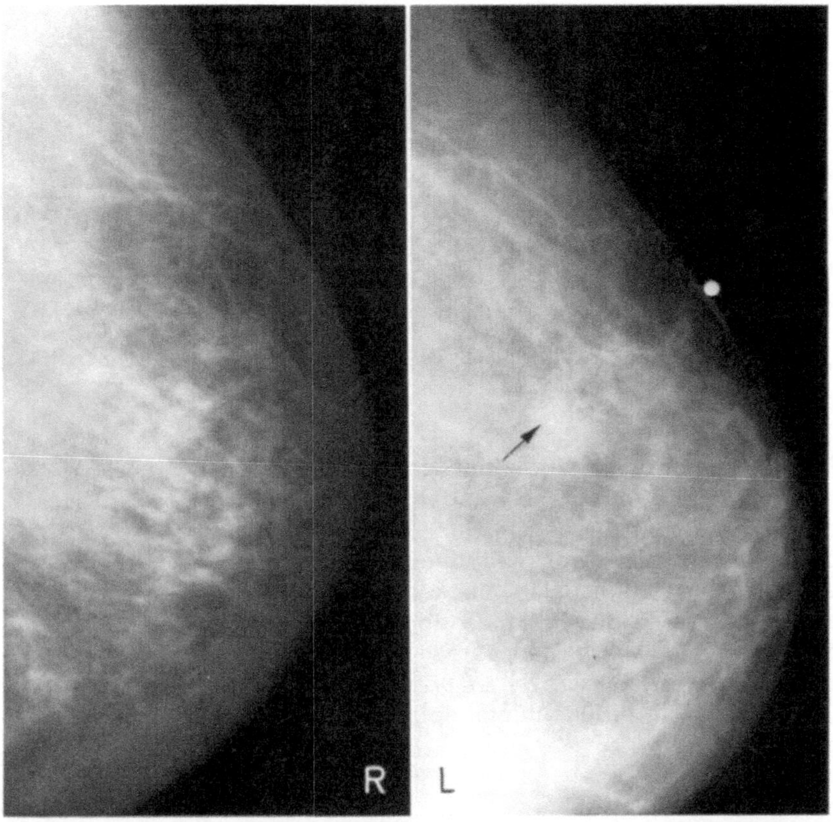

196

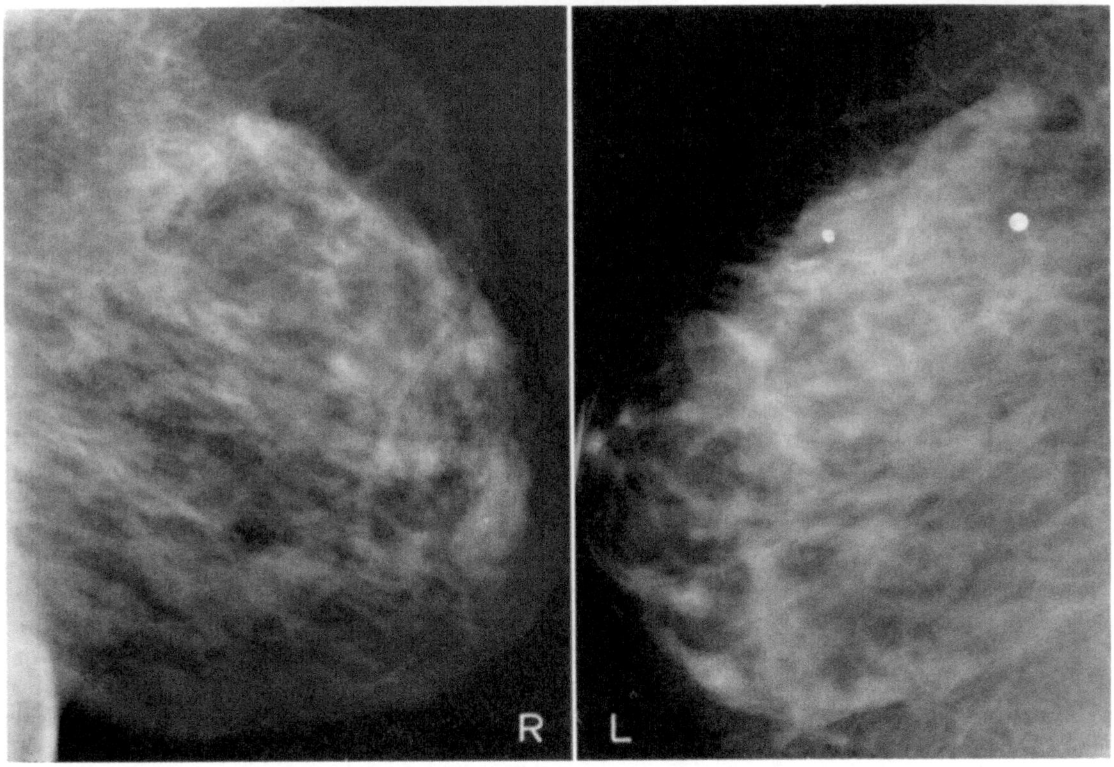

197

Fig. 198. Infiltrating duct cell carcinoma, right breast. Cancer was suspected clinically in the right breast because of a palpable mass. This is not seen roentgenographically, but slight skin thickening and distortion are visible, with blurring of details due to edema. *These changes can be appreciated by comparison with the left breast*, which is involved with diffuse ductal epithelial hyperplasia

Fig. 199. Infiltrating duct cell carcinoma, right breast. A tumor, per se, is not visible. Hyperplastic fibrosis and edema are present only in the right breast, best appreciated when compared with the opposite side. Cancer in such a hyperplastic, fibrous breast may be masked. The left ductal pattern suggests epithelial hyperplasia. A lump was felt by this patient in her right breast for only one week. The clinician could palpate a mass 2 cm in diameter, adherent to the surrounding tissues and displacing the nipple. In these circumstances, the clinical findings should take precedence

198
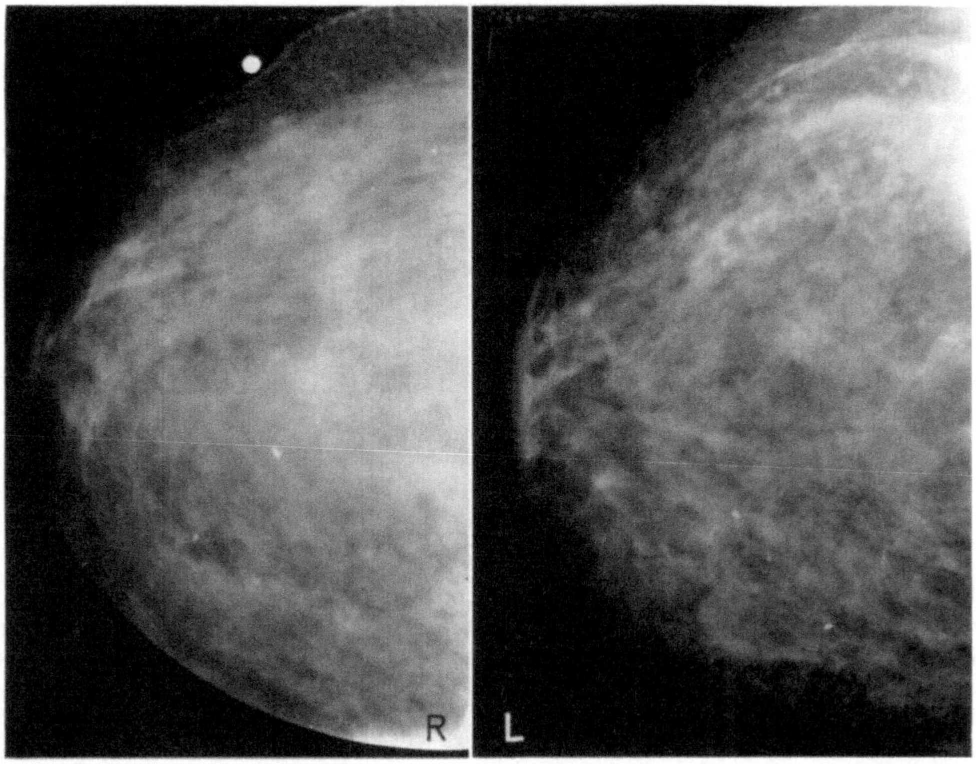

199
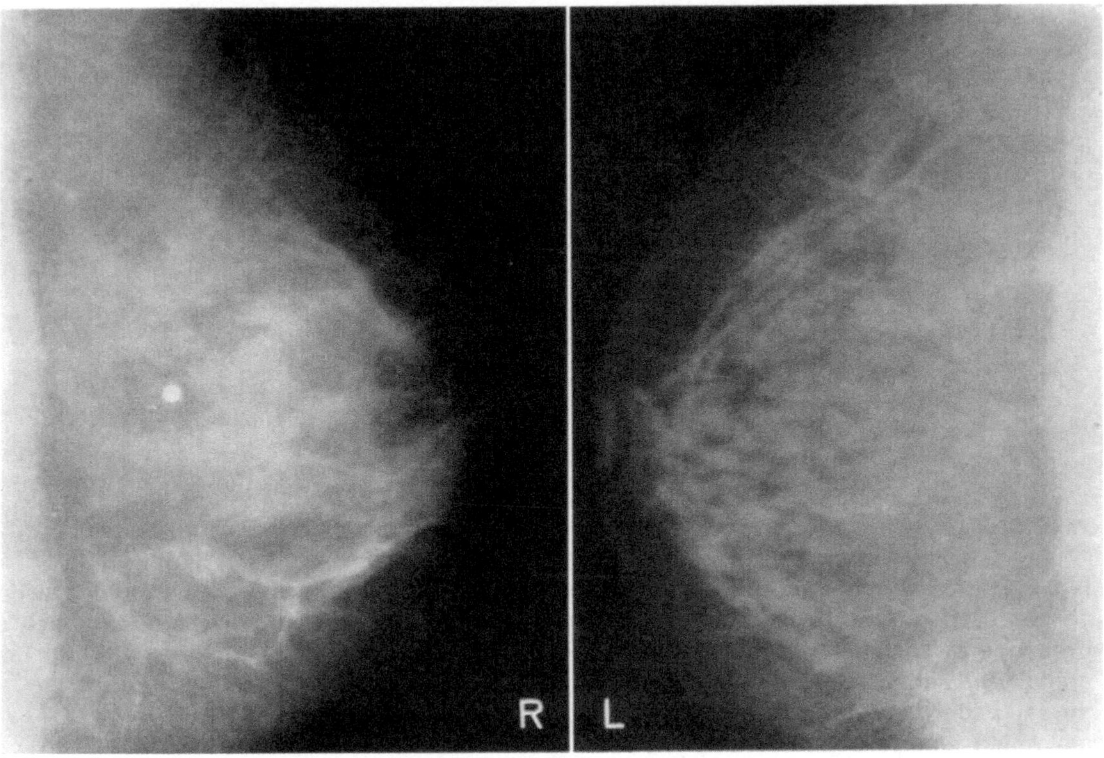

Fig. 200. Advanced infiltrating duct cell cancer. A tumor per se is not visualized, but the skin edema should always raise the suspicion of cancer, and was obvious even to the clinician. A mass was palpable, the nipple was retracted, and the skin was red and swollen

Fig. 201. Advanced infiltrating duct cell carcinoma. This 82 year old patient knew she had a growing mass in her breast for 8 months. The red, thick skin suggested an "inflammatory" carcinoma to the clinician, and the thickened skin alerted the roentgenologist to the cancer

Fig. 202. Advanced infiltrating duct cell cancer. Recognition is based chiefly on the presence of secondary signs of skin thickening and edema. The cancer itself is spread widely in areas of sclerosing adenosis which tend to obscure tumor tissue

Fig. 203. Infiltrating duct cell cancer, widely permeated with extensive edema which almost obscures the scirrhus with its dendritic extensions (arrow)

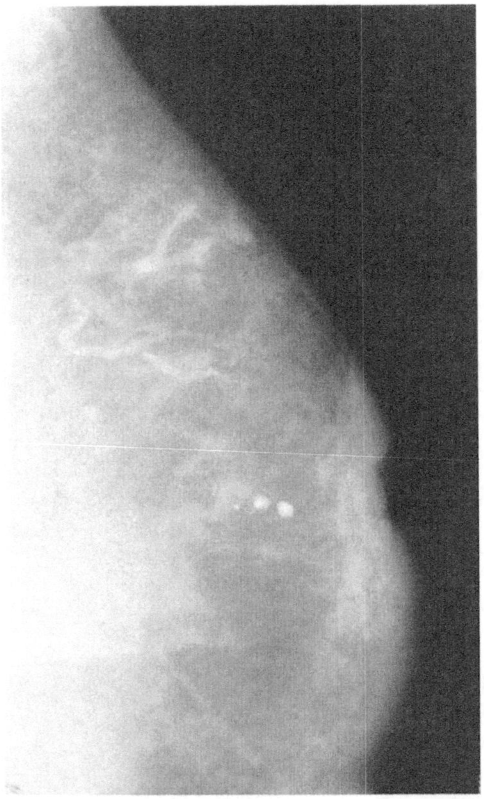
200

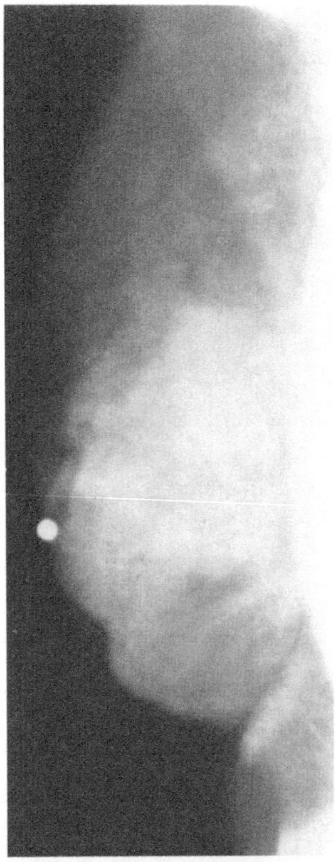
201

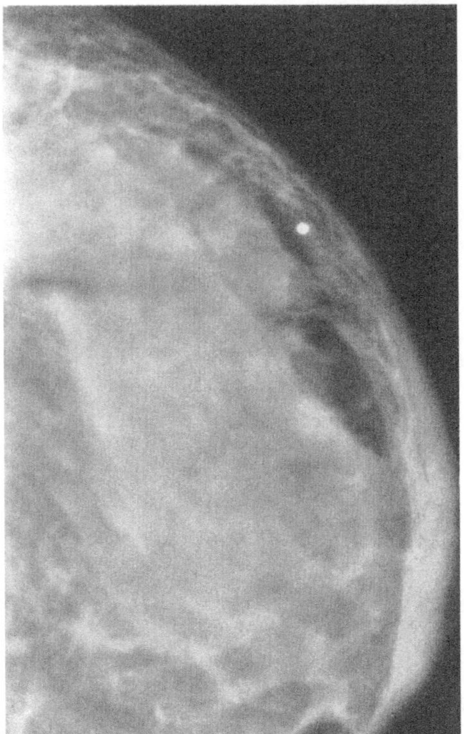
202

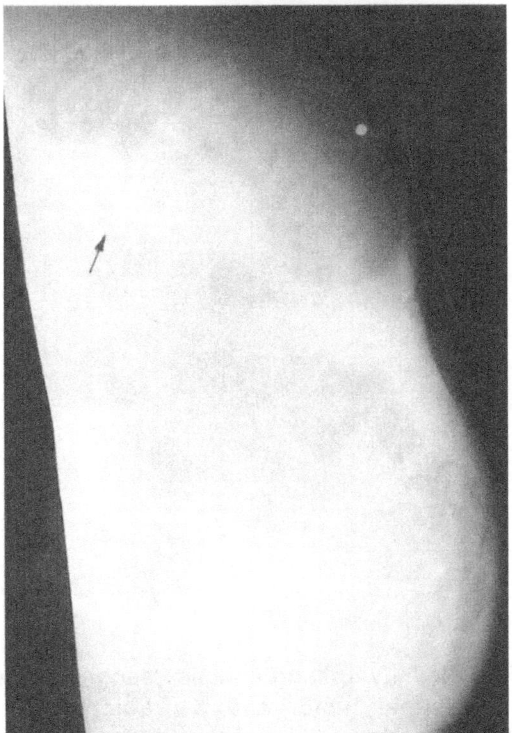
203

Fig. 204. "Inflammatory" cancer, right breast, 8 months postpartum. The edema and widespread lymphangiectasis blur the structural details, better appreciated by comparison with details of opposite (left) breast

Fig. 205. Lymphangiectasis secondary to mediastinal tumor and X-irradiation. The edema and swelling of the skin and breast tissue blur structural details

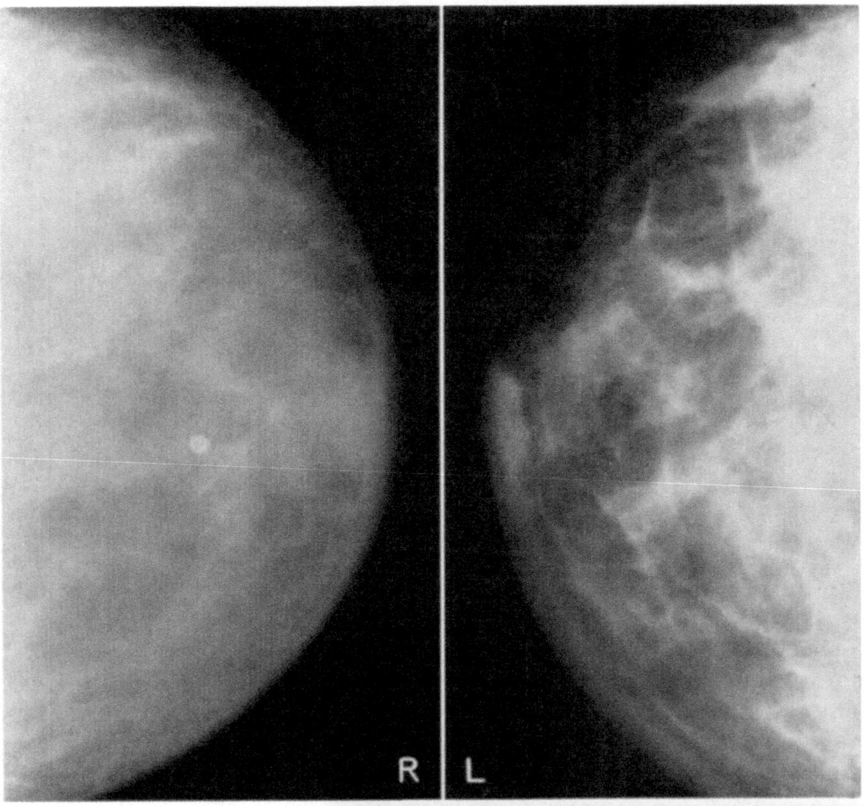

204

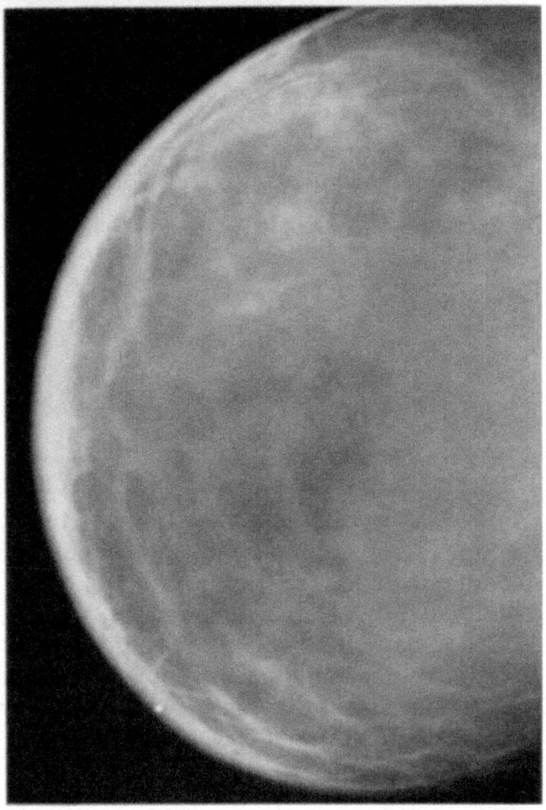

205

Fig. 206. Bilateral infiltrating duct cell cancers, clinically recognized only on right. The irregularly-outlined solitary non-palpable mass on left (arrow) was correctly suspected as cancer by roentgenologist

Fig. 207. Microcalcifications shown in tissue section. Roentgenogram of thin section of tissue shows widespread intraductal microcalcifications of duct cancer as bizarre-shaped particles with irregular outlines. They are disseminated but closely spaced along the course of ducts or clustered in sequestered aggregates

Fig. 208. Infiltrating duct cell cancer, non-palpable. Several clustered, irregularly-shaped microcalcifications are seen in areas of mazoplasia cystica and sclerosing adenosis. The suggestion of the presence of cancer based merely on the finding of a few bizarre calcified spicules was confirmed by the pathologist, who found a cancer 8 mm in diameter which was not suspected clinically. Inset magnifies the particles 5 ×

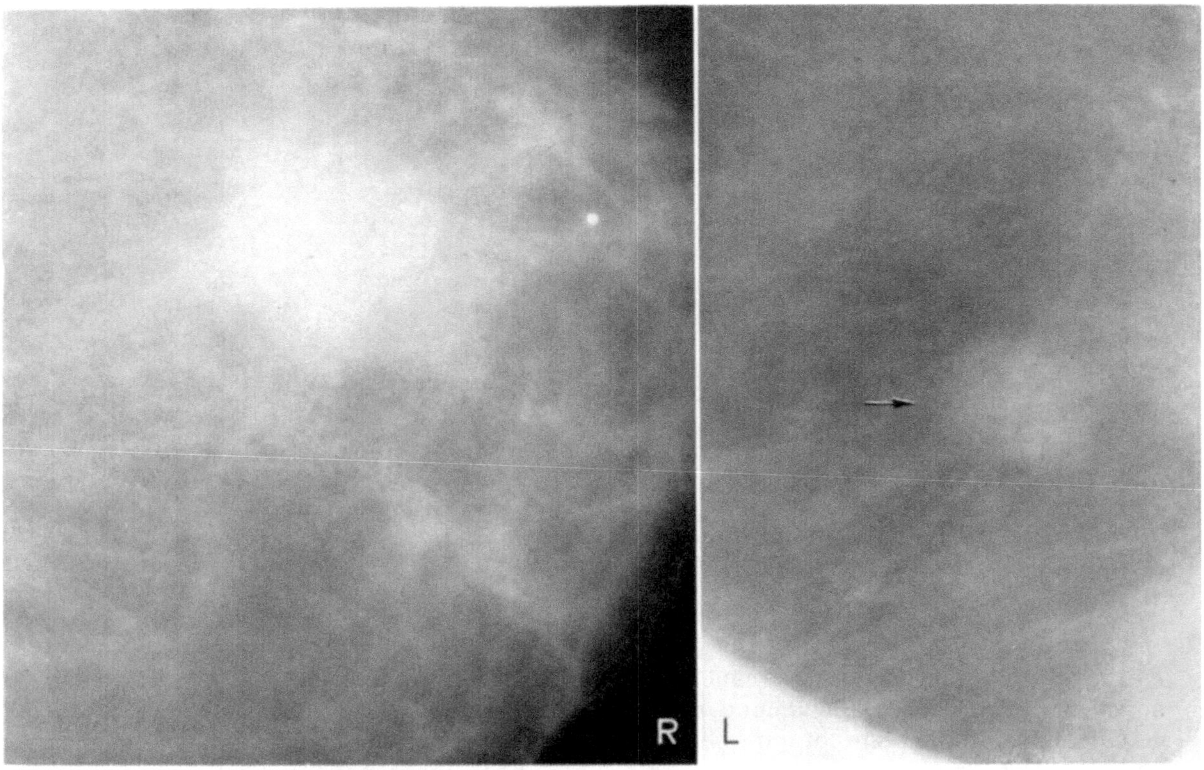

206

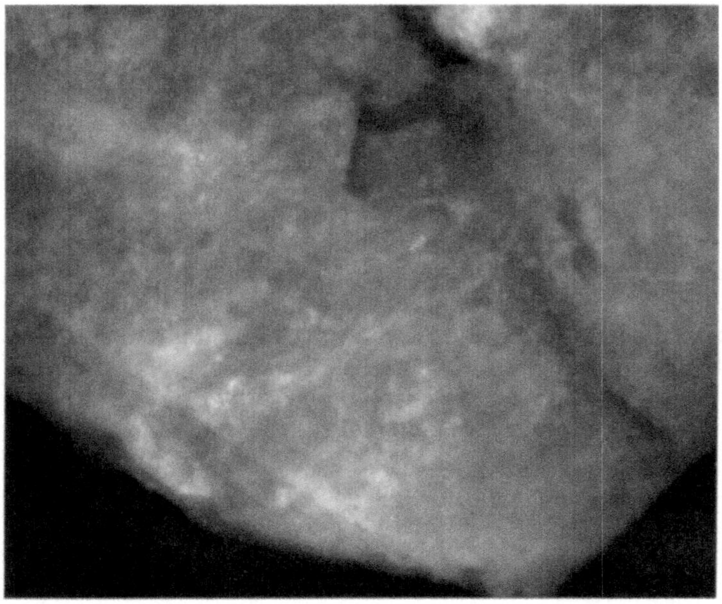

207

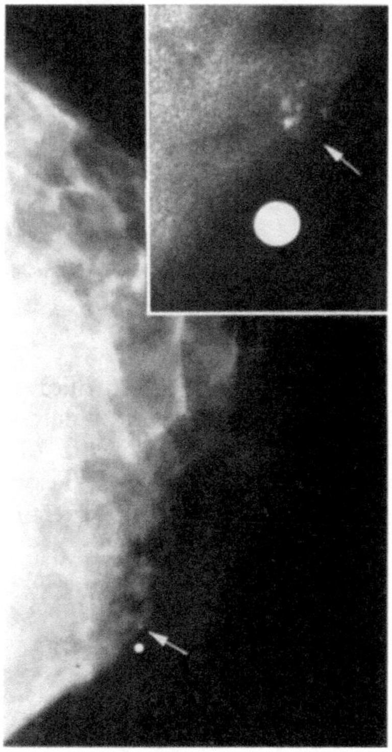

208

Fig. 209. Infiltrating duct cell cancer. A small cluster of irregularly-shaped microcalcifications marks site of non-palpable cancer. Two months postpartum, this 34 year old patient felt a "lumpiness" not regarded as significant by the clinician

Fig. 210. Infiltrating duct cell carcinoma. In an area of adenosis, only an aggregate of microcalcifications indicates the presence of cancer. Inset magnified 3×

Fig. 211. Infiltrating duct cell cancer. Extensive reticulated, lacy calcium deposits mark site of cancer as the only positive X-ray sign. This 59 year old patient complained of local pain, but no palpable tumor was present

Fig. 212. Infiltrating duct cell carcinoma. Widespread microcalcifications are present in a breast widely involved in ductal epithelial hyperplasia, adenosis, and duct ectasia. An aggregate of microcalcifications, edema, and skin thickening (arrows) in an area of symptoms localized by this 46 year old patient led the radiologist to suspect the presence of cancer in spite of the surgeon's skepticism. The pathologist confirmed the presence of an infiltrating duct cell cancer with metastasis to 4 of 19 nodes

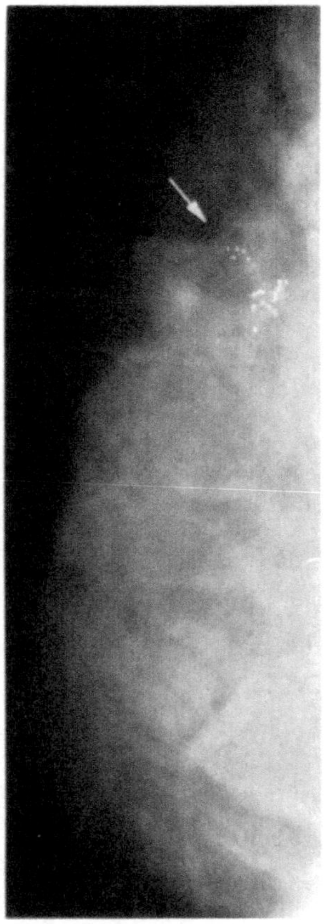
209

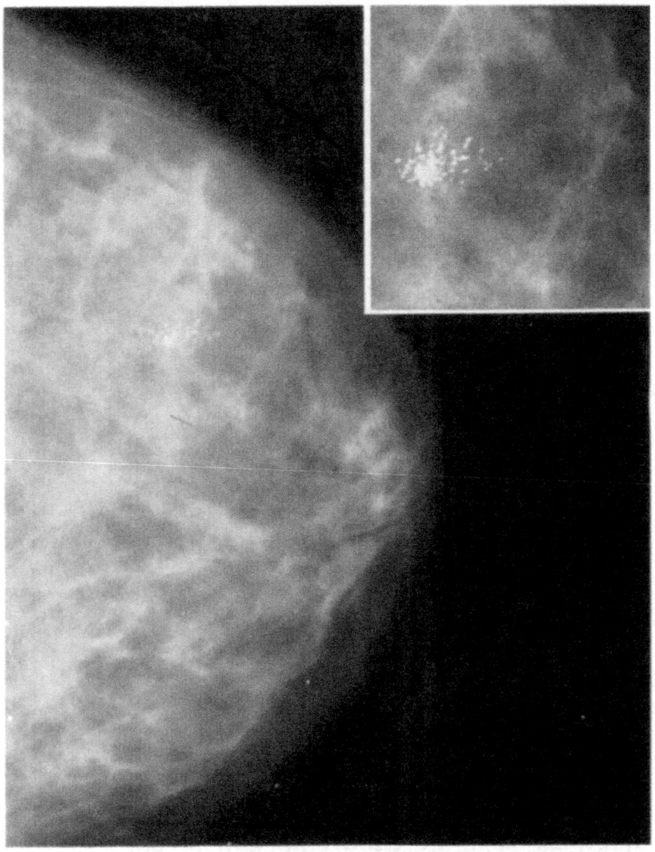
210

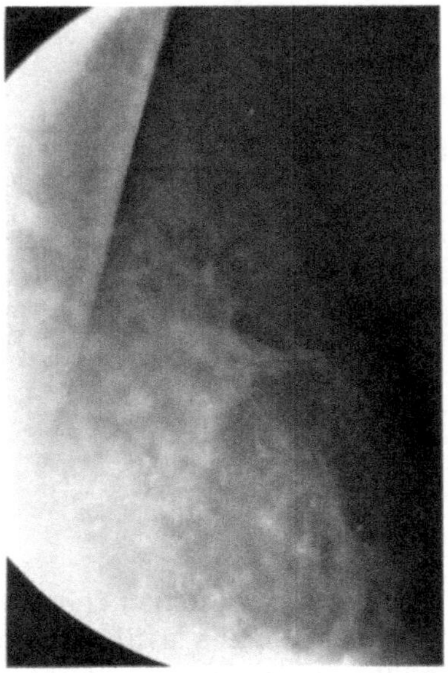
211

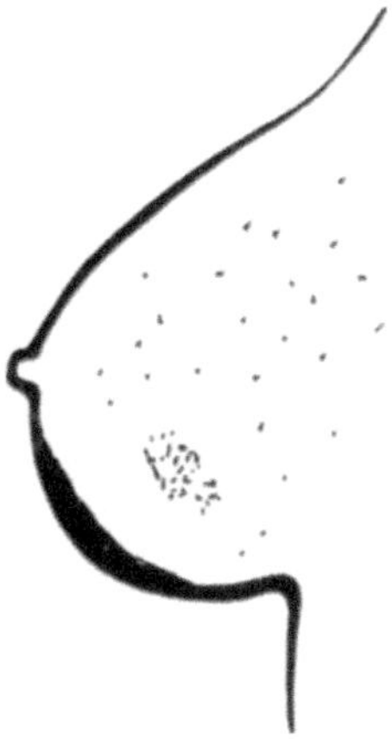

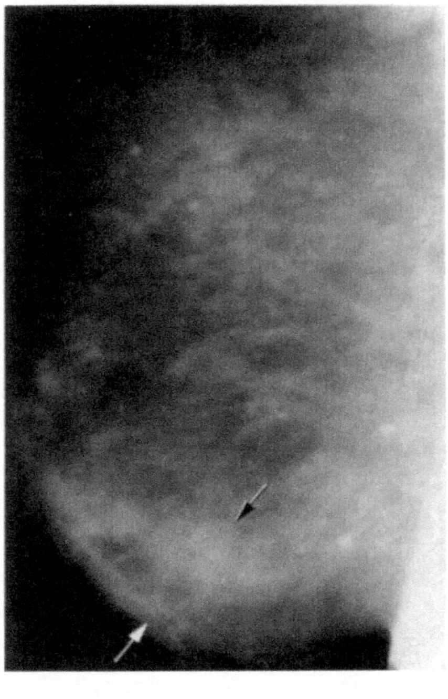
212

Fig. 213. Infiltrating duct cell carcinoma. No palpable tumor was present and no isolated mass was visible, but the scattered microcalcifications were sufficient to suggest an X-ray diagnosis of cancer

Fig. 214. Medullary cancer. Smooth margins resembling those of a benign lesion may sometimes be associated with this type of cancer

Fig. 215. Medullary carcinoma. The circumscribed tumor resembles a fibroadenoma. An isolated lesion like this in a woman over 45 years of age should always be suspected as a cancer until proven otherwise

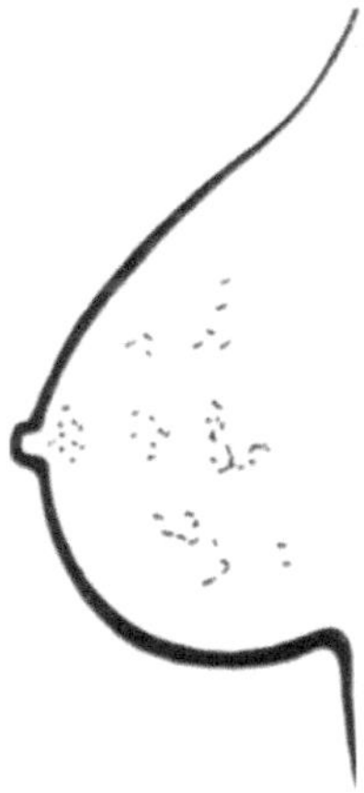

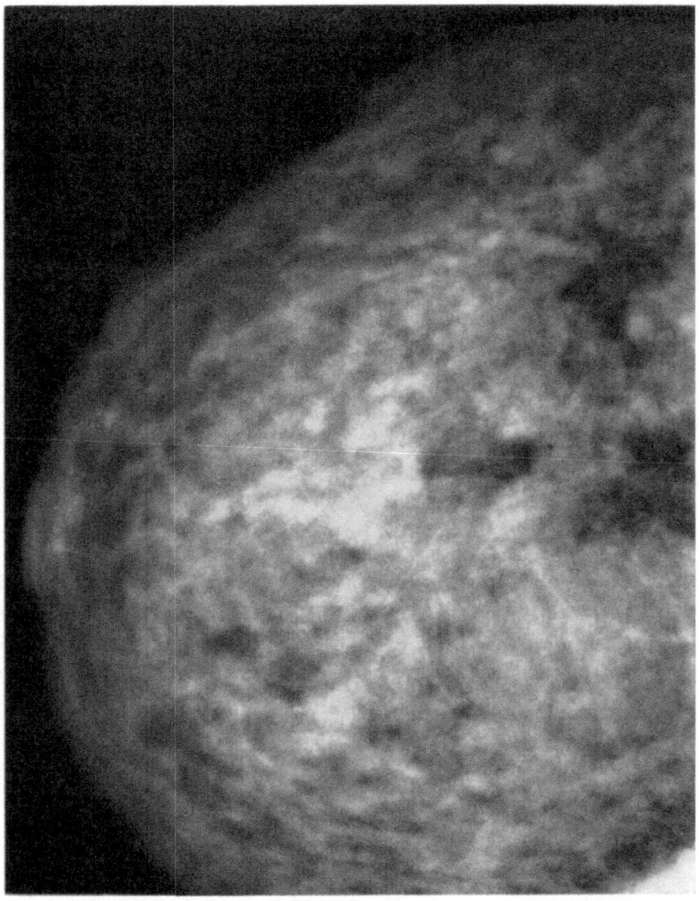

213

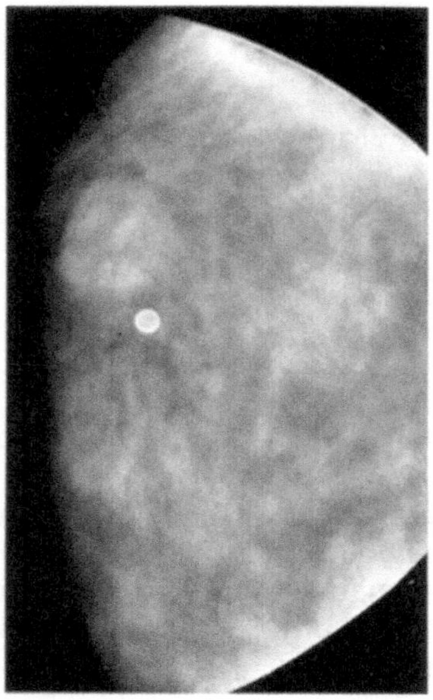

214

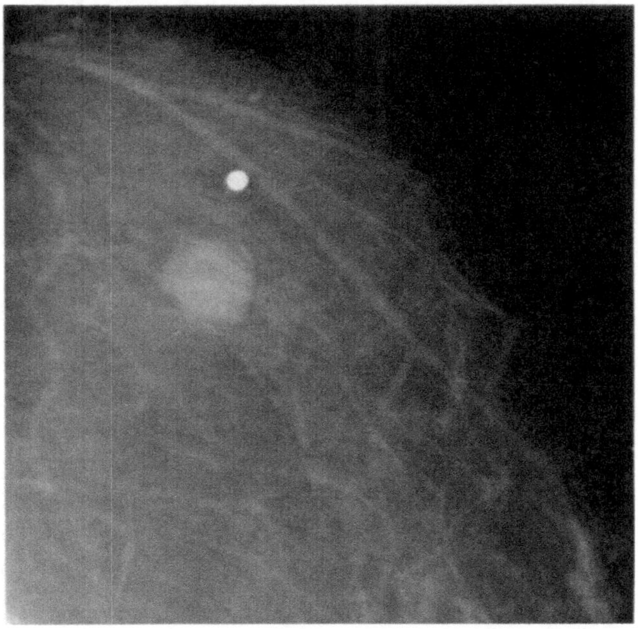

215

Fig. 216. Medullary carcinoma. Although it may not be palpable, any isolated double-contoured mass with sinuous margins seen on the X-ray film of a woman 47 years of age must first be suspected of being malignant

Fig. 217. Medullary carcinoma. This isolated, notcned, smooth-walled cancer resembles a fibroadenoma or a cyst. The lesion was palpable and regarded as benign. It measured 2 cm in diameter on palpation, but only 8 mm in diameter on the X-ray film and on gross section

Fig. 218. Small medullary carcinoma (arrow). The small, globoid, irregularly-marginated tumor is adjacent to a palpable cyst (under skin marker). Cancer was not suspected clinically

Fig. 219. Medullary cancer. An isolated, lobulated, smoothly-contoured mass in a 68 year old woman should first be regarded as cancer instead of a fibroadenoma, which it resembles

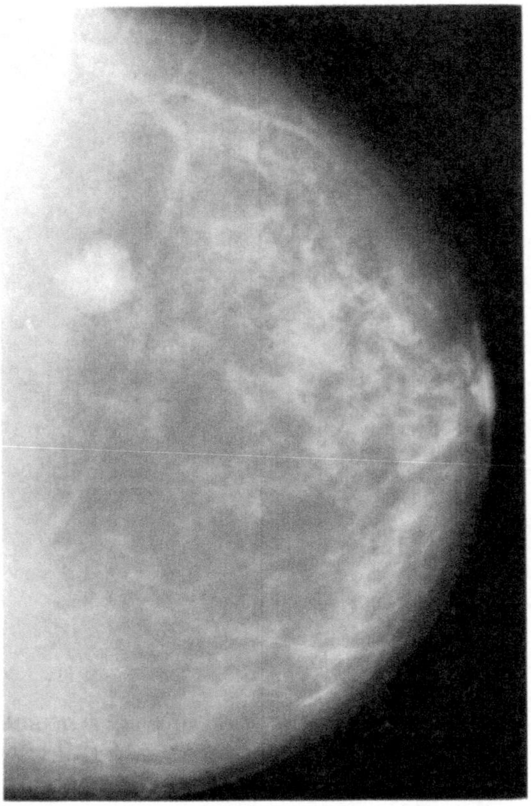

216

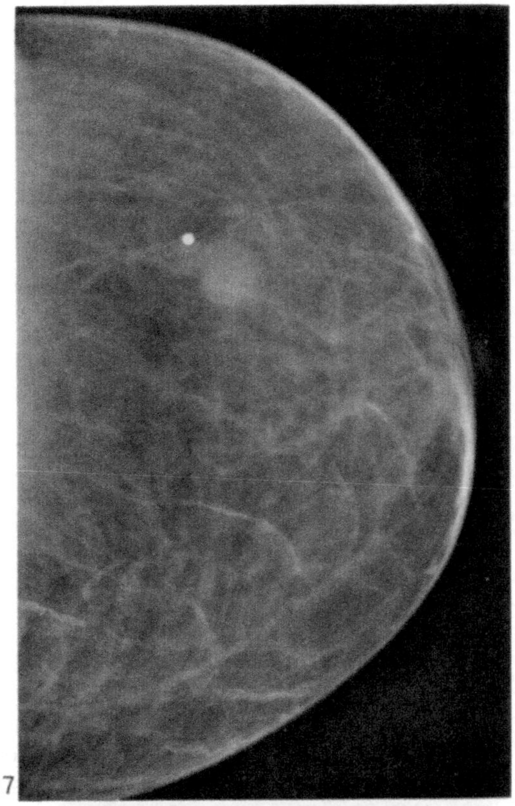

217

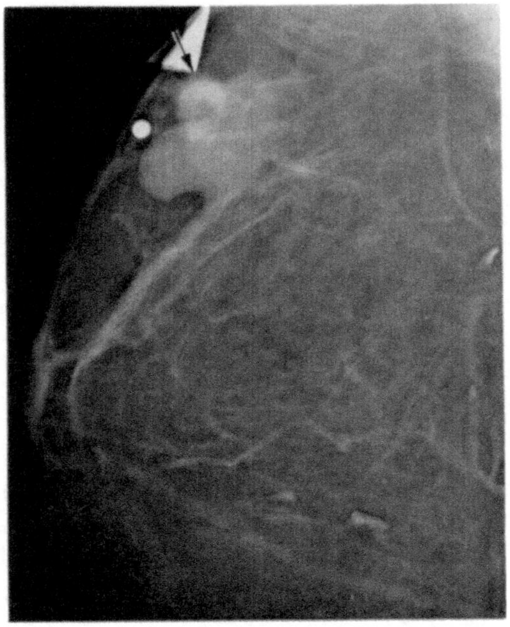

218

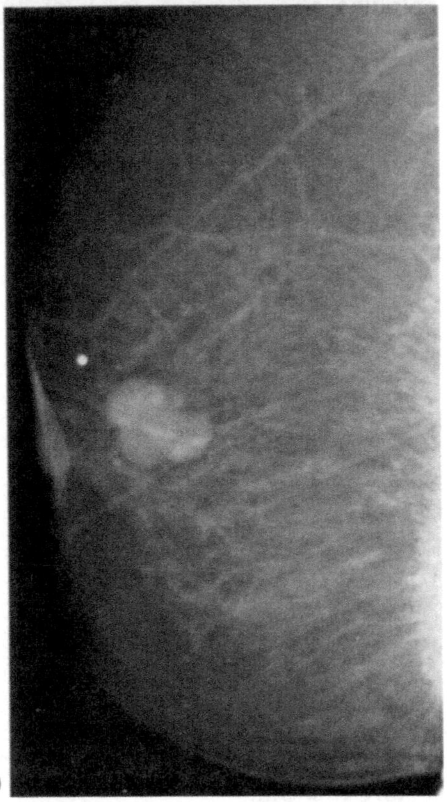

219

Fig. 220. Medullary cancer. The sharp undulating margins of the mass resemble those of a benign lesion, but a few short spicules raise the suspicion of cancer

Fig. 221. Medullary carcinoma. An isolated tumor whose margins are sharp and smooth, but sinuous and irregularly spiculated, was correctly suspected to be malignant

Fig. 222. Medullary cancer. A small nonpalpable tumor, with blurred, notched margins and sentinel strands, is present. This suggests cancer rather than a cyst or a fibroadenoma

Fig. 223. Medullary cancer. Some spiculations of the margin will resemble those of a scirrhus. Thickening is due to perifocal edema

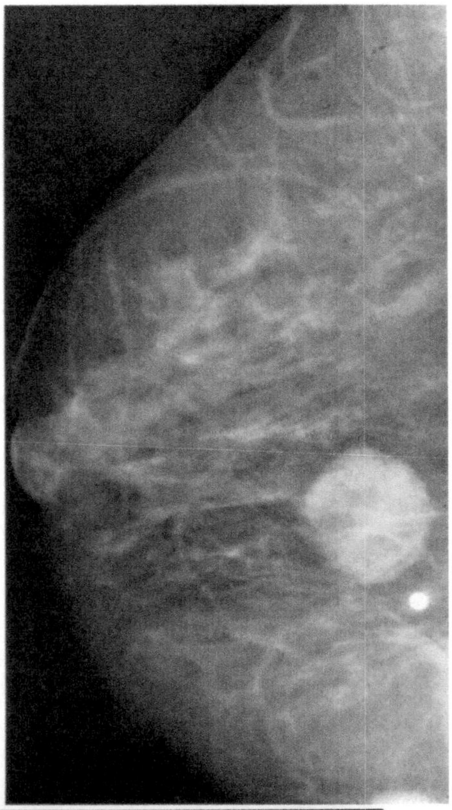

220

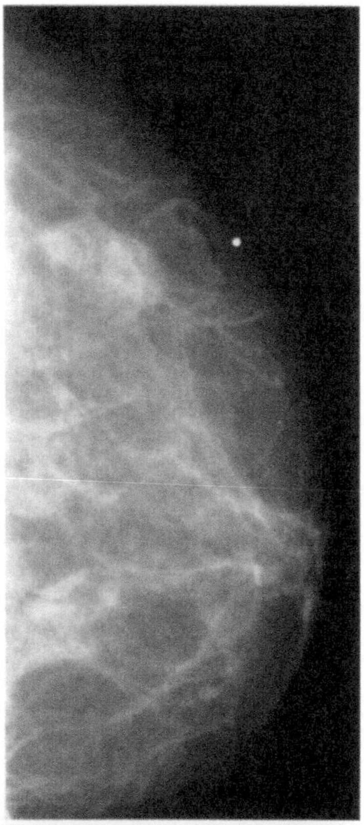

221

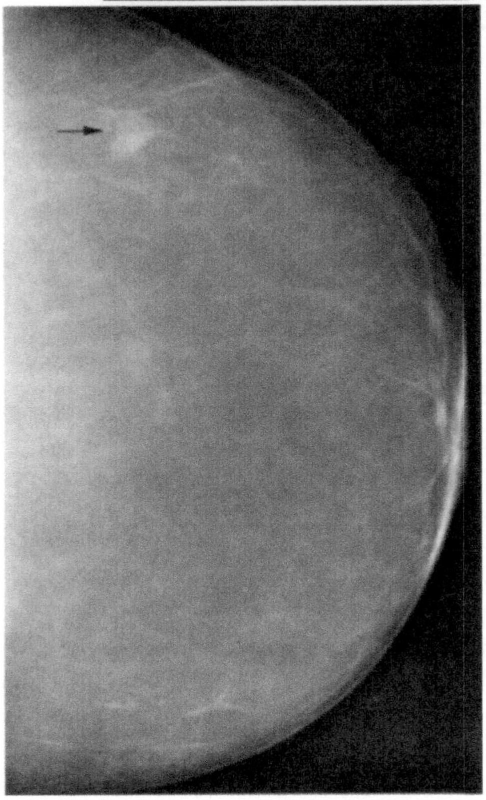

222

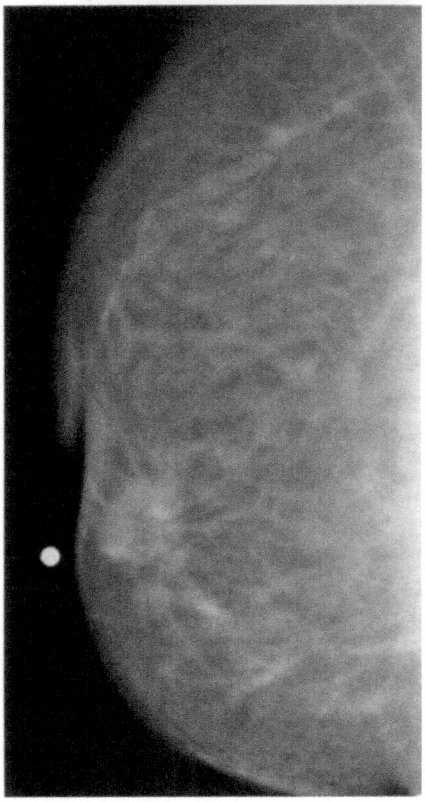

223

Fig. 224. Medullary cancer. The irregular, spiculated margins resemble a scirrhus. Edematous blurring of details and engorgement of vessels are seen around the mass

Fig. 225. Medullary cancer. Comet-tail extensions are present with thickening of adjacent skin due to perifocal edema

Fig. 226. Medullary carcinoma. An isolated mass with notching of its undulating borders (arrows) in a 52 year old woman suggests cancer rather than a fibroadenoma or multilocular cyst, which it resembles

Fig. 227. Medullary cancer. Some of these lesions may have many short spiculated extensions and almost resemble a scirrhus

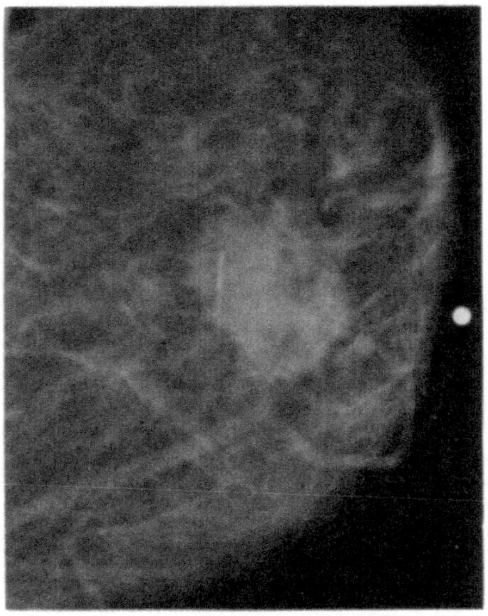
224

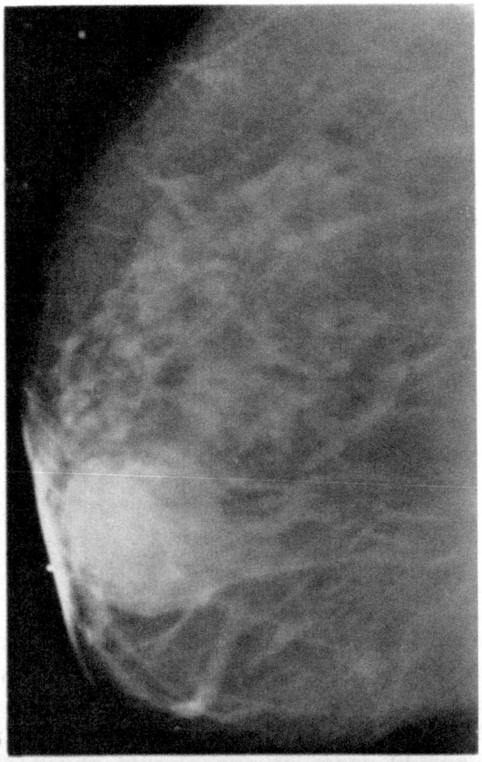
225

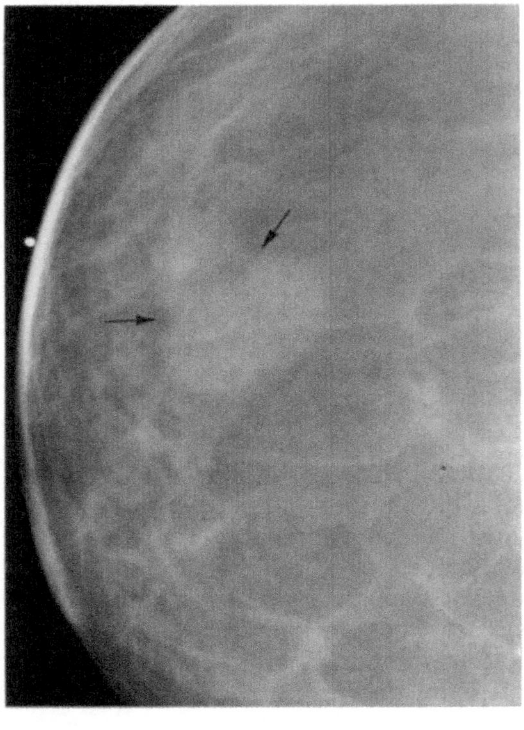
226

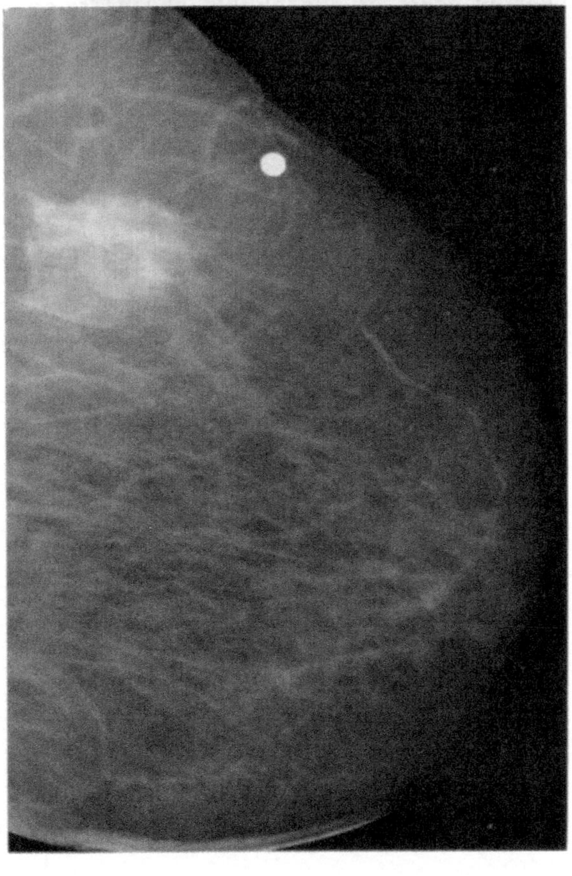
227

Fig. 228. Medullary cancer. A noduiar mass with relatively smooth, sinuous borders may closely resemble a fibroadenoma or a cyst; but an isolated lesion like this in a woman over 40 years of age should always raise the question of cancer

Fig. 229. Medullary cancer. An isolated mass with a sinuous, relatively smooth border, portions of which are lost in a field of adenosis, may be a medullary cancer even though it resembles a fibroadenoma or a cyst

Fig. 230. Two medullary cancers. The undulating, blurred margins are due to incomplete encapsulation and edema

Fig. 231. Medullary cancer. An isolated tumor with sinuous, notched borders may suggest medullary cancer in spite of its resemblance to a multilocular cyst, an intracystic papilloma, or a bosselated fibroadenoma. Such lesions found in women over 40 years of age merit diagnostic resection without delay

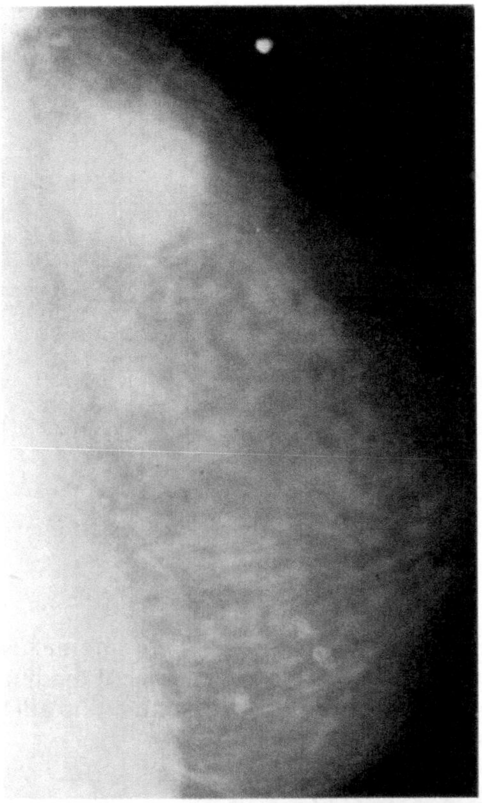

228

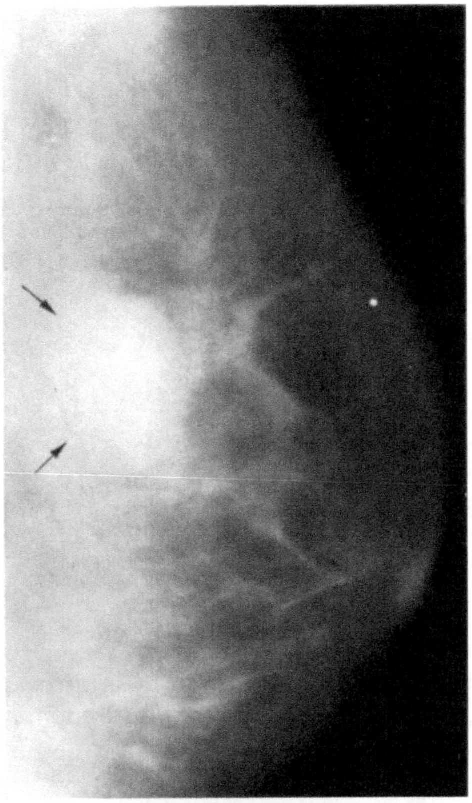

229

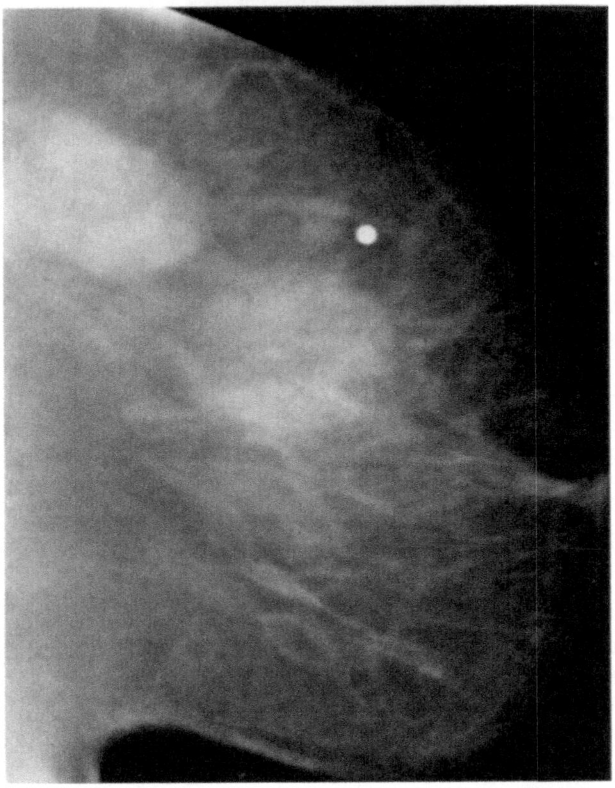

230

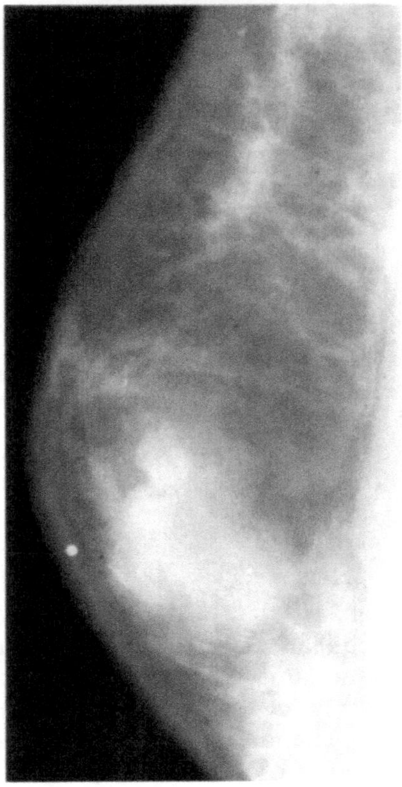

231

Fig. 232. Large medullary cancer. The smooth, sinuous margins (arrows) are barely visible due to perifocal edema which includes the adjacent skin

Fig. 233. Large medullary carcinoma. These lesions may resemble cysts, but the blurred, wavy margins and thickening of the adjacent skin suggest malignancy

Fig. 234 A
Medullary cancer. The cancer has occurred in an area of adenosis which partly accounts for the indistinct margins. Perifocal edema and vascular turgescence add to the blurring of structural details

B
Opposite breast for comparison

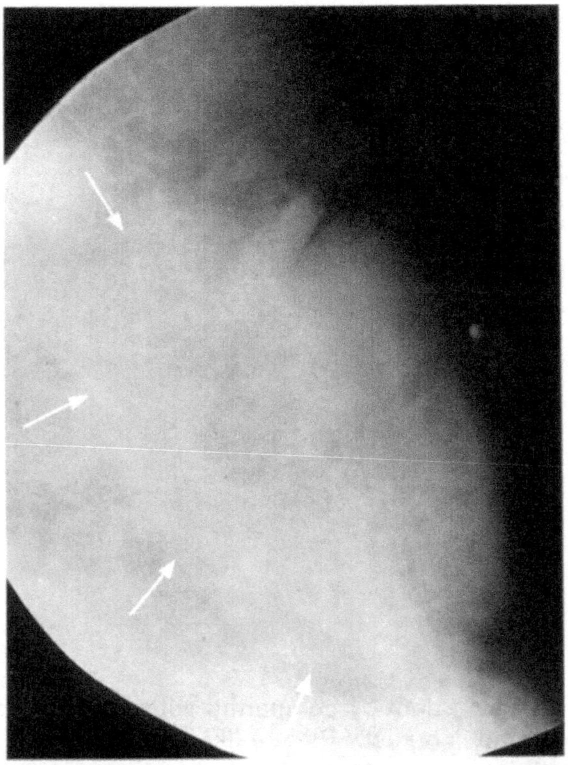

232

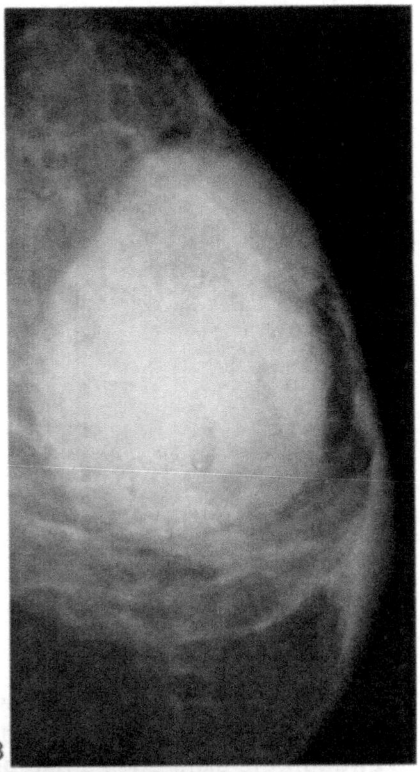

233

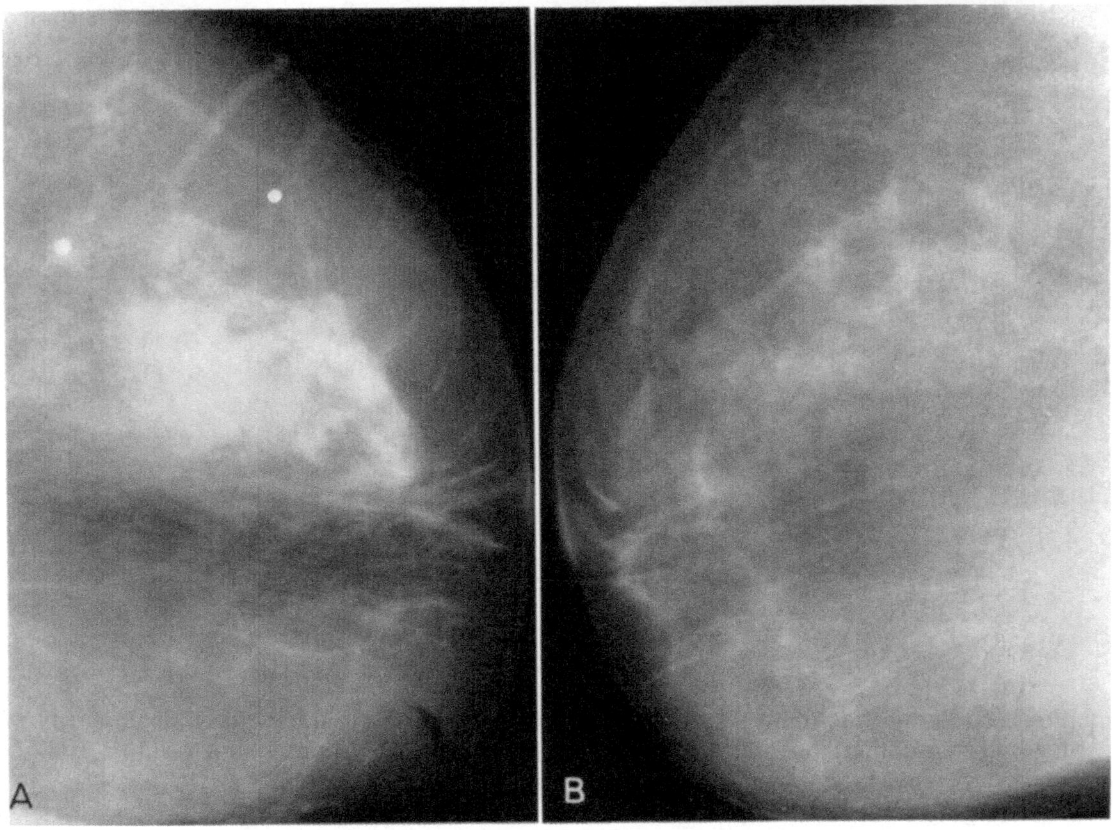

234

Fig. 235. Large medullary cancer, left breast. Mass 8 cm in diameter had ulcerated through the skin. Edema has blurred all the structural details of the breast, better evident by comparing with details of opposite breast. Plaque-like calcifications in both breasts are located in fibroadenomata

Fig. 236. Localized lobular carcinoma. The irregularly-outlined lesion tugs on trabeculae (arrow), and there is perifocal edema with engorgement of the vessels

Fig. 237. Lobular cancer. Irregularity of the margins is the sole index of this malignancy

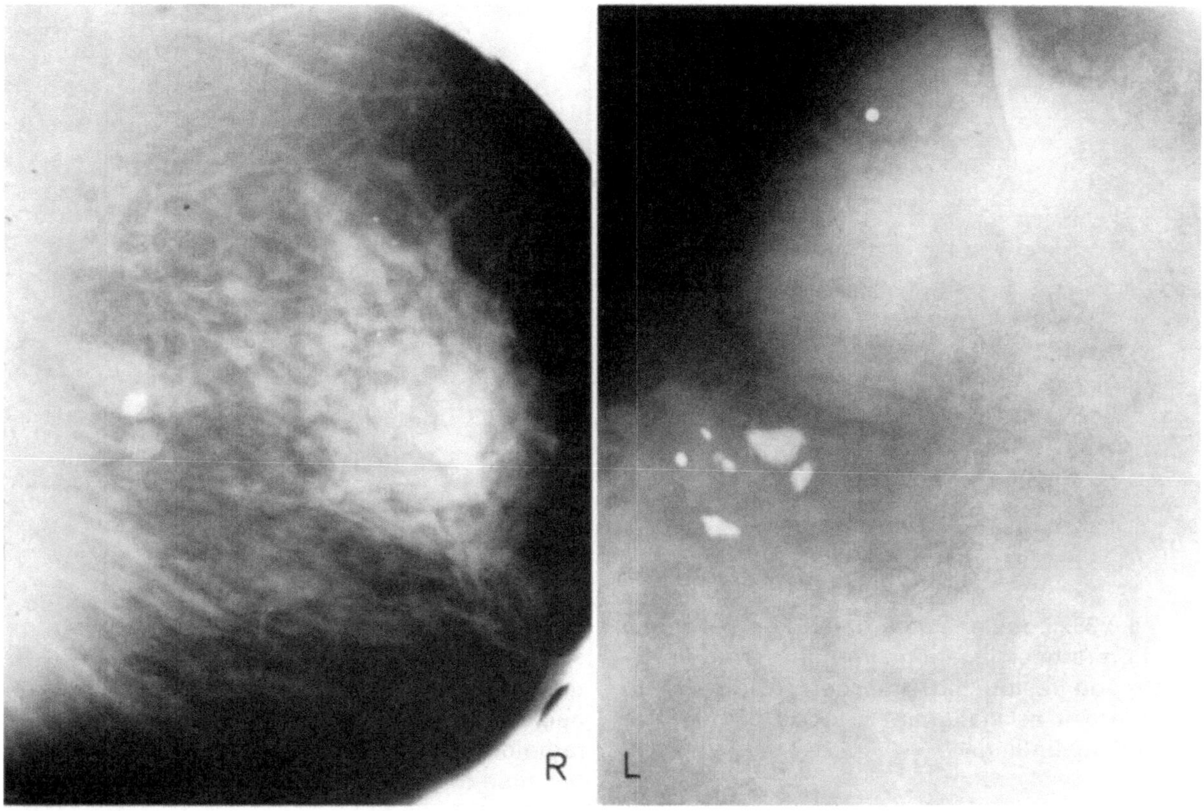

235

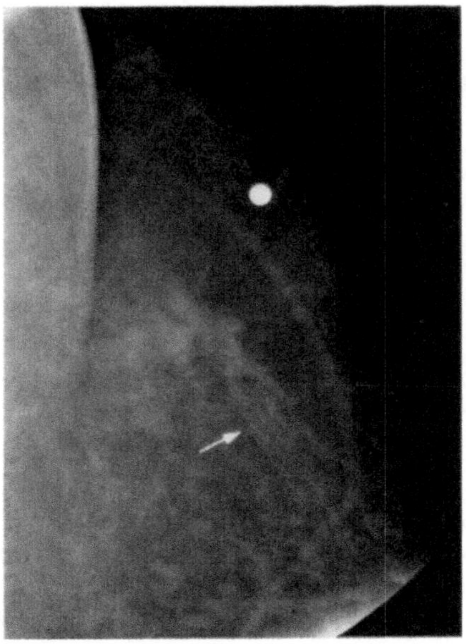

236

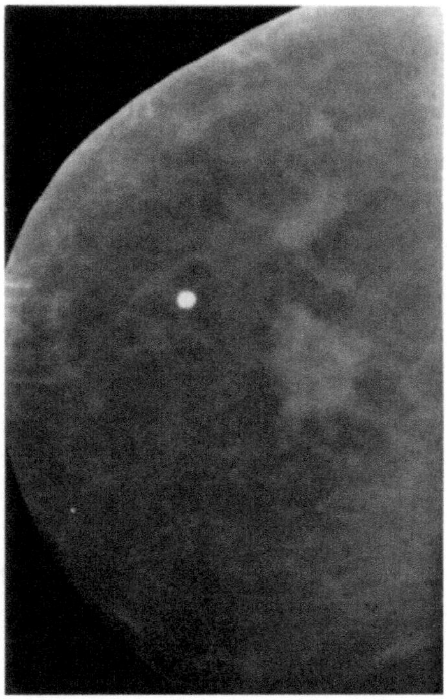

237

Fig. 238. Lobular carcinoma. The presence of microcalcifications in an irregularly-shaped lesion led the roentgenologist to regard it as malignant in spite of negative clinical findings

Fig. 239. Lobular cancer. In a field of adenosis with "epithelial pearls" (arrow head) the presence of carcinoma was not suspected on physical examination; but the radiologist, with foresight, advised biopsy because of blurring of details due to edema

Fig. 240. A
Infiltrative lobular carcinoma. No palpable tumor was present. Punctate calcifications (arrows) were the basis for the X-ray report of cancer

B
The pathologist could not find the tumor and its calcifications until they were demonstrated for him on an X-ray film of tissue (1 and 2) removed at operation

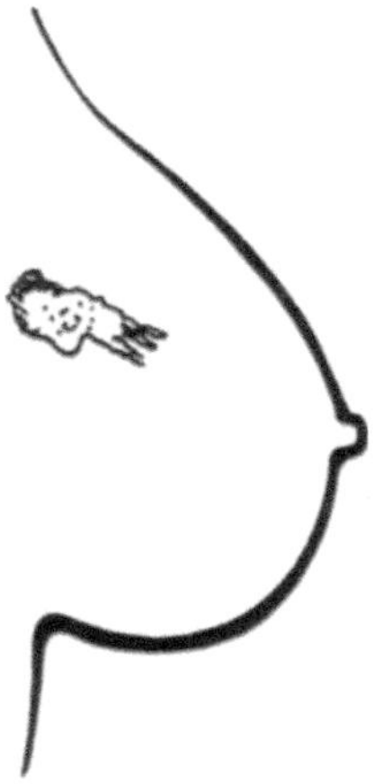

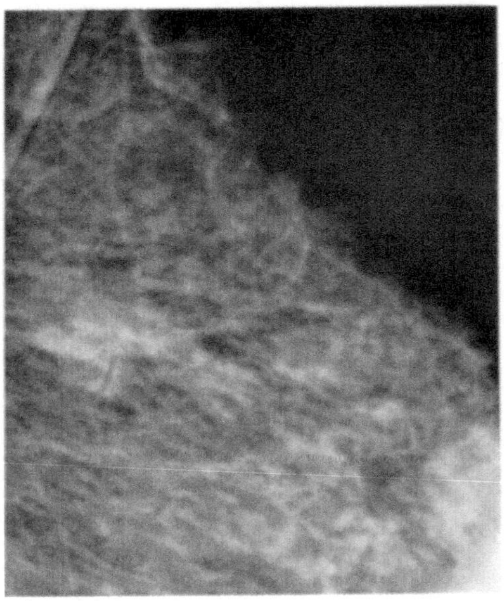

238

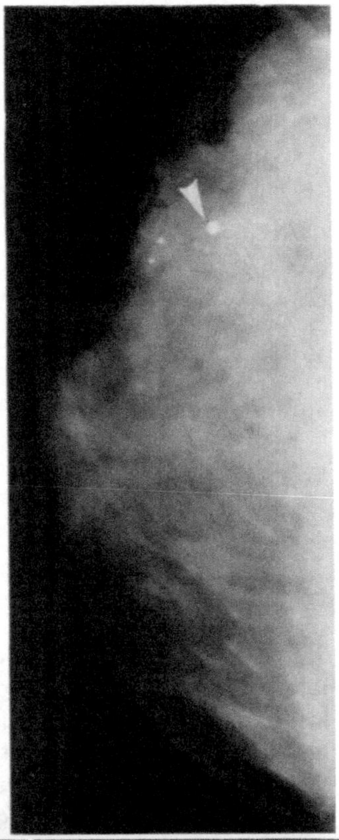

239

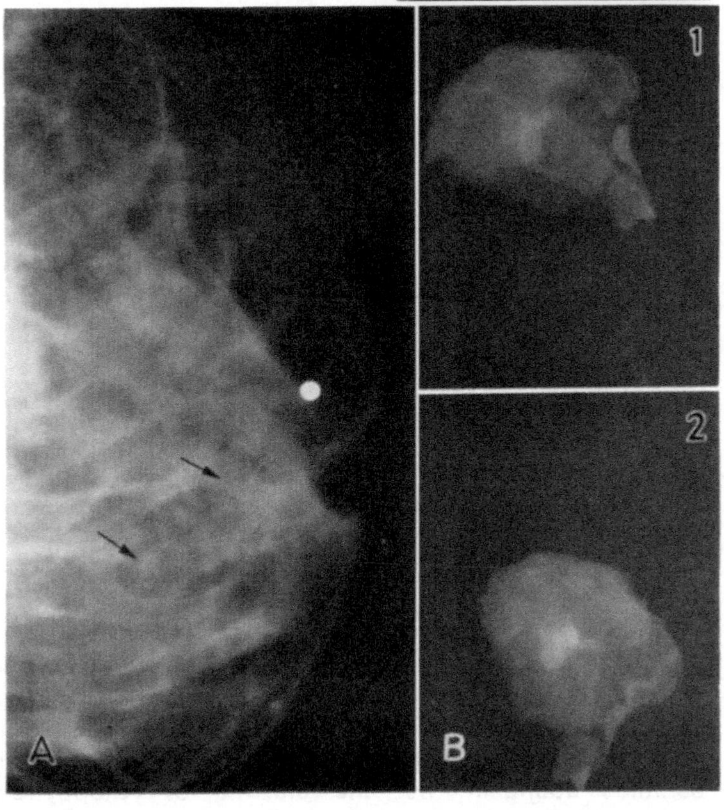

240

Fig. 241A—C. Lobular carcinoma in situ, left breast. A Normal right breast. B The increased density of lobular parenchyma in left breast where patient complained of a "burning" sensation (arrow head); the prominence of the neighboring vessels, better determined by comparing similar area in (A); and the disruption of architectural elements in the tail of the breast seen in a spot film of the axilla (C) were the bases for suspecting the presence of cancer

Fig. 242. Lobular carcinoma, right breast. A mass was palpable in the right breast at the site of the skin marker. The poorly defined zone of homogeneous density resembles adenosis; but the blurring of details due to edema, best appreciated by comparing film of opposite breast, is sufficient evidence in a woman past 40 years of age to suggest the possibility of cancer. Biopsy revealed lobular carcinoma

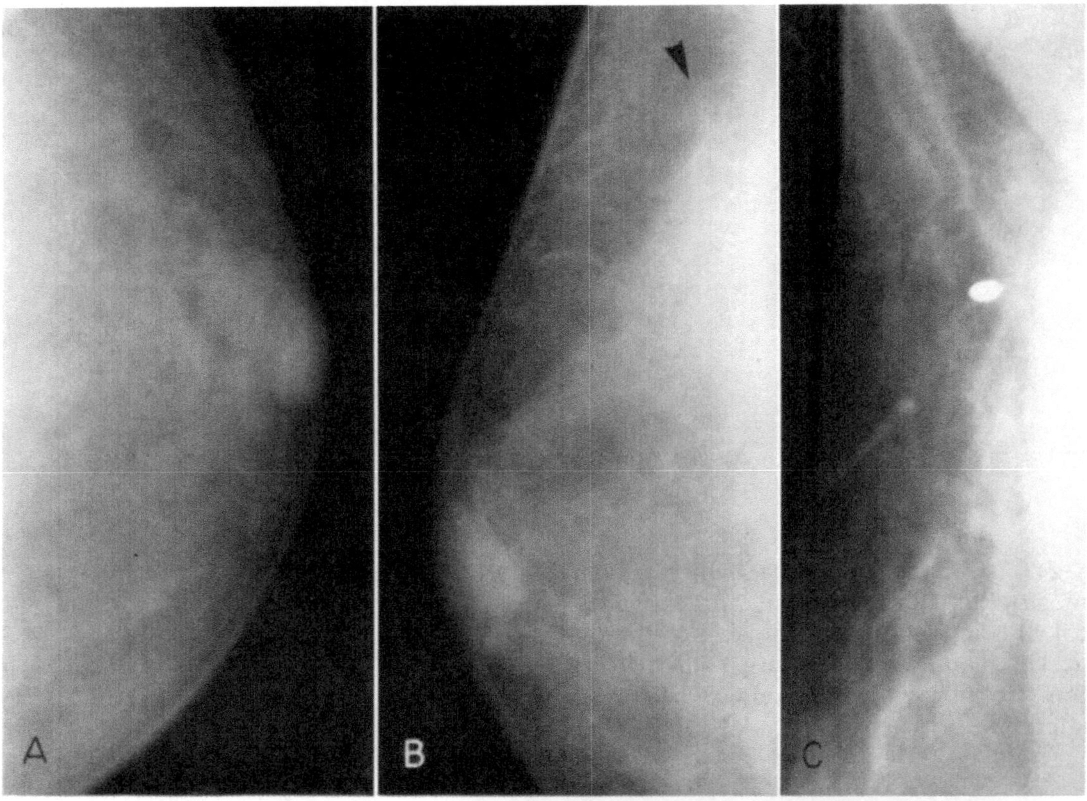

241

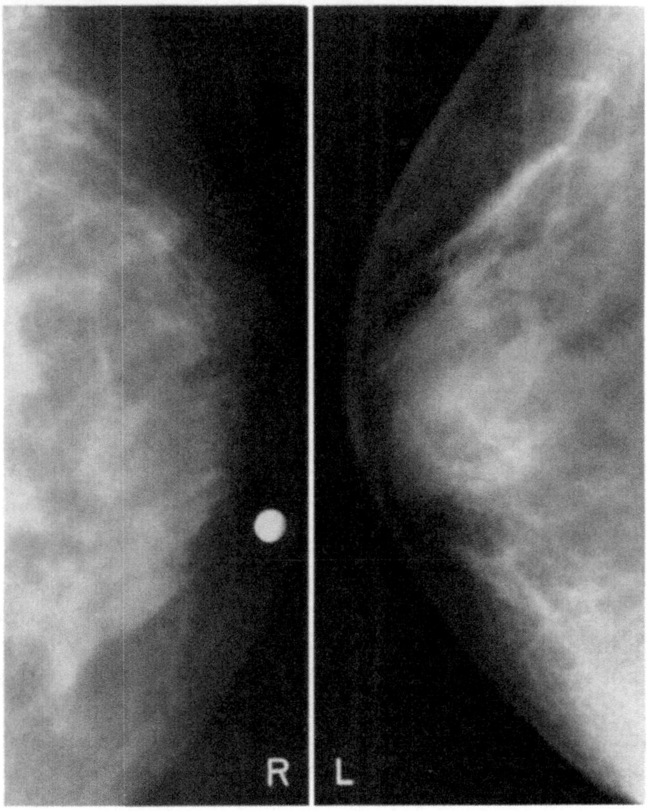

242

Fig. 243. Lobular carcinoma, right breast. The structural derangement and the perifocal blurring edema of the cancer under the skin marker on right are evident only when the film of the opposite breast is compared

Fig. 244. Lobular carcinoma, left breast. The cancer is difficult to recognize because lobular fibrous hyperplasia is present in both breasts, and the only additional distinguishing diagnostic features are the distortion of the breast architecture, prominence of the neighboring vessels, and generalized edema in the left breast. These features are more evident when the structures on the right side are compared. The palpable mass, localized by the skin marker, was not the cancer — which was found several centimeters distant (arrow)

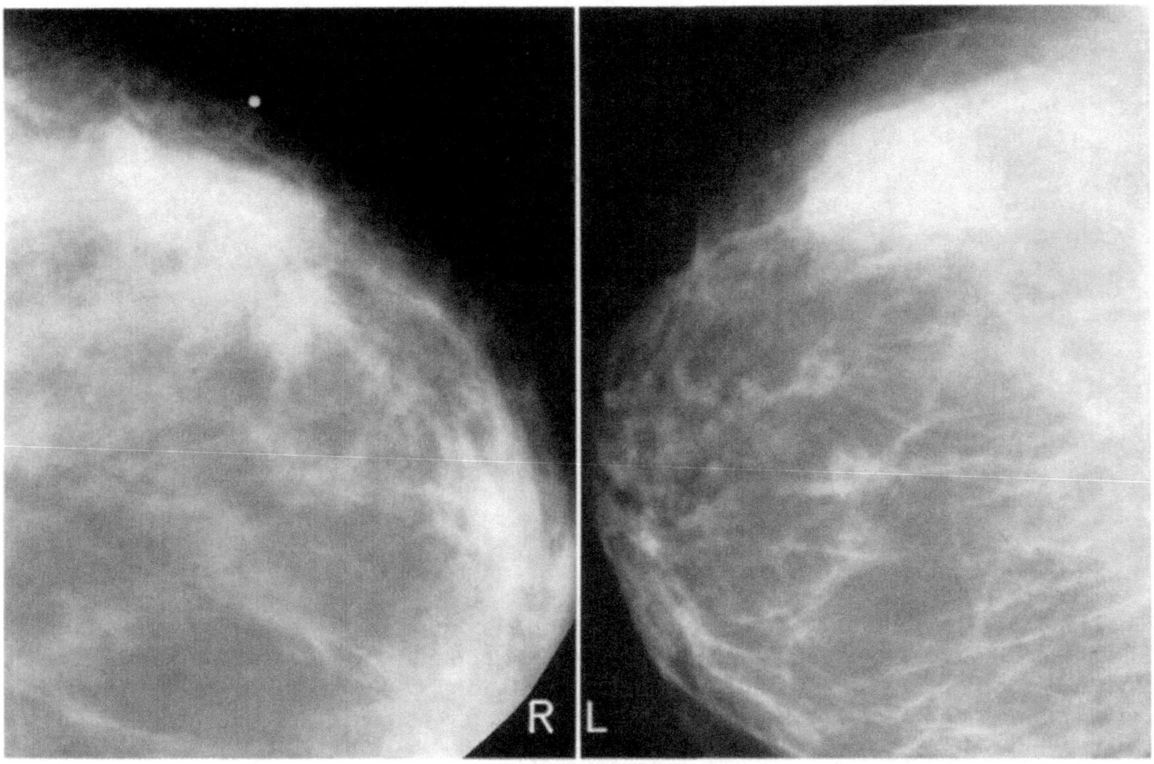

243

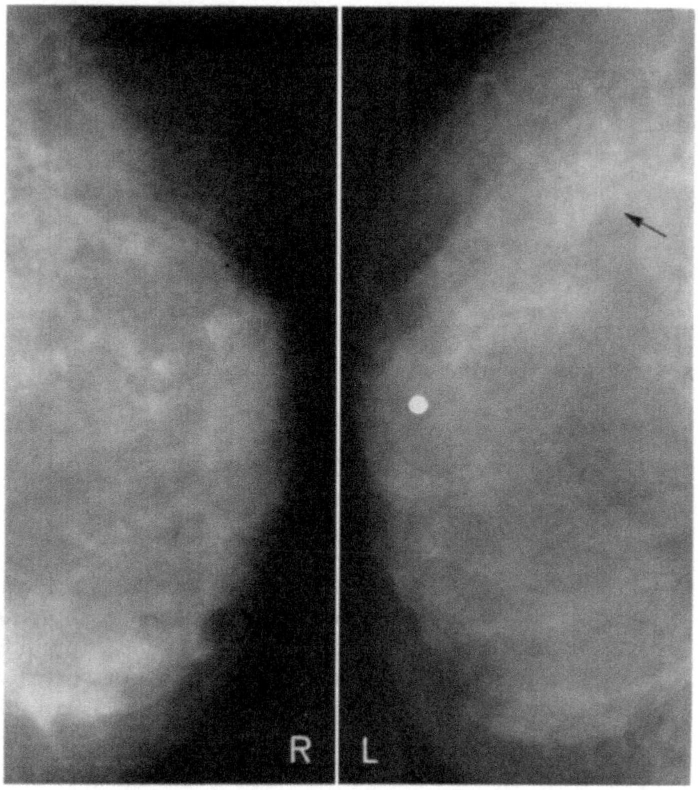

244

Fig. 245. Lobular caroinoma, left breast. The bilateral sclerosing adenosis and hyperplastic fibrosis are asymmetrical. Only the denser, more compact tissue of the left breast where the 58 year old patient complained of pain aroused the suspicion of lobular oareinoma. Both nipples weie slightly retracted (under skin markers). The slight, localized thickening of the skin of the left breast was not appreciated clinically

Fig. 246. Lobular carcinoma, left breast. Diffuse adenosis and mazoplasia fibrosa are present in both breasts of this 25 year old patient. Localized pain at site of skin marker was present in left breast although multinodularity was palpable bilaterally. An X-ray diagnosis of cancer was not made but was suspected because of edematous blurring of structures in the left breast. It is in such circumstances that most diagnostic errors occur. The patient's symptoms were an additional basis for the fortunate decision to do a biopsy

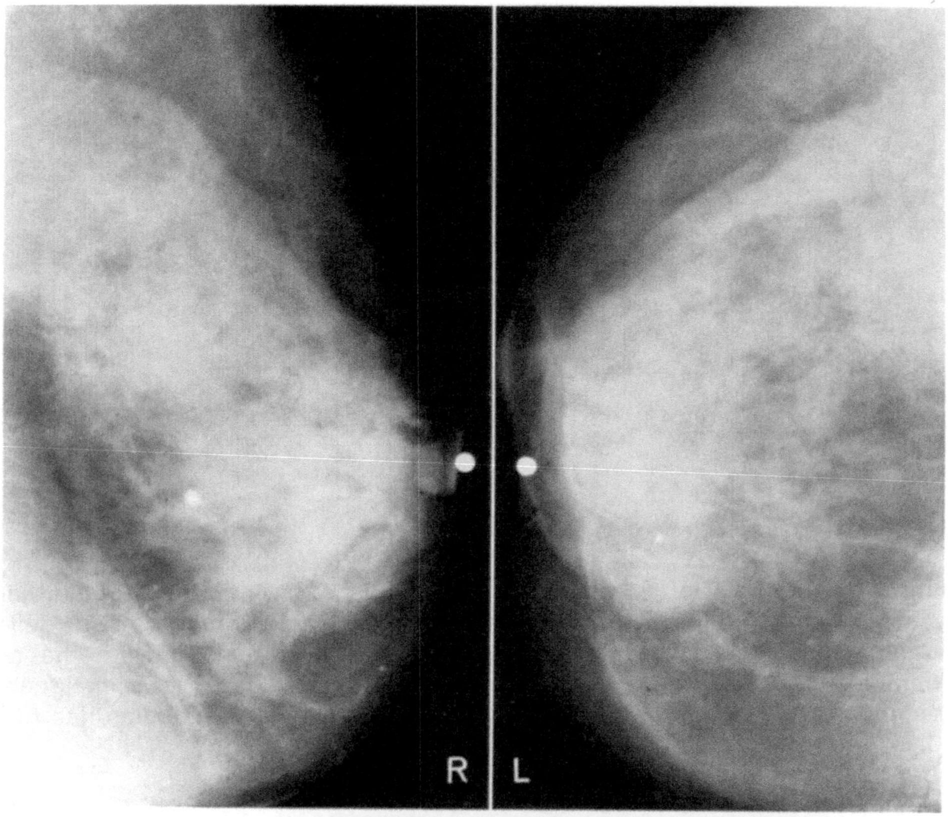

245

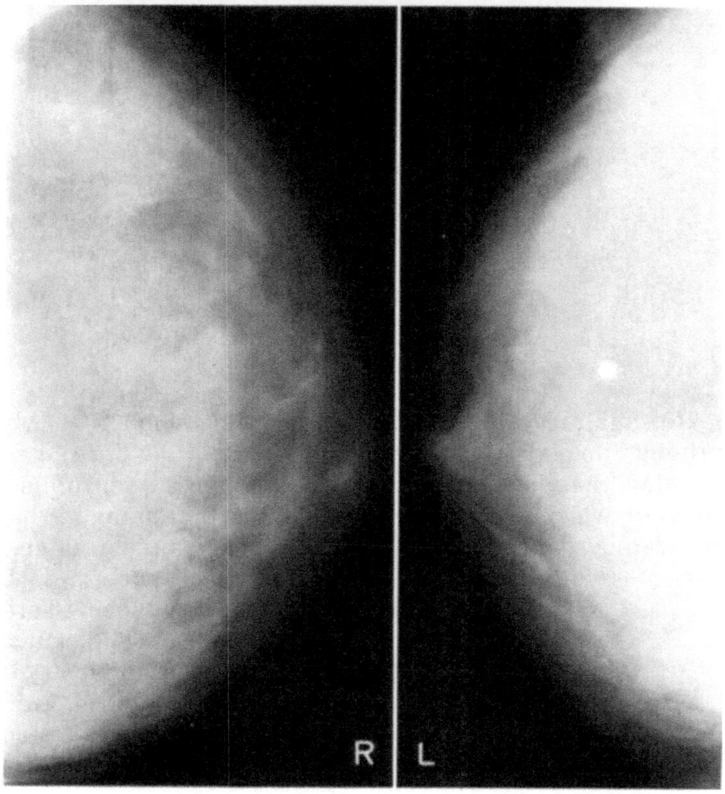

246

Fig. 247. Infiltrative lobular carcinoma with scirrhus. the radiating thin fibrous strands tugging on all the surrounding tissues identified the scirrhous aspects of this lesion

Fig. 248. Infiltrative lobular cancer with scirihous invclution. The delioate dendritio strands issuing from the margins of the lesion identify it as malignant. The infiltration from the lobules has formed a discoid mass

Fig. 249. Infiltrative lobular carcinoma with scirrhous involution. Increased density, spiculated margins, traction on perifocal structures which are blurred and edematous, identify the malignant nature of this lesion

Fig. 250. Lobular cancer. A mass with dendritic margins (arrow heads) suggests a scirrhous cancer. A separate, hard, nontender mass was palpable lower in the breast under the skin marker. A lobular cancer was thus found in a clinically unsuspected area, and a cyst was found where the clinician suspected cancer. Both breasts of this 40 year old patient were diffusely involved with adenosis and mazoplasia cystica. Detection of cancer in such breasts is difficult

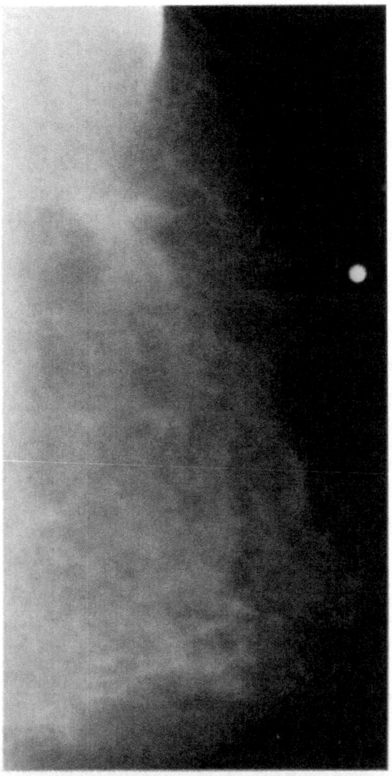

247

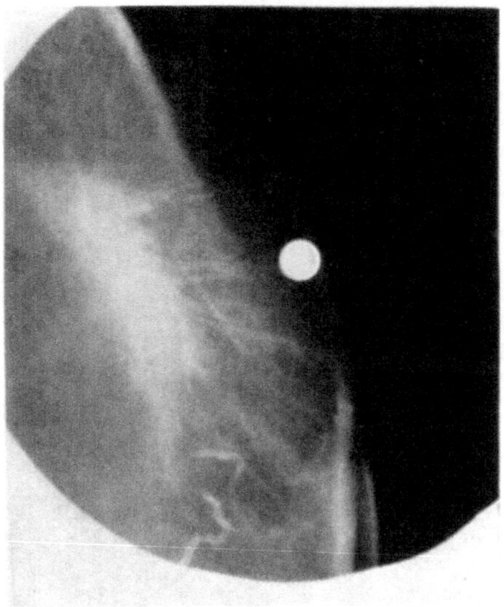

248

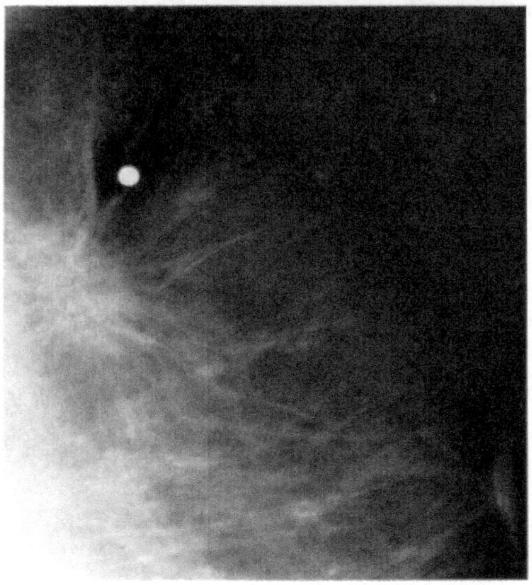

249

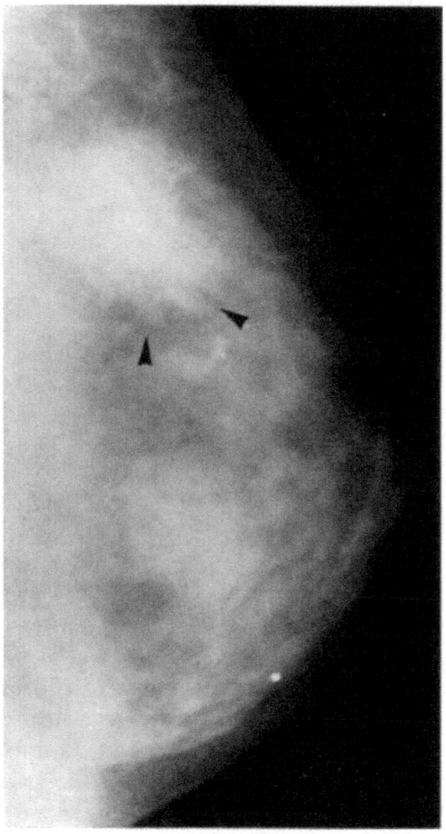

250

Fig. 251. Bilateral lobular cancers. Cancer was suspected clinically only in the left breast, but was recognized in both breasts by the roentgenologist. The irregularly-shaped tumor in the left breast and the distorted pattern in the upper right breast, together with edema involving the skin, led to X-ray diagnosis of cancer in both breasts

Fig. 252. Paget's disease. Excoriated nipple and thickening of skin were noted clinically. Two secondary scirrhous cancers (arrows) are present

Fig. 253. Paget's disease. Microcalcifications in ducts close to the nipple and a scirrhous cancer (arrow) deeper in the breast are visible. Patient had slight excoriation of the nipple

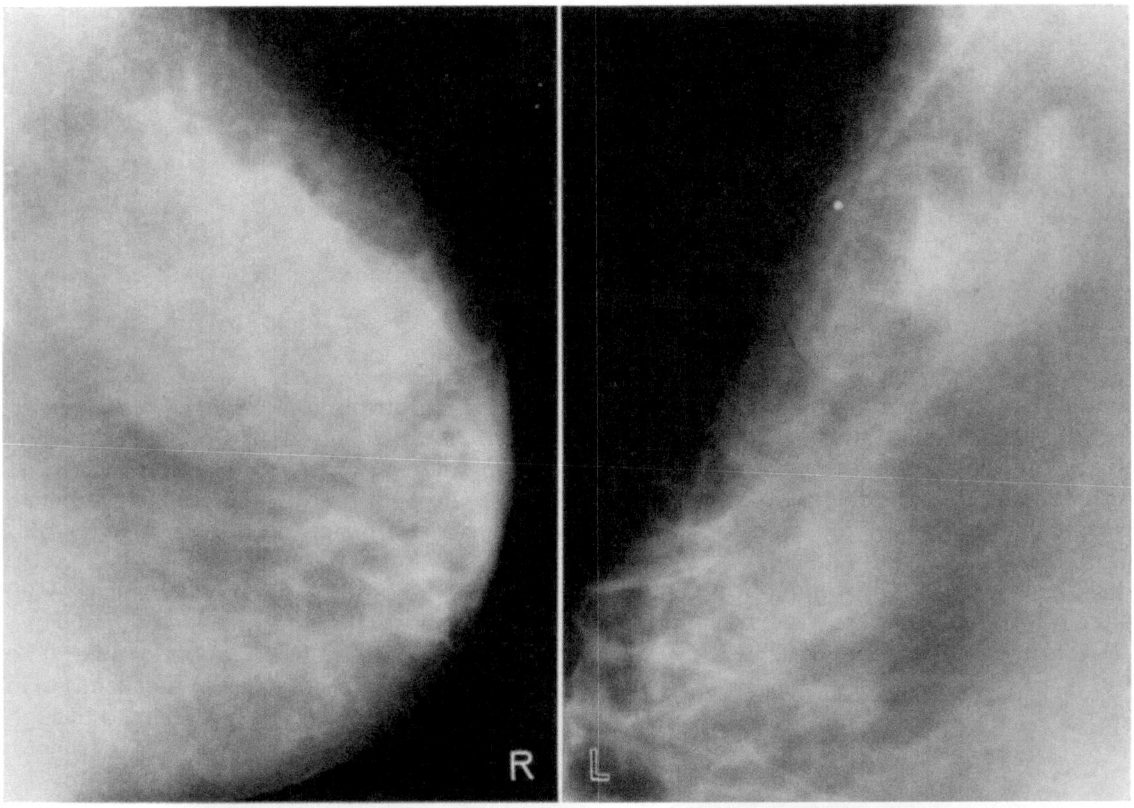

251

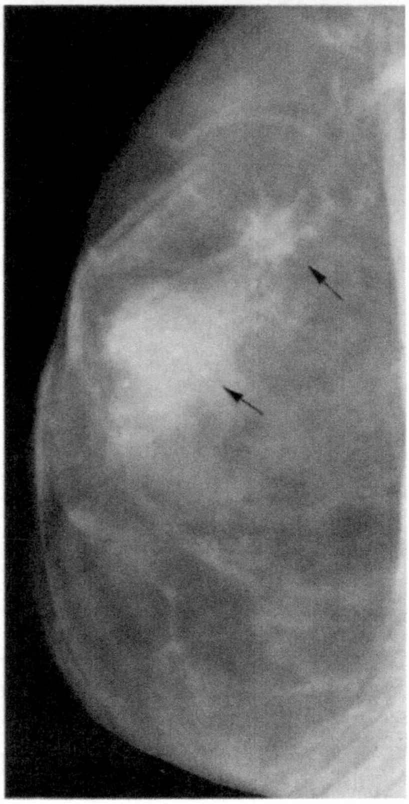

252

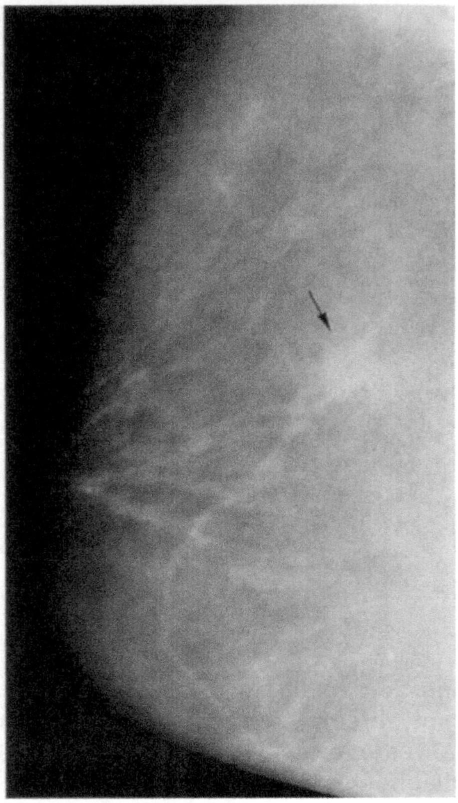

253

Fig. 254. Infiltrating duct cell cancer (scirrhus), male breast. An isolated mass with fuzzy margins suggests cancer, especially if associated with progressive nipple inversion. This 69 year old man first noted a lump in the breast and nipple inversion three weeks prior to examination. The axillary lymph nodes were free of metastasis

Fig. 255. Infiltrating duct cell carcinoma with scirrhus, male breast. A dense, poorly encapsulated mass with irregularity of some portions of its margins suggests cancer in a 61 year old male

Fig. 256. Infiltrating duct cell cancer, male breast. An isolated irregularly-outlined mass in a 75 year old male suggests cancer. The nipple was retracted, and localized skin edema is visible on the X-ray film, although it was not noted clinically

Fig. 257. Infiltrating duct cell carcinoma, male breast. A poorly defined mass in a 72 year old male should always suggest the diagnosis of cancer

Fig. 258. Infiltrating duct cell carcinoma, male breast. A mass, indistinctly outlined in a 72 year old male, is sufficient to suggest the presence of cancer

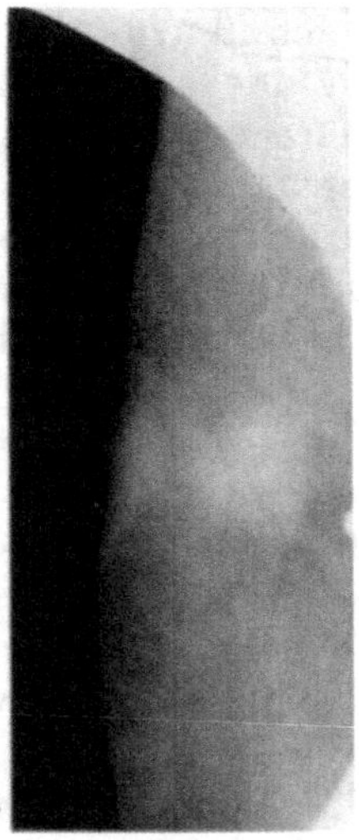
254

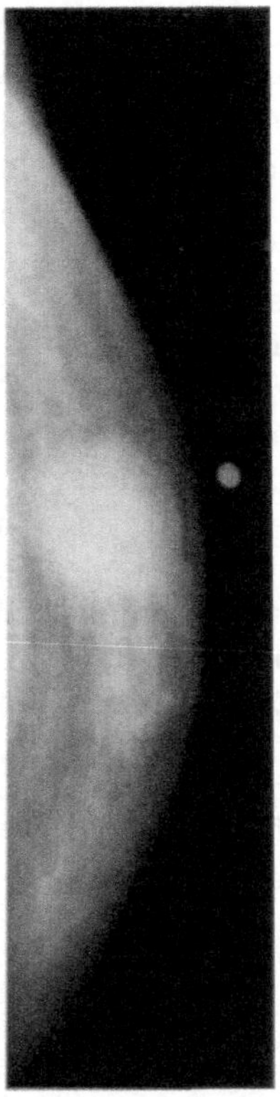
255

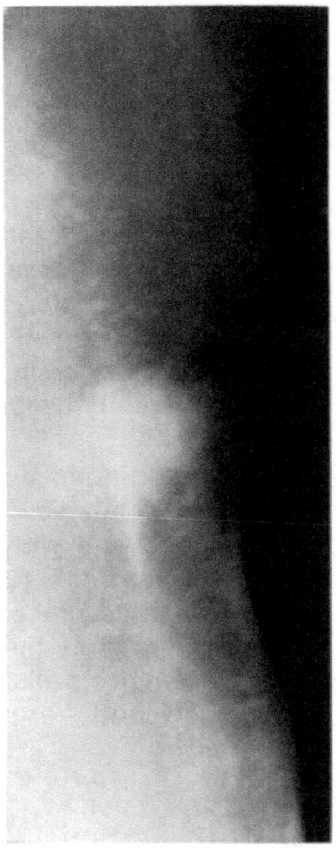
256

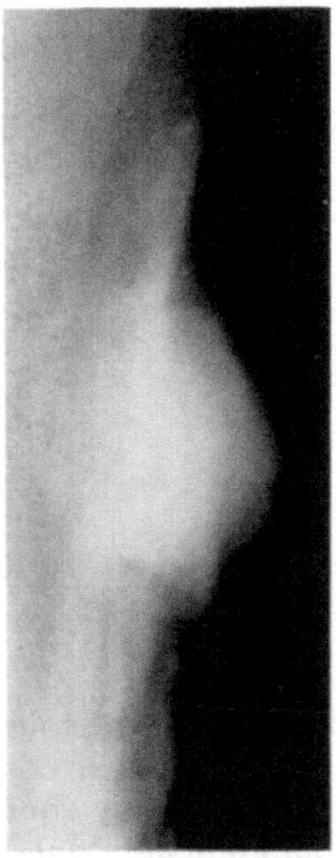
257

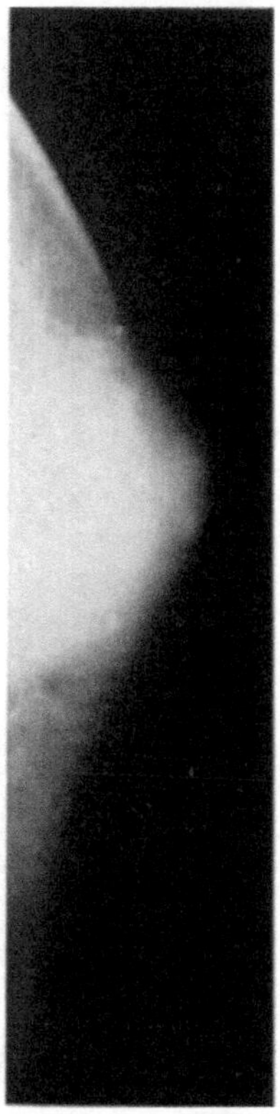
258

Fig. 259. Infiltrating duct cell cancer with scirrhus, male breast. A dense, smoothly-contoured oval-shaped mass usually indicates a benign lesion; but the slight thickening of the overlying skin in a 55 year old male suggested the possibility of cancer. The patient had noted the mass for three months. It was movable, nontender, and seemed to fluctuate, suggesting a cyst to the clinician. The pathologist reported it to be a scirrhous carcinoma with metastasis to 4 of 20 axillary lymph nodes

Fig. 260. Infiltrating duct cell cancer, male breast. An isolated ovoid mass, not smoothly contoured and with fuzzy outlines, in a swollen breast of a 63 year old male, suggested possible cancer. Although the mass had been noted by the patient for only two weeks, extensive axillary lymph node metastasis was found

Fig. 261. Infiltrating duct cell cancer, male breast. An uneven density with irregular margins, retracting the overlying edematous skin, suggested cancer in this 59 year old male. No axillary lymph nodes were involved even though the patient was aware of an enlarging breast for 14 months

Fig. 262. Intracystic papillary carcinoma, male breast. A smoothly-contoured ovoid mass such as this suggests a benign lesion. It was first noted by this 69 year old male six months earlier. It became smaller during the succeeding three months, then began to enlarge again. Biopsy of any mass in a male over 50 years of age, even if it appears benign, is always advisable

Fig. 263. Intracystic papilloma. An isolated tumor with sinuous margins and a comet tail (arrows) resembles a medullary cancer, from which it was differentiated only by biopsy

Fig. 264. Intracystic papillary carcinoma. An isolated lobate mass might be a bosselated fibroadenoma, a conglomerate cyst, a medullary cancer, or an intracystic papillary carcinoma, as in this case. Slight blurring of the perifocal structural details inclined the roentgenologist to suspect a medullary cancer, and he advised biopsy

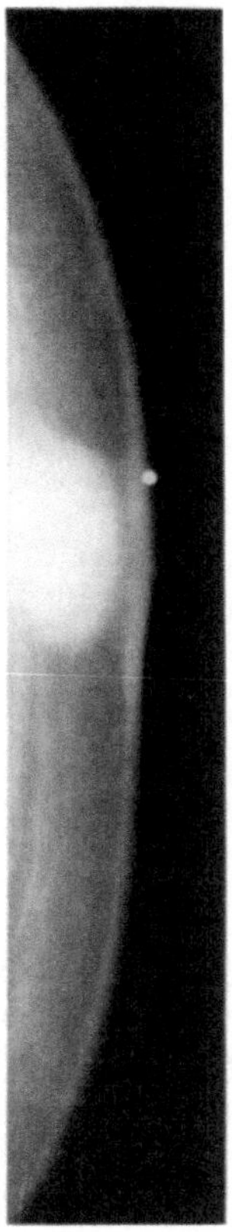
259

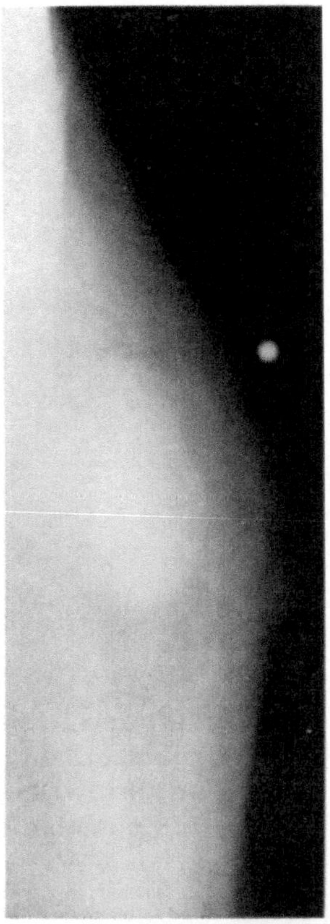
260

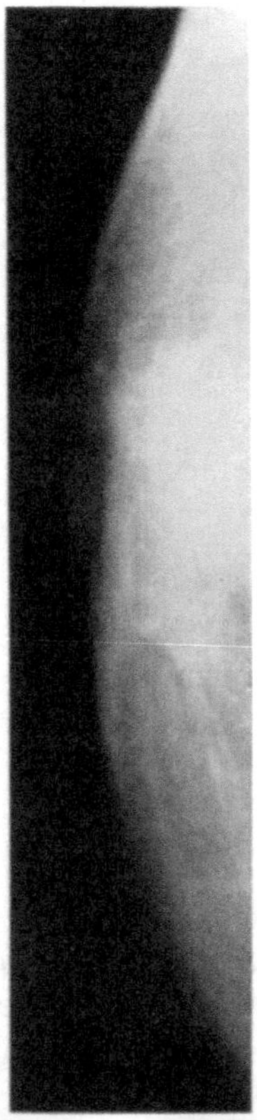
261

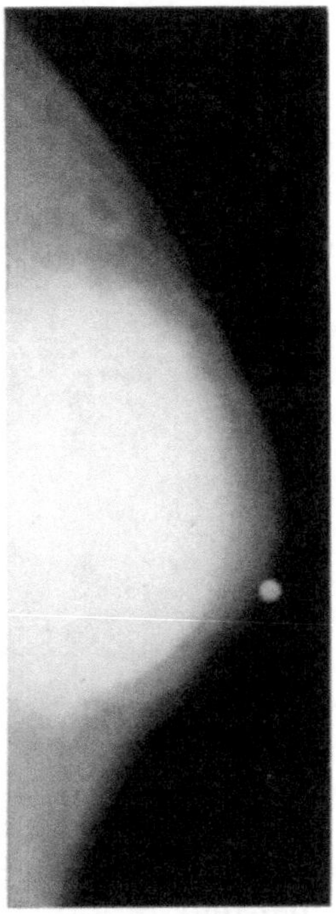
262

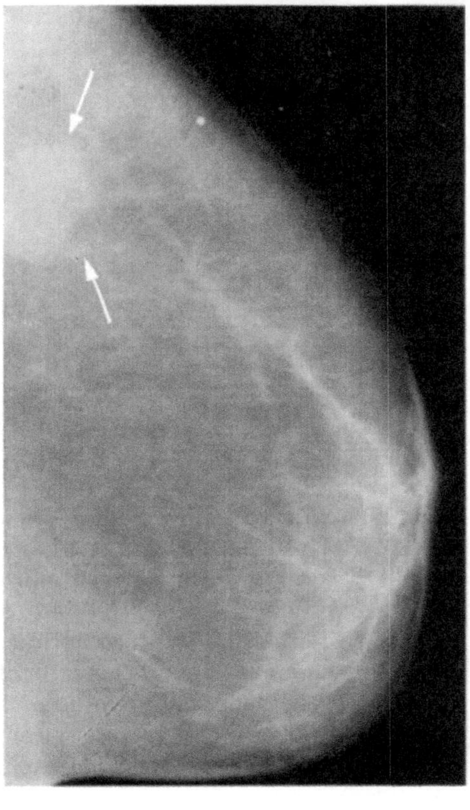
263

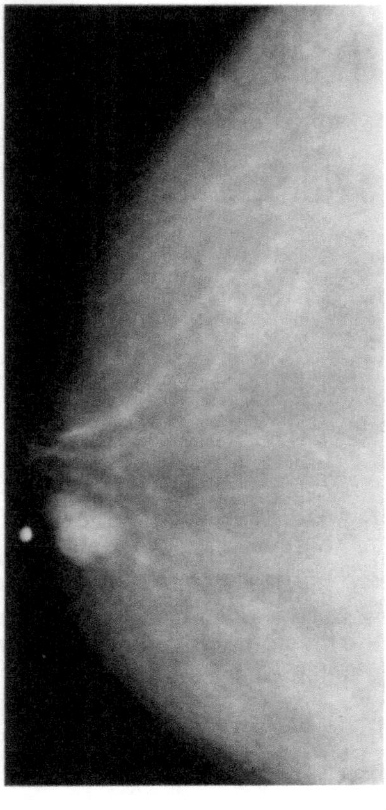
264

Fig. 265. Intracystic papillary carcinoma. An isolated, irregularly-contoured mass with blurring of structural details due to perifocal edema is usually a scirrhous or medullary cancer. In this case, the lesion was an intracystic papillary carcinoma

Fig. 266. Intracystic papillary cancer. An isolated circumscribed mass with a comet-tail extension (arrow) suggested an imperative biopsy for possible cancer

Fig. 267. Intracystic papillary carcinoma. A solitary notched mass (arrow) with blurred borders due to perifocal edema is usually a medullary carcinoma, but in this case the lesion proved to be an intracystic papillary carcinoma

Fig. 268. Intracystic papillary carcinoma. The opaque skin marker is projected over the lesion, the sharp margins of which are notched anteriorly and prolonged into a comet-like tail posteriorly, suggestive of cancer. The microcalcifications in the lower breast marked the area of another infiltrative duct cell cancer. The edema of the skin and prominence of the vessels are obvious

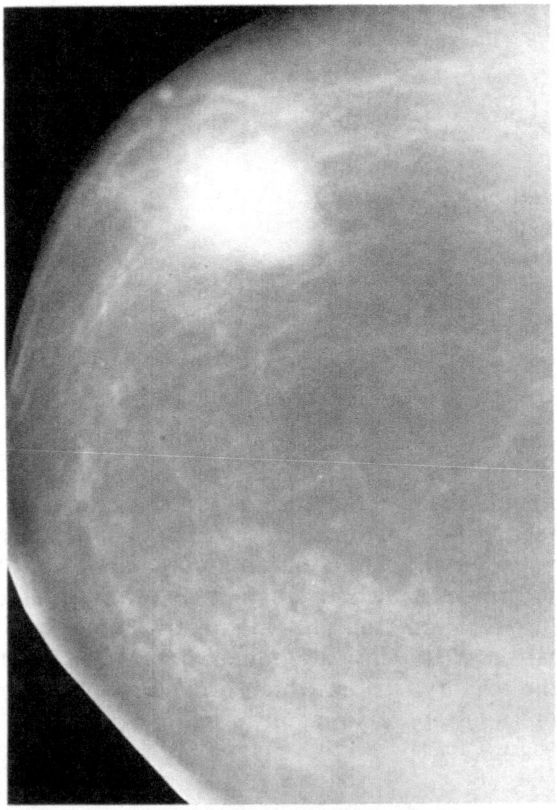

265

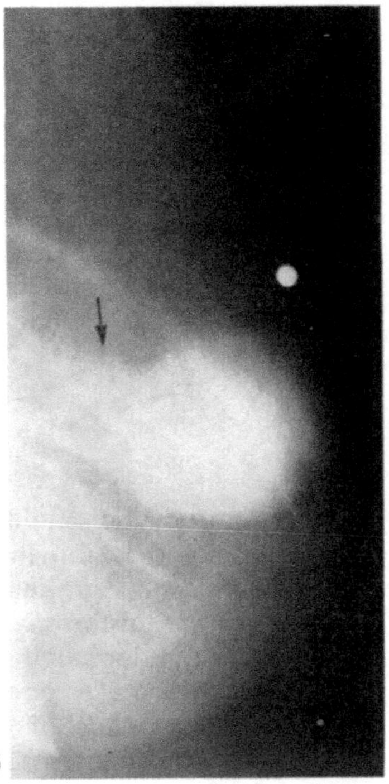

266

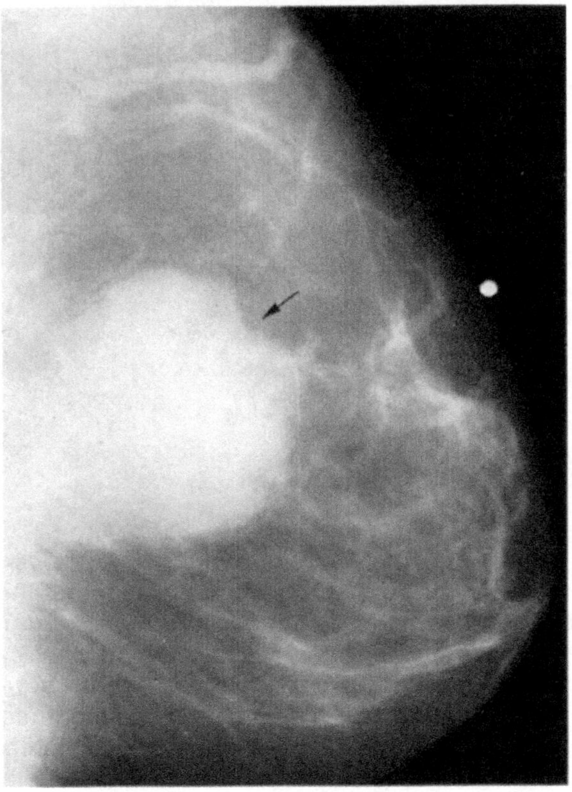

267

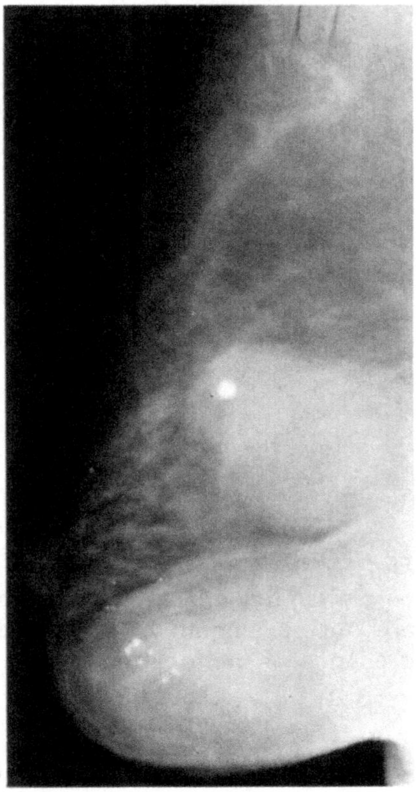

268

Fig. 269. Intracystic papillary carcinoma. A large isolated lesion in the breast of a 79 year old woman suggests cancer, especially if portions of the margin are irregular and diffuse granular calcification is present. A large cystic mass containing necrotic material with patches of calcification was found. In spite of metastasis to the axillary nodes, this patient lived four years after radical mastectomy

Fig. 270. Large mucinous carcinoma. An isolated mass in the breast of a 62 year old woman with smooth but sinuous and notched margins suggests a cancer, especially when associated with dilated superficial veins. A medullary cancer or a cystic papillary adenocarcinoma may resemble this lesion, which proved to be a mucinous, gelatinous, large-cell carcinoma

Fig. 271. Mucinous carcinoma. These cancers often resemble cysts, but their borders are not so smooth or distinct due to the presence of perifocal edema

Fig. 272. Mucinous carcinoma (arrow). The blurred margin of the lesion is the only stigma of malignancy differentiating it from the smooth, spherical, neighboring cysts of greater density. All three lesions were close to the chest wall in a breast diffusely implicated with adenosis. Note prominence of superficial veins

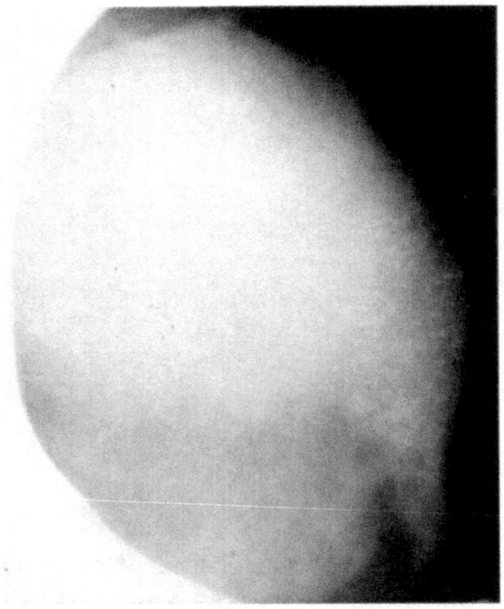

269

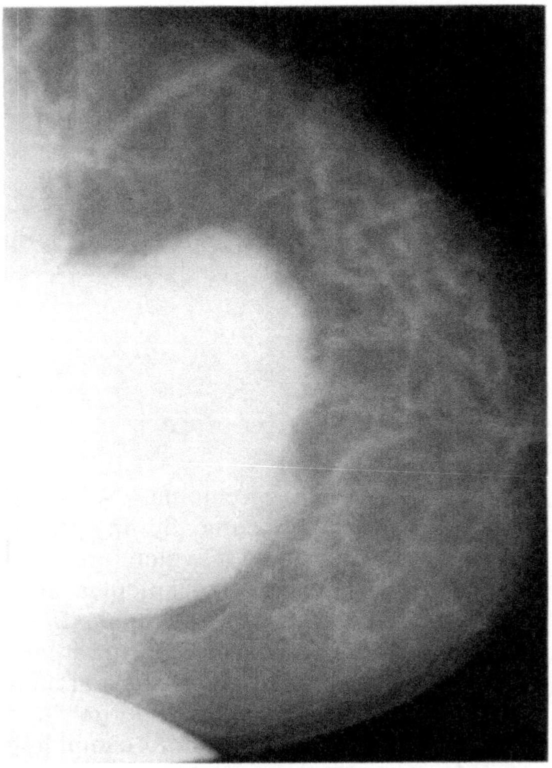

270

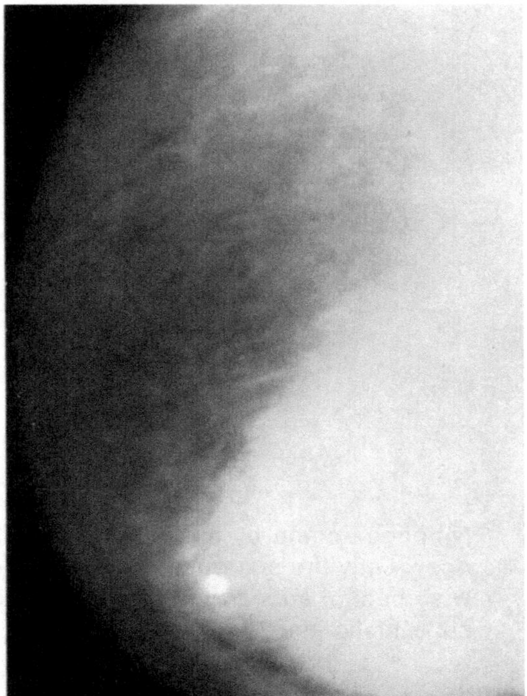

271

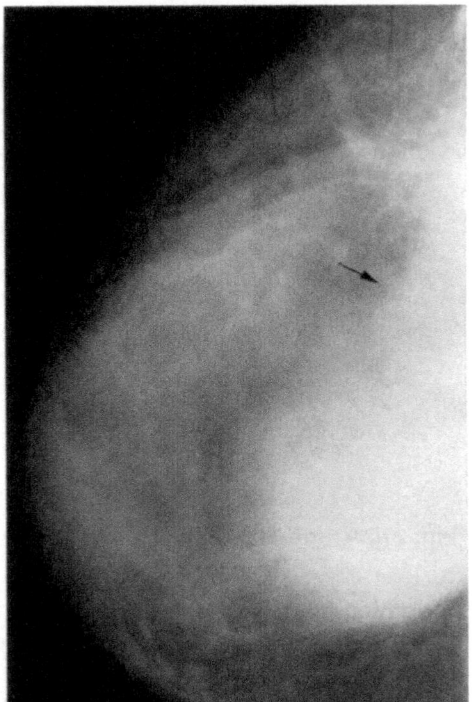

272

Fig. 273. Mucinous carcinoma. A small lesion is partially obscured by an area of adenosis, the margins of which are only faintly visible. The radiating spicules suggest a scirrhus. Note the sentinel strand (arrow), possibly due to edema in the perifocal interstitial tissue. Mucinous carcinomas are usually depicted as larger and cystic, but here is a small lesion resembling a scirrhus

Fig. 274. Lymphosarcoma. An irregularly contoured solitary mass suggests a malignant process. In this case, lymphosarcoma was found

Fig. 275 A and B. Lymphosarcoma.

A

Biopsy of cervical lymph nodes of this 40 year old woman established a diagnosis of lymphosarcoma two years earlier, but a mass in the right breast only recently became palpable. This was established as lymphosarcoma by the pathologist after biopsy. Only the sinuous border of this otherwise benign appearing mass suggests possible malignancy.

B

Two years after intensive radiation therapy, only residual fibrosis and edema are visible

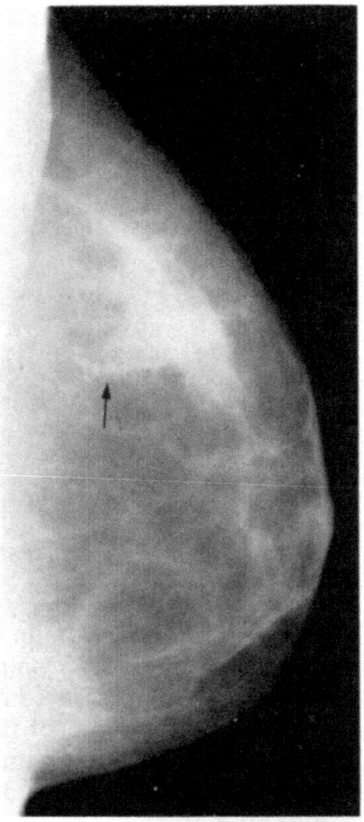

273

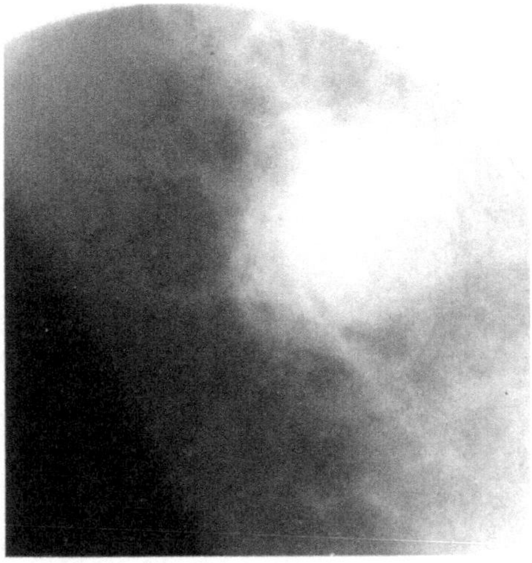

274

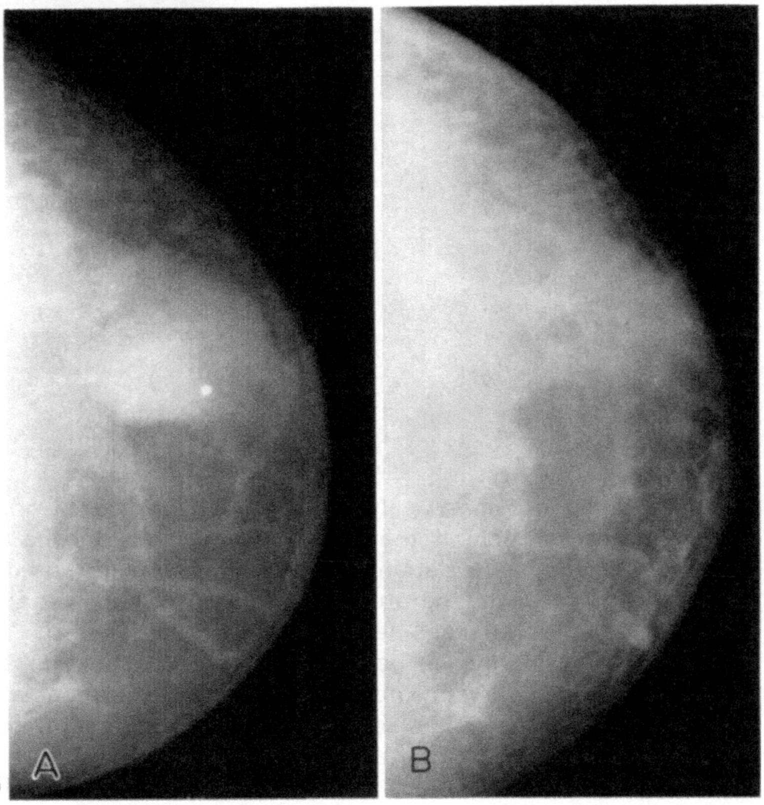

275

Fig. 276. Lymphosarcoma. A palpable mass at site of skin marker has an irregular contour and there is blurring of detail due to edema. Biopsy was suggested and established the diagnosis of lymphosarcoma

Fig. 277. Fibrosarcoma. In the left breast of this 41 year old woman a freely movable nontender mass was palpable and thought to be a cyst. An isolated mass with sinuous borders in a woman of this age suggested a possible cancer to the roentgenologist. A fibrosarcoma was diagnosed by the pathologist

Fig. 278. Lymphosarcoma. A palpable nodule in the left breast behind the nipple was checked regularly by the patient's physician for 20 years before mammography was done. A smoothly-contoured mass near the nipple was found, resembling a benign lesion. Because the patient was known to have metastatic lymphosarcoma elsewhere, however, biopsy was advised, and lymphosarcoma was found

Fig. 279. Lymphosarcoma. A nontender mass in the left breast (under the skin marker) was discovered by this 39 year old woman two weeks earlier. The clinician palpated an "indefinite" mass about 4 cm in diameter. An area of increased density due to edema, with localized disruption of breast architecture, suggested possible cancer to the roentgenologist. A lymphosarcoma was found by the pathologist

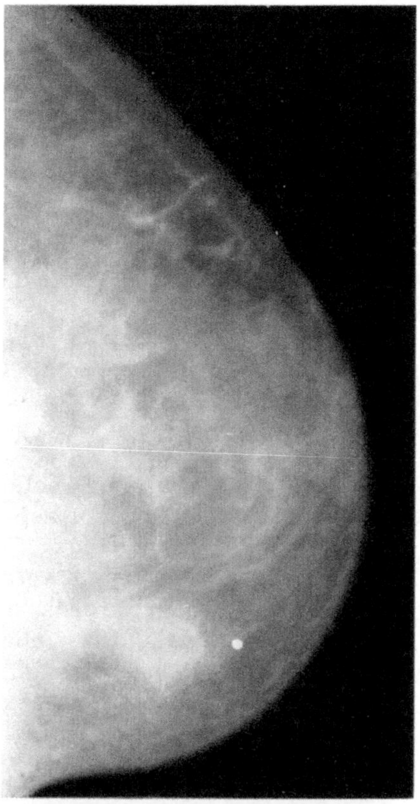
276

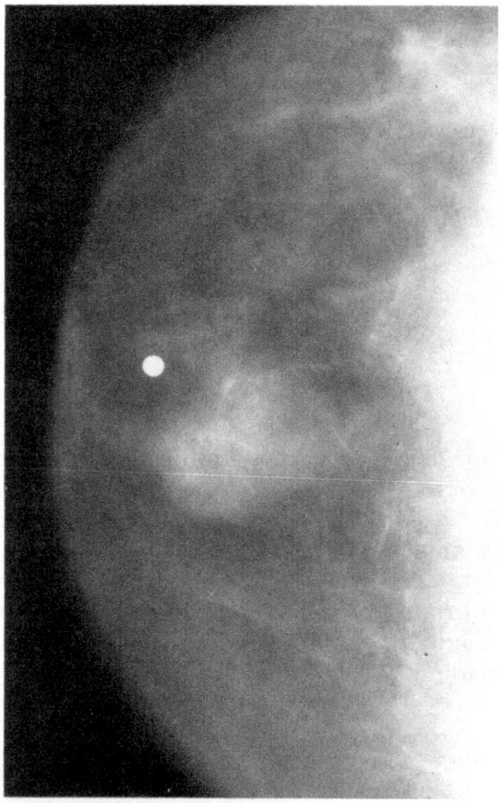
277

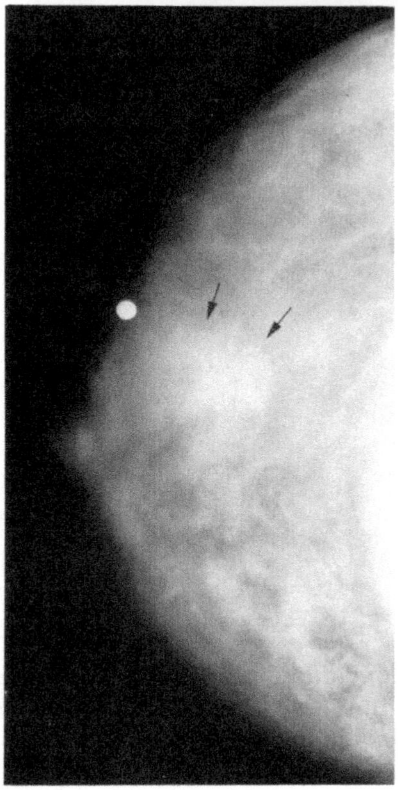
278

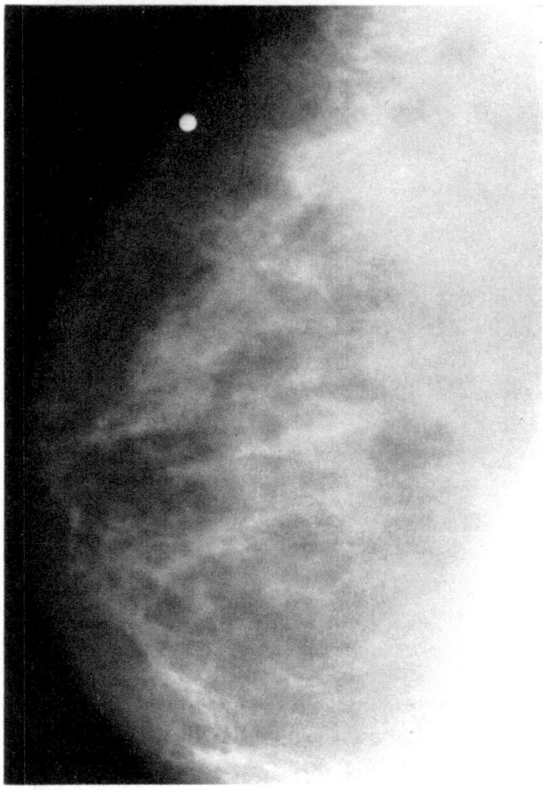
279

Fig. 280 A and B. Noninfiltrating duct cell cancer.

A

A small scirrhus (arrow) in area of pain (site of skin marker) was not palpable and not recognized by the roentgenologist. The group of distended, cancer-filled ducts leading to the lesion was not appreciated

B

Nine months later, a tumor palpable at the site of skin marker corresponds with enlargement of the scirrhus. The swollen ducts leading to the scirrhus were now more distended with cancer cells and clearly recognized. This patient was alive and well six years after a radical mastectomy, when no evidence of axillary metastasis was found

Fig. 281. Bilateral infiltrating duct cell comedo cancers, advanced and recognized (left), unsuspected clinically (right). Aggregates of microcalcifications distributed among dilated ducts (right) signified cancer to the radiologist despite absence of palpable mass. The pathologist found this to be a comedo form of duct cell cancer

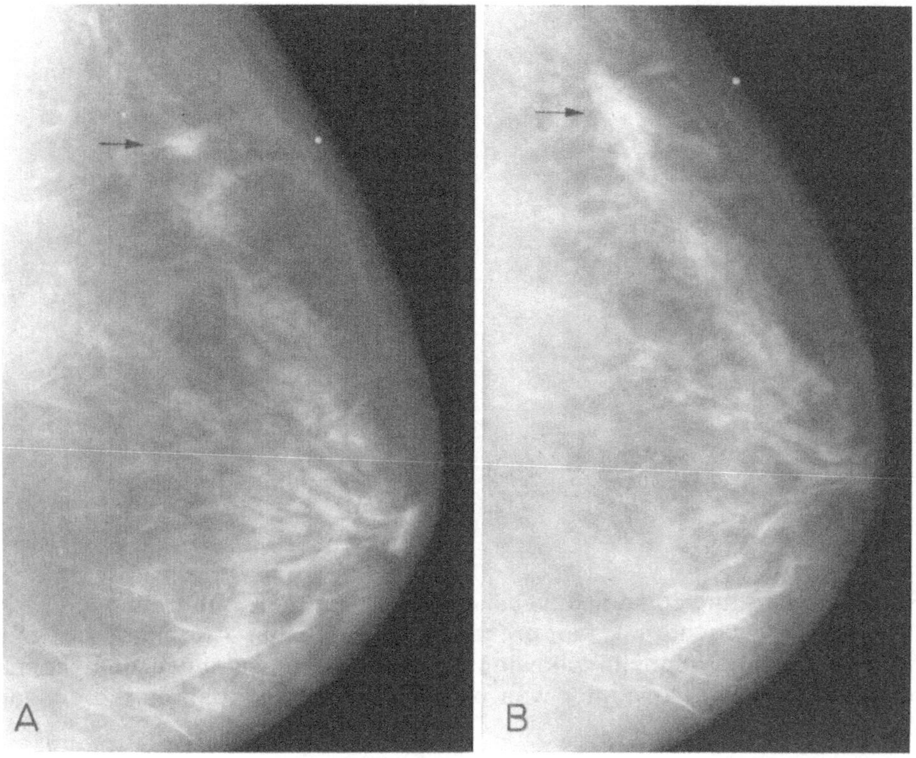

280

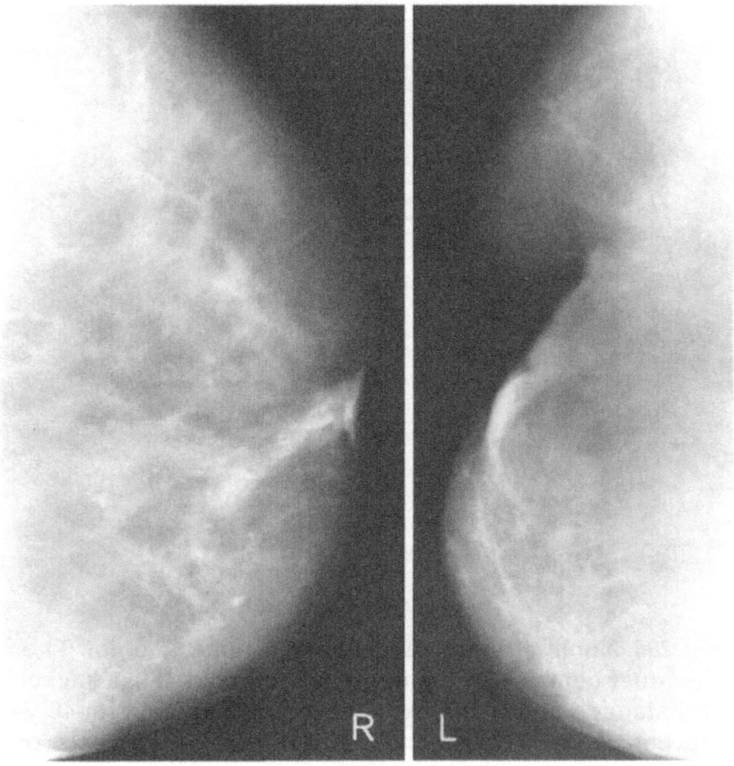

281

Fig. 282. Infiltrating comedo duct cell cancer. Diagnosis is based on the presence of granular calcium deposits following course of ducts (arrows). No tumor was palpable

Fig. 283. Infiltrating comedo duct cell carcinoma. Aggregates of microcalcifications stream along a duct complex to establish the diagnosis in the absence of a palpable tumor

Fig. 284. Noninfiltrating papillary carcinoma. The duct complex in the upper right breast is distended and ballooned, and suggested the possibility of cancer to the roentgenologist. The clinician palpated only a plaque-like thickening which he thought was benign. In a 48-year-old woman the hyperplastic fibrosis of the left breast is excessive

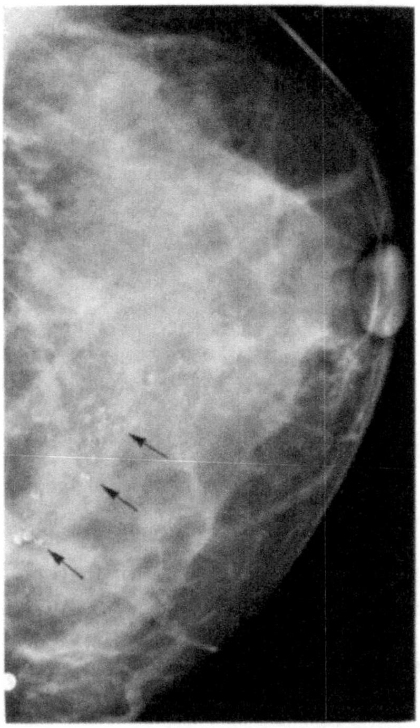

282

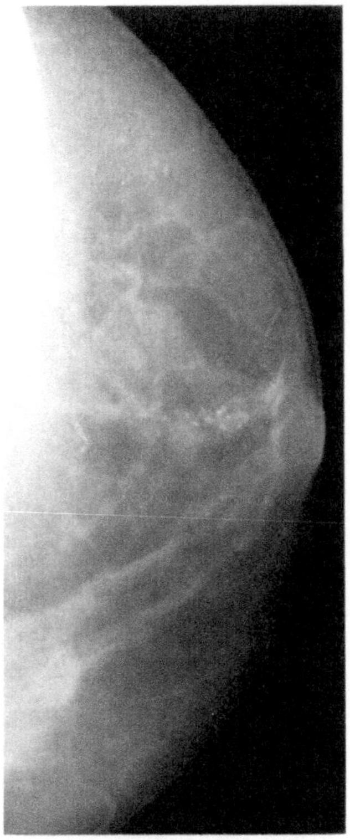

283

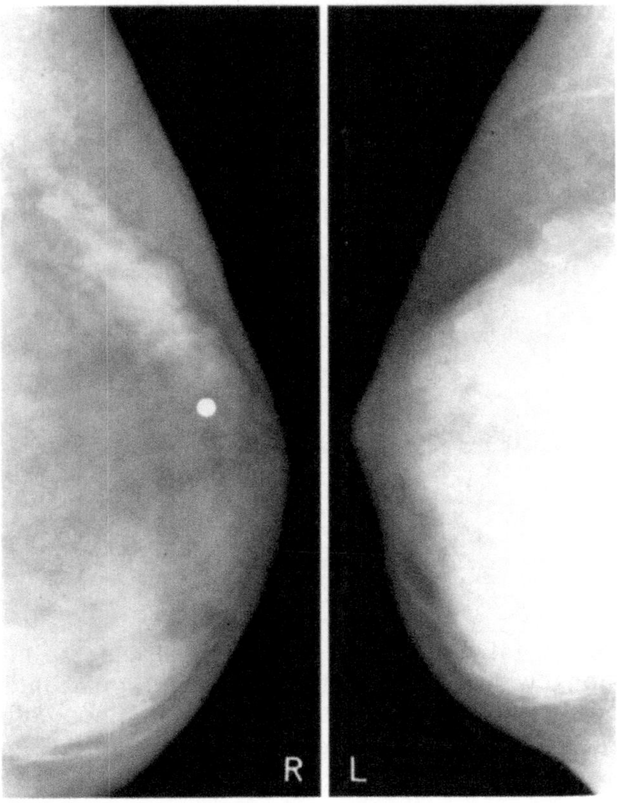

284

Fig. 285. Infiltrating papillary duct cell carcinoma with early scirrhus. An irregularly-defined density with perifocal edema involving the nearby skin measures 1.5 cm in diameter. Except for the adjacent thickened skin, the appearance of this lesion could be confused with fat necrosis

Fig. 286. Infiltrating papillary duct cell carcinoma. A small, smoothly-contoured but angular mass, resembling a scirrhus, may be discerned only with care in a field of ductal hyperplasia and sclerosing adenosis (arrows)

Fig. 287. Infiltrating papillary duct cell carcinoma with scirrhus, left breast. Distortion and swelling of the trabeculae under the skin marker, with blurring of details due to edema, mark the site of cancer, palpable as a mass with larger dimensions than those on the mammogram. Pseudo-encapsulation with a smooth angular margin is present. Comparison with film of opposite (right) breast aids diagnosis

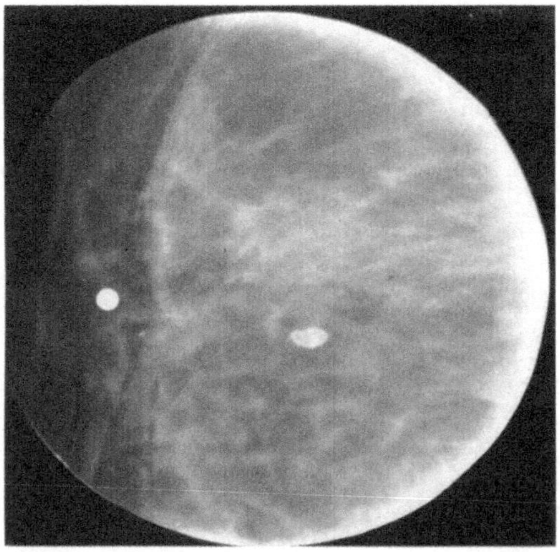

285

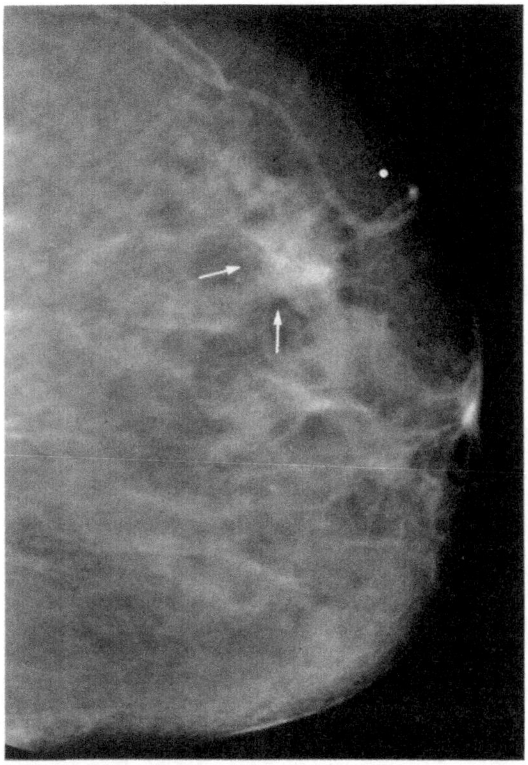

286

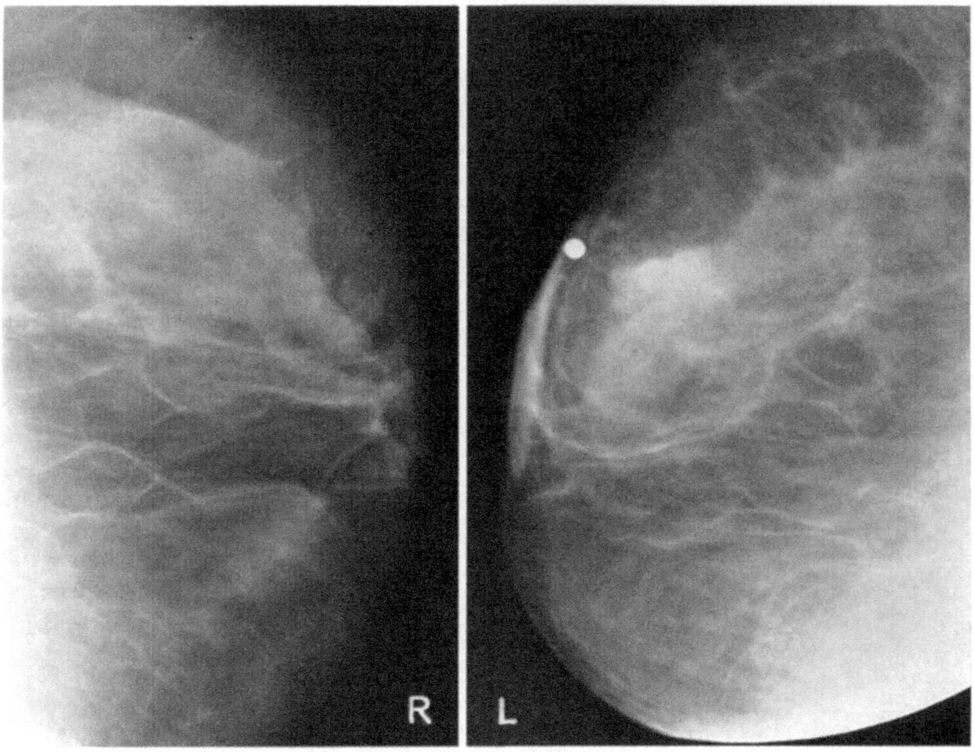

287

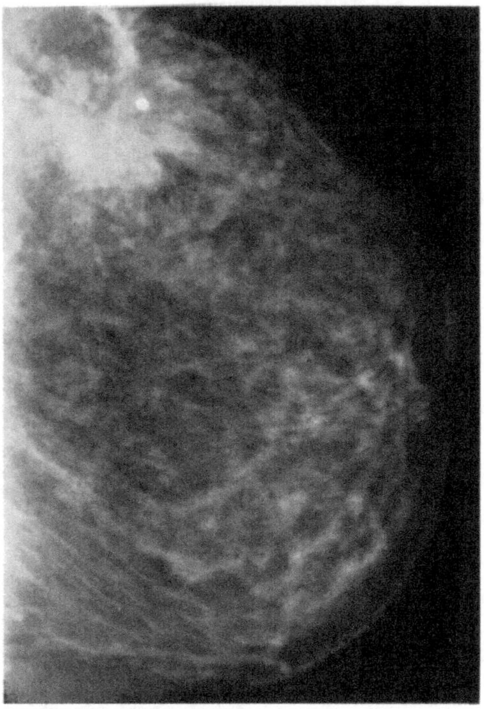

Fig. 288. Infiltrating papillary duct cell carcinoma. The margins of a nodular mass are blurred because of the surrounding edema. The ducts, swollen with tumor tissue, may be seen leading into the angular contoured tumor

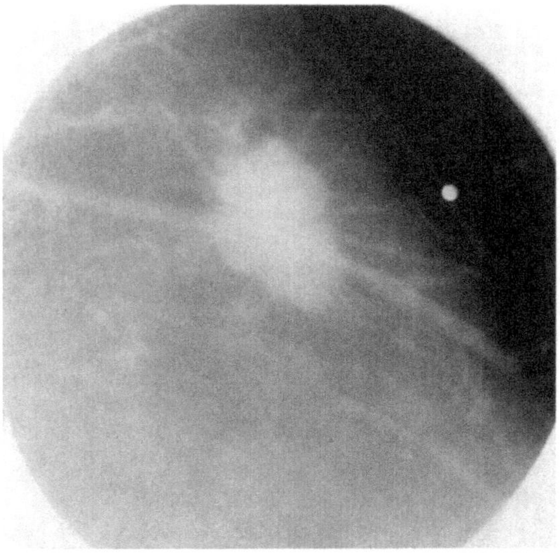

Fig. 289. Infiltrating papillary duct cell carcinoma. An ovoid circumscribed mass with fine fibrous radiating strands, perifocal edema, and vessel engorgement is visible

VIII Miscellaneous

1. Mondor's Disease

The diagnosis of palpable cord-like lesions which appear in the breast is not easy. We have seen cysts, localized secretory disease, plasma cell mastitis, and carcinoma present as such cord-like masses. Occasionally they are the result of thrombosed veins, or the so-called "Mondor's disease."

The characteristic clinical appearance of mammary thrombophlebitis was described as early as 1869 by Fagge. However, there is some reason to believe that the condition was due to scleroderma, as originally seen in a patient described by Addison in 1854. In 1922, Fiessinger and Mathieu reported three cases without biopsy, and attributed the condition to thrombophlebitis. In 1931, Williams, and in 1932, Daniels, also reported cases in which chest pain and dyspnea were presenting symptoms.

These sporadic reports were not widely known until 1939, when the condition was popularized by Henri Mondor of Paris. He reported cases with histologic confirmation and called the condition "string phlebitis of the breast." It has since been given his eponym.

Subcutaneous phlebitis may result from generalized or localized infection, trauma, or operation. The patient will usually notice some discomfort in the breast, often associated with a palpable, tender cord. The examining physician will sometimes see a puckering of the skin over the area of involvement, and the suspicion of an underlying malignant lesion may arise. Thrombosis of veins occurs most commonly in the outer quadrants of the breast, as do most other lesions.

Pathologically, the lesion is that of thrombophlebitis and periphlebitis. The thrombosis associated with endophlebitis is seen in the earliest phase of development and not only in advanced cases (Fig. 290).

2. Lipoma

The detection of lipomas is usually easy. An area of radiolucency bounded by a thin, smooth wall of fibrous envelope is easily discerned on the mammogram (Fig. 291).

3. Skin Lesions

Skin lesions, like *verruca*, *angioma*, *sebaceous cysts* and *epidermoid cysts* may simulate intramammary lesions roentgenographically, and often offer diagnostic difficulties unless resolved by the findings of a preliminary physical examination, which should always be included as part of the X-ray study (Figs. 292—297).

4. "Brassiere Breast"

Tight-fitting brassieres will sometimes set up an inflammatory reaction in the region of the inframammary fold. The localized skin thickening over areas of dysplasia where the patient localizes her complaints may lead to a faulty diagnosis, unless all the circumstances have been properly appraised. We have been calling these syndromes "brassiere breast" (Fig. 298).
Care must be exercised, however, not to overlook a bona fide cancer which may occur in this area (Figs. 299, 300).

Fig. 290 A and B. Thrombophlebitis.

A
This 42 year old patient was aware of the presence of a strand of painful, tender, beaded nodules extending from the areola toward the axilla. The arrow points to the beaded nodularity along the cord-like lesion which was palpable over the upper lateral aspect of the breast

B
The roentgenogram shows the presence of a tortuous varicose-like infiltration corresponding to the palpable cord, confirmed by the pathologist as thrombophlebitis. The six lead markers were placed on the skin corresponding to the palpable cord and follow the course of the thrombosed vein

Fig. 291. Lipoma. A lipoma is easily recognized by its lucency, in contrast with the dense tissue of adenosis which obscures part of its thin fibrous envelope

Fig. 292. Skin verruca (arrow)

290
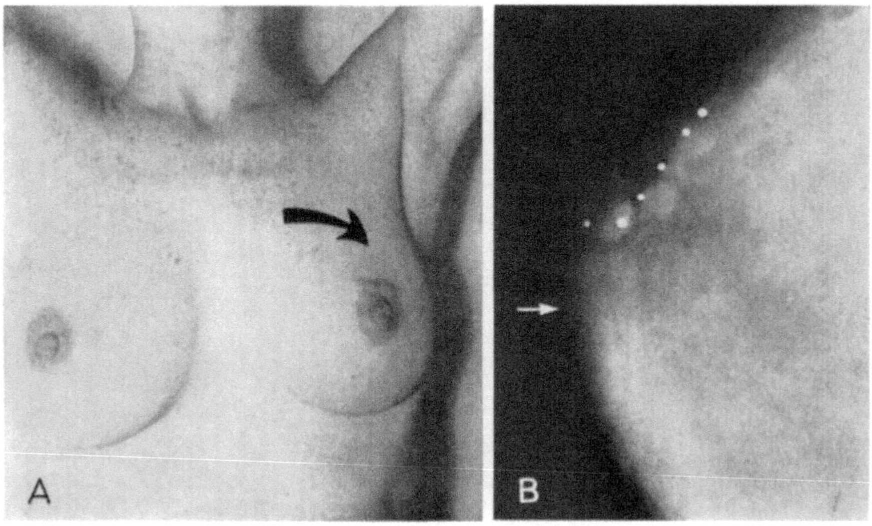

291
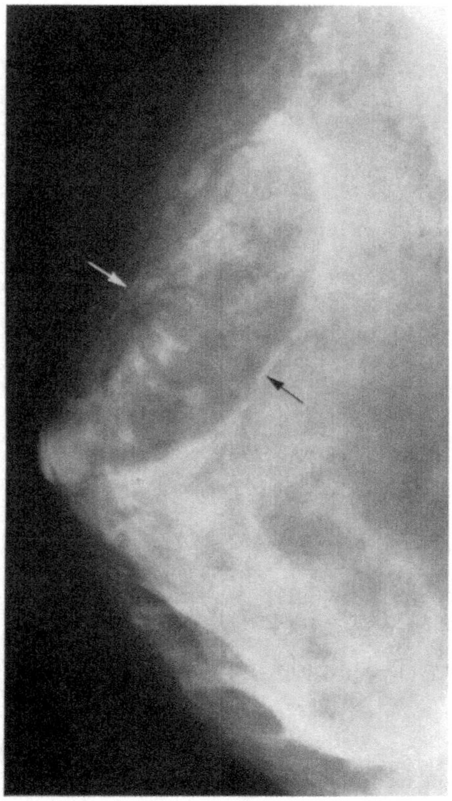

292
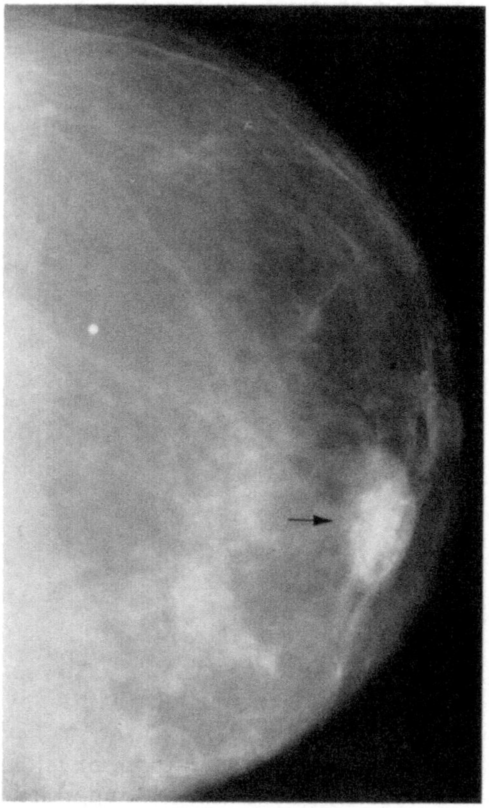

Fig. 293. Keloid. This skin lesion was obvious on physical examination

Fig. 294. Angioma of skin

Fig. 295. Epidermoid cyst in a 19 year old girl. Only by correlation with physical examination is this lesion likely to be suspected. The findings of the physical examination should always be appraised

Fig. 296. Epidermoid cyst

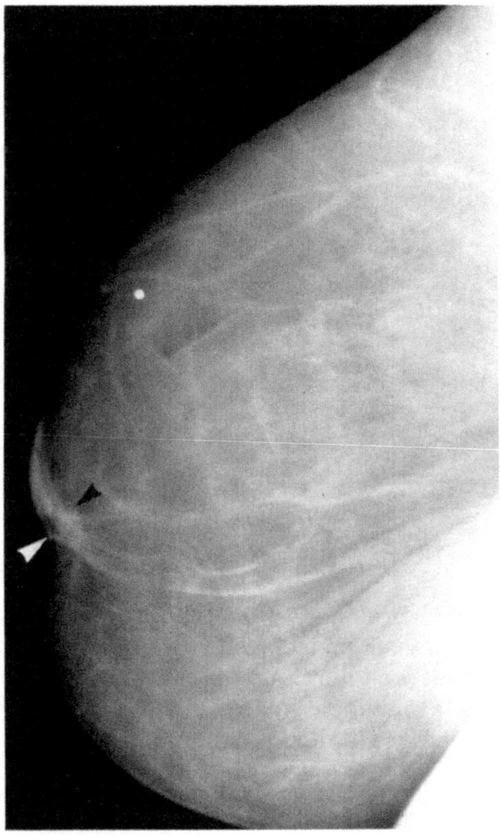
293

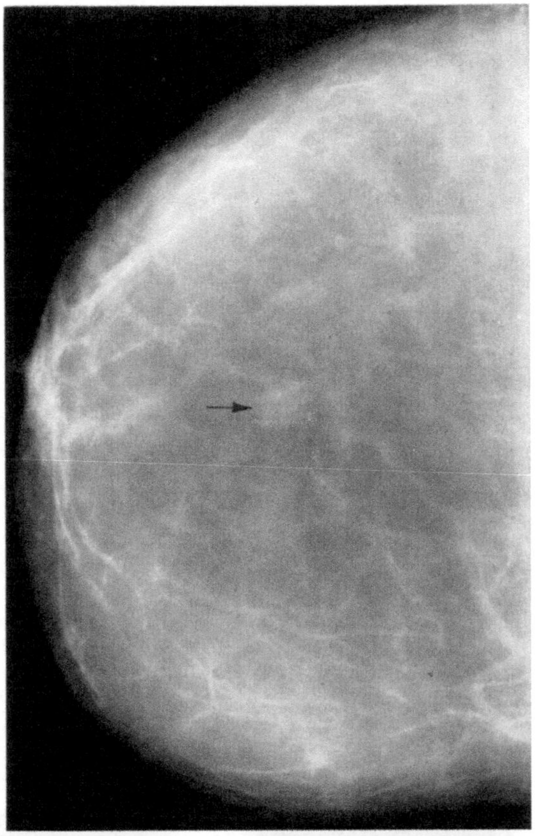
294

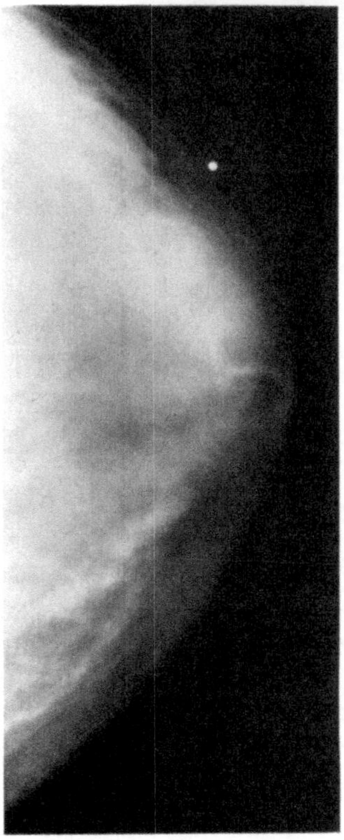
295

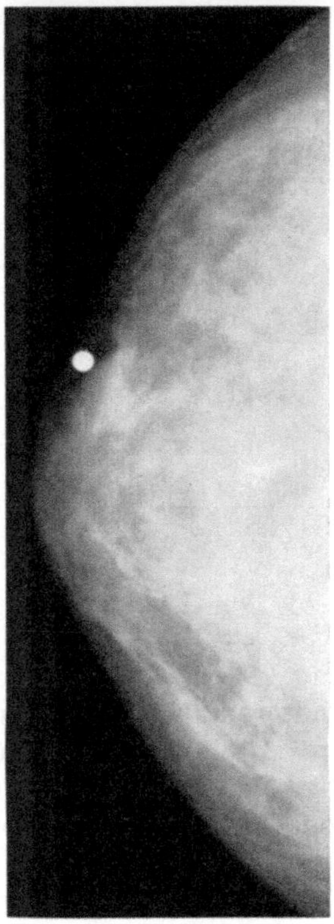
296

Fig. 297. Sebaceous cyst. Clinical examination alone established the diagnosis

Fig. 298. "Brassiere breast." Ill-fitting brassieres may set up a chronic irritation against the chest wall just below the breast, resulting in a palpable mass (arrow) that not infrequently simulates cancer

Fig. 299. Infiltrating duct cell cancer. The diagnosis is based on the presence of a mass of increased density with irregular margins in a field of edema including the nearby skin (compare with Fig. 298)

Fig. 300. Infiltrating duct cell cancer with scirrhus. Perifocal fibrous spicules are present around scirrhus blurred by edema which involves the skin. Localized skin thickening like that seen at the lower edge of the breast is occasionally the result of irritation from a tight-fitting brassiere

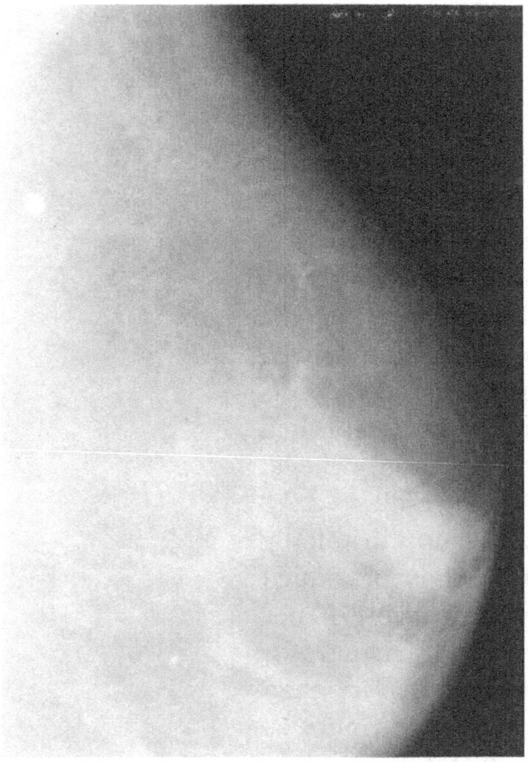

297

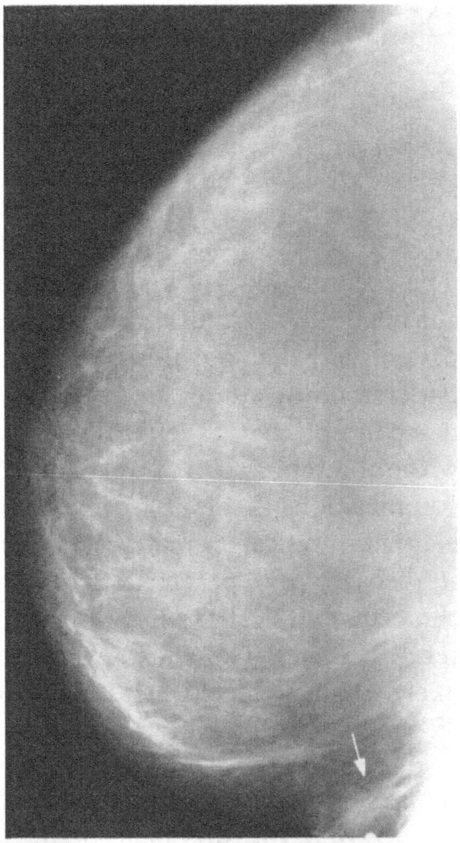

298

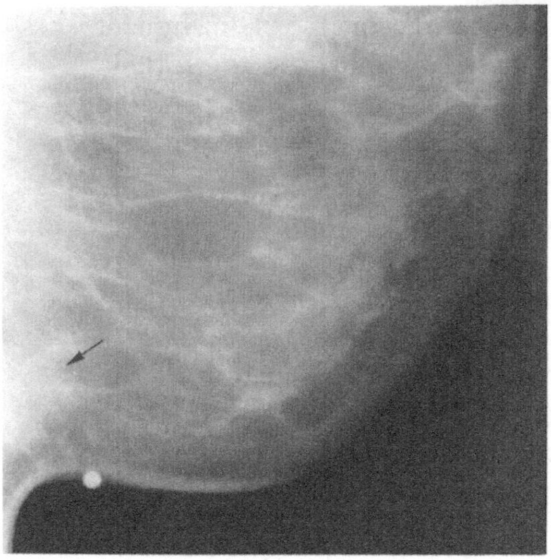

299

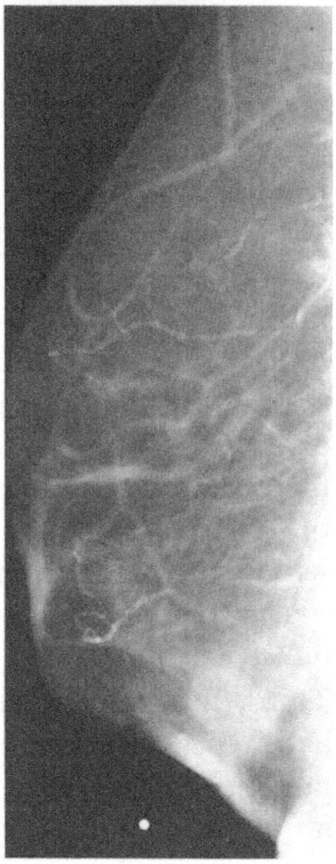

300

IX Medico-Legal Implications

The roentgenologist who makes a mammographic examination automatically assumes certain special responsibilities to the patient and the consulting physician, facts which are not well understood or appreciated. Unless everyone concerned accepts the concept that a definitive diagnosis cannot be established without a biopsy, it is possible for iatrogenic, medical, or legal complications — alone or in combination — to result.

Neither physical examination, mammography, nor histologic studies are 100 per cent definitive. In the hands of skilled clinicians physical examination of the breast is probably 70 per cent accurate. The most experienced roentgenologist is not likely to make a correct diagnosis of cancer in more than 85 per cent; and the best-trained pathologist will err as much as 10 per cent in the diagnosis of cancer from his histologic studies. When one adds to this inchoate situation the errors of surgeons in resecting the involved tissue and the faulty selection of tissues by the pathologist for the discovery of malignant lesions, it is obvious that all physicians must try to work in concert, while at the same time exerting every effort to avoid a depressing iatrogenic effect on the patient which might lead to unpleasant legal complications.

What steps might be taken to obviate such complications?

First, the roentgenologist would be well advised to familiarize himself with what the consulting physician or surgeon has found on physical examination and *what he has told the patient.*

Second, he should make his own physical examination. If the patient has an area to which she localizes symptoms, or if there is a questionable, palpable tumor, even if asymptomatic, the radiologist might affix a minute lead marker (B-B shot) with Scotch tape to the skin over the area to make it easy for him to pay particular attention to the area when he scans the films.

Third, he should verify the accuracy of the projections. We have repeatedly witnessed roentgenologists struggling to interpret films which failed to project properly the area of the breast in question. With a lead marker in place, the roentgenologist can easily detect improper projection.

Next arises the difficulty of reconciling the clinical and roentgenographic findings. If they concur, the accuracy of the diagnosis reaches beyond 90 per cent. If there is a difference, then a biopsy is the only proper course to follow. This is a two-fold admonition to surgeons and radiologists alike. If the surgeon finds a condition he believes should be subjected to histologic verification, the radiologist should automatically support this belief even if the X-ray findings fail to support such a conclusion. Conversely, if the roentgenologist suspects or concludes that the lesion is malignant, the surgeon should be ready to carry out a diagnostic resection even though he might demur in the diagnosis.

A small percentage of infiltrating duct cell cancers will not be palpable, but their presence will be revealed to the roentgenologist by minute calcium particles. In these circumstances, not only may the surgeon be loath to operate, but if he consents, he does not know where to find the lesion. He must depend upon the roentgenologist to localize the area for him.

The roentgenologist should also assume the responsibility of checking the success of the surgeon's operation by making X-ray examinations of the removed tissue, thus assuring by the demonstration of microcalcifications in the specimen that the field of involvement has actually been resected.

Finally, the roentgenologist must see to it that the pathologist makes his histologic studies in those areas of the tissue that contain these microcalcifications. If an error of diagnosis and treatment ensues because these steps were not strictly adhered to, the patient might raise legal questions of malpractice.

One of the most difficult situations to arise occurs when a cancer is present but is not recognized either by the roentgenologist or the clinician, and the latter accepts the X-ray report as definitive. The only protection the roentgenologist may have in these circumstances is to incorporate in his report, either in its body or as a footnote, a statement to the effect that a margin of error is inherent in his findings and that they must not ever be construed as definitive. Because of the great respect the public has for the specialty of roentgenology, a belief is generally held that the X-ray report is totally accurate. Thus, if a roentgenologist's opinion turns out to be faulty, his proficiency seems to be more susceptible to legal action than is that of the clinician or surgeon.

How can the footnote or statement concerning X-ray diagnostic fallibility be couched? We habitually state something like this: "In the light of localized symptoms or a palpable mass, even if not suspected by us to be malignant, if you do not propose an immediate biopsy, you would be foresighted to keep this patient under strict surveillance and repeat the examination again in three to six months."

When such a statement is included in the X-ray report, the patient is given the best attention humanly possible and to a large extent the roentgenologist is freed from the threat of legal action. It is obvious that only by close communication and collaboration between the clinician, surgeon, roentgenologist, and pathologist can the patient be assured of the utmost to be offered by the medical profession for the earliest detection of breast cancer. By the same token, care is thus taken to protect all the involved physicians from misguided malpractice complaints.

Suggested Reading

Adair, F. E.: Plasma cell mastitis. Arch. Surg. **26**, 735—749 (1933).

Baclesse, F., Willemin, A.: Atlas of Mammography. Paris: Librairie des Facultes 1967.

Black, J. W., Young, B.: A radiological and pathological study of the incidence of calcification in diseases of the breast and neoplasms of other tissues. Brit. J. Radiol. **38**, 596—598 (1965).

Brodie, Sir Benjamin C.: Clinical lectures on surgery; Lecture 24: On serocystic tumors of the breast, p. 206—214. Philadelphia: Lee & Blanchard 1846.

Buttenberg, D., Werner, K.: Die Mammographie. Technik-Röntgenatlas-Statistik. Stuttgart: Friedrich-Karl Schattauer 1962.

Byrne, R. N., Foxx, W., Gershon-Cohen, J.: Periodic postoperative mammography. Int. Surg. **50**, 415—420 (1968).

Cheatle, G. L., Cutler, M.: Tumors of the Breast. Philadelphia: J. B. Lippincott Co. 1931.

Collins, V. P., Loeffler, R. K., Tivey, H.: Observations on growth rates of human tumors. Amer. J. Roentgenol. **76**, 988—1000 (1956).

Cooper, Sir Astley: The Anatomy and Diseases of the Breast. Philadelphia: Lee & Blanchard 1845.

Copeland, M. M., Scott, W. G.: Mammography: a progress report. Amer. J. Surg. **116**, 57—61 (1968).

Dobretsberger, W.: Die isodensische Weichteilaufnahme (Fluidogramm). Radiologe **5**, 28—35 (1965).

Dominguez, C. M.: Estudio radiológico de los calcificadores. Bol. Soc. Anat. Rayologica **1**, 175 (1930).

Egan, R. L.: Mammography. Springfield, Ill.: C. C Thomas 1964.

— Technologist Guide to Mammography. Baltimore, Md.: The Williams & Wilkins Co. 1968.

— Roles of mammography in the early detection of breast cancer. Cancer (Philad.) **24**, 1197—1200 (1969).

Espaillat, A.: Contribution à l'étude radiographique du sein normal et patologique. Thése Paris, No 417. Paris: Librairie Arnette 1933.

Farrow, J. H.: Clinical considerations and treatment of in situ lobular breast cancer. Amer. J. Roentgenol. **102**, 652—656 (1968).

— Current concepts in the detection and treatment of the earliest of the early breast cancers. Cancer (Philad.) **25**, 468—477 (1970).

Feinleib, M., Garrison, R. J.: Interpretation of the vital statistics of breast cancer. Cancer (Philad.) **24**, 1109—1116 (1969).

Feinstein, A. R.: A new staging system for cancer and reappraisal of "early" treatment and "cure" by radical surgery. New Engl. J. Med. **279**, 747—753 (1968).

Fink, R., Shapiro, S., Lewison, J.: The reluctant participant in a breast cancer screening program. Publ. Hlth Rep. (Wash.) **83**, 479—490 (1968).

Foulds, L.: The experimental study of tumor progression. Cancer Res. **14**, 327—329 (1954).

— The histologic analysis of mammary tumors of mice. J. nat. Cancer Inst. **17**, 701—711 (1956).

Friedman, A. K., Askovitz, S. I., Berger, S. M., Dodd, G. D., Fisher, M. S., Lapayowker, M. S., Moore, J. P., Parlee, D. E., Stein, G. N., Pendergrass, E. P.: A cooperative evaluation of mammography in 7 teaching hospitals. Radiology **86**, 886—891 (1966).
Gershon-Cohen, J.: Chap. on Breast roentgenography. In: Classic Descriptions in Diagnostic Roentgenology, vol. I, p. 414—420. Springfield, Ill.: C. C Thomas 1964.
— Self-examination and the detection of early breast cancer. Pa. Med. **70**, 75 (1967).
— Should methods of detecting breast cancer be changed? Postgrad. Med. **45**, 84—89 (1969).
— Medical and legal implications of mammography (Editorial). Surg. Gynec. Obstet. **130**, 347—348 (1970).
— Berger, S. M.: Mastography. Radiol. Clin. N. Amer. **1**, 115—143 (1963).
— — Curcio, B. M.: Breast cancer with microcalcifications: diagnostic difficulties. Radiology **87**, 613—622 (1966).
— — Delpino, L., Curcio, B. M.: Mammography: some remarks on technique. Radiol. Clin. N. Amer. **3**, 389—401 (1965).
— — Klickstein, H. S.: Roentgenography of breast cancer moderating concept of "biologic predeterminism." Cancer (Philad.) **16**, 961—964 (1963).
— Borden, A. G. B., Hermel, M. B.: Mammometry: simple diagnostic aid in breast cancer. Radiology **92**, 1371—1372 (1969).
— Hermel, M. B.: Modalities in breast cancer detection: xeroradiography, mammography, thermography, and mammometry. Cancer (Philad.) **24**, 1226—1230 (1969).
— — Birsner, J. W.: Advances in mammographic technique. Amer. J. Roentgenol. **108**, 424—427 (1970).
— — Murdock, M. G.: Priorities in breast cancer detection. New Engl. J. Med. **283**, 82—85 (1970).
— Ingleby, H.: Roentgenography of unsuspected carcinoma of the breast. J. Amer. med. Ass. **166**, 869—873 (1958).
— — Berger, S. M., Forman, M., Curcio, B. M.: Mammographic screening for breast cancer. Results of a 10-year survey. Radiology **88**, 663—667 (1967).
— — Hermel, M. B.: Roentgenographic diagnosis of calcification in carcinoma of the breast. J. Amer. med. Ass. **152**, 575—577 (1953).
— — — Calcification in secretory disease of the breast. Amer. J. Roentgenol. **76**, 132—135 (1956).
— — — Occult carcinoma of the breast; the value of roentgenography. Arch. Surg. **70**, 385—389 (1955).
— Strickler, A.: Roentgenologic examination of the normal breast. Its evaluation in demonstrating early neoplastic changes. Amer. J. Roentgenol. **40**, 189—201 (1938).
— Yiu, L. S.: Mammography of thrombophlebitis: Surgery **53**, 657—661 (1963).
— — Berger, S. M.: The diagnostic importance of calcareous patterns in roentgenography of breast cancer. Amer. J. Roentgenol. **88**, 1117—1125 (1962).
Gilbertsen, V. A.: The potentiality for survival enhancement by expeditious detection of neoplastic diseases. Experience of the Cancer Detection Center of the University of Minnesota. Progr. Clin. Cancer **2**, 48—67 (1966).
— Detection of breast cancer in a specialized cancer detection center. Cancer (Philad.) **24**, 1192—1195 (1969).
Goyanes, J., Gentil, F., Guedes, B.: Sobre la radiografía de la glandula mamaria y su valor diagnóstico. Arch. esp. Oncol. **2**, 111—142 (1931).

Griesbach, W. A.: Screening for breast carcinoma. Oncology **23**, 167—171 (1969).
Gros, C. M.: Les cancers occultes du sein et la radiographie. Mem. Acad. Chir. **79**, 742—745 (1953).
— Les Maladies du Sein. Paris: Masson & Cie. 1963.
— Méthodologie. J. Radiol. Électrol. **48**, 638—655 (1967).
— Le Gal, Y., Burg, S.: Aspect radiologique des tumeurs phylloides. Bull. Ass. franç. Cancer **40**, 460—462 (1953).
— Sigrist, R.: La radiographie de la glande mammaire. J. belge Radiol. **35**, 226—268 (1952).
— — The roentgen differential diagnosis between chronic mastitis and breast carcinoma. Fortschr. Röntgenstr. **80**, 50—65 (1954).
Harrison, E. G., Jr., Witten, D. M.: Occult or unsuspected breast carcinoma. GP **31**, 78—88 (1965).
Hermel, M. B., Gershon-Cohen, J., Byrne, R. N.: Mammographic technique: need for routine spot roentgenograms. Amer. J. Roentgenol. **105**, 880—884 (1969).
Ingleby, H., Gershon-Cohen, J.: Comparative Anatomy, Pathology, and Roentgenology of the Breast. Philadelphia: Univ. of Pa. Press 1960.
Lane, N., Goksel, H., Salerno, R. A., Haagensen, C. D.: Clinicopathologic analysis of the surgical curability of breast cancers: a minimum ten-year study of a personal series. Ann. Surg. **153**, 483—498 (1961).
Lasky, H. J.: A new mammographic technic. Radiology **91**, 381—383 (1968).
Leborgne, R.: Diagnóstico de los procesos patológicos de la mama por la radiografía con la inyeccíon de medios de contrasta. Obstet. Ginec. lat.-amer. **7**, 551—561 (1944).
— Diagnosis of tumors of the breast by simple roentgenography. Calcifications in carcinoma. Amer. J. Roentgenol. **65**, 1—11 (1951).
Levitan, L. H., Witten, D. M., Harrison, E. G., Jr.: Calcification in breast disease; mammographic-pathologic correlation. Amer. J. Roentgenol. **92**, 29—39 (1964).
Masson, P.: Traité de Pathologie Médicale, vol. 2, p. 280. Paris: N. Maloine 1923.
Mausner, J. S., Shimkin, M. B., Moss, N. H., Rosemond, G. P.: Cancer of the breast in Philadelphia hospitals, 1951—1964. Cancer (Philad.) **23**, 260—274 (1969).
Minagi, H., Tennant, J. C., Youker, J. E.: Coning and breast compression. An aid in mammographic diagnosis. Radiology **91**, 379—381 (1968).
Missakian, M. M., Witten, D. M., Harrison, E. G., Jr.: Mammography after mastectomy; usefulness in search for recurrent carcinoma of breast. J. Amer. med. Ass. **191**, 1045—1048 (1965).
Moertel, C. G., Soule, E. H.: The problem of the second breast: a study of 118 patients with bilateral carcinoma of the breast. Ann. Surg. **146**, 764—771 (1957).
Moore, O. S., Foote, F. W., Jr.: The relatively favorable prognosis of medullary carcinoma of the breast. Cancer (Philad.) **2**, 635—641 (1949).
Moszkowicz, L.: Sexual cycle, mastopathy, and tumor growth in the breast. Langenbecks Arch. klin. Chir. **144**, 138—161 (1927).
Muntean, E.: Die Röntgenuntersuchung der Mamma. Radiologe **5**, 22—28 (1965).
Paget, J.: On disease of the mammary areola: preceding cancer of the mammary gland. St Bart. Hosp. Rep. **10**, 87—89 (1874).
Paschetta, V.: Étude radiologique de la glands mammaire. Bull. Soc. Radiol. Méd. France **19**, 346—348 (1931).

Picard, J. D., Desprez-Curely, J. P.: Le diagnostic radiologique des affections tumorales du sein. Sem. Hôp. Paris **33**, 1472—1481 (1957).
— — Rouquette, C.: Place de la mammographie parmi les éléments du prognostic des cancers du sein. Bull. Ass. franç. Cancer **46**, 621—633 (1959).
Pisani, G., Malaspina, A., Savino, G.: Diagnostica radiologica del cancro della mammella. Minerva med. 162 pp. (1960).
Proceedings of the Seventh Annual Seminar of the Detection of Breast Cancer, May 3—4, 1968, St. Louis, Mo. Cancer (Philad.) **23**, 761—891 (1969).
Proceedings Symposium Européen de Radiologie Mammaire, Strasbourg, July 1—3, 1966. J. Radiol. Électrol. **48**, 615—816 (1967).
Progress Report of Committee for Study of Breast Cancer of Philad. Co. Med. Soc., June 30, 1960. Philad. Med. **56**, 1007—1011 (1960).
Quezada, J. J.: Radiología de la mama. El Medico M. **13**, 41—48 (1963).
Reclus, P.: La maladie kystique des mamelles. Bull. Soc. anat. Paris **58**, 428—433 (1883).
— La maladie kystique des mamelles. Rev. Chir. (Paris) **3**, 761—775 (1883).
Robbins, G. F., Berg, J. W.: Bilateral primary breast cancers. Cancer (Philad.) **17**, 1501—1527 (1964).
Ronnen, J. F. v.: Plain roentgenography of the breast. Amsterdam: Academic Press 1956.
Ruzicka, F. F., Jr., Kaufman, L., Shapiro, G., Perez, J. V., Grossi, C. E.: Xeromammography and film mammography: a comparative study. Radiology **85**, 260—269 (1965).
Salomon, A.: Beiträge zur Pathologie und Klinik des Mammakarzinoms. Langenbecks Arch. klin. Chir. **101**, 573—668 (1913).
Samuel, E.: Soft-tissue radiology of the breast. Proc. roy. Soc. Med. **56**, 770—772 (1963).
Schimmelbusch, C.: Das Fibroadenom der Mamma. Langenbecks Arch. klin. Chir. **44**, 102—116 (1892).
— Das Cystadenom der Mamma. Langenbecks Arch. klin. Chir. **44**, 117—134 (1892).
Schwartz, A. M., Siegelman, S. S.: Non-palpable carcinoma in fibrocystic disease of the breast. Surg. Gynec. Obstet. **126**, 94—98 (1968).
Scott, W. G.: Mammography and the training program of the American College of Radiology. Amer. J. Roentgenol. **99**, 1002—1008 (1967).
Seemann, H. E., Lubberts, G.: Films for soft-tissue radiography. Med. Radiogr. Photogr. **41**, 18—20 (1965).
Seidman, H.: Cancer of the breast. Statistical and epidemiological data. Cancer (Philad.) **24**, 1355—1378 (1969).
Semb, C.: Pathologico-anatomical and clinical investigations of fibroadenomatosis cystica mammae and its relation to other pathological conditions in mammae, especially cancer. Acta chir. scand. **64** (Suppl. 10), 1—484 (1928).
Shapiro, S., Strax, P., Venet, L., Fink, R.: The search for risk factors in breast cancer. Amer. J. publ. Hlth **58**, 820—835 (1968).
Shepard, T. J., Crile, G., Jr., Strittmatter, W. C.: Roentgenographic evaluation of calcifications seen in paraffin block specimens of mammary tumors. Radiology **78**, 967—969 (1962).
Shimkin, M. B.: Cancer of the breast. Some old facts and new prospectives. J. Amer. med. Ass. **183**, 358—361 (1963).
Snyder, R. E.: Mammography and lobular carcinoma in situ. Surg. Gynec. Obstet. **122**, 255—260 (1966).
Stanton, L., Lightfoot, M. A.: Obtaining proper contrast in mammography. Radiology **87**, 111—115 (1966).

Stevens, G. M., Weigen, J. F.: Survey mammography as a case-finding method for routine and postmastectomized patients. A 5-year study. Cancer (Philad.) **24**, 1201—1205 (1969).

Stewart, F. W.: Tumors of the Breast. Washington, D.C.: Armed Forces Inst. Path., sect. 9, fasc. 34 (1950).

Strax, P., Oppenheim, A.: New apparatus for mass screening in mammography. Amer. J. Roentgenol. **102**, 941—945 (1968).

— Venet, L., Shapiro, S., Gross, S.: Mammography and clinical examination in mass screening for cancer of the breast. Cancer (Philad.) **20**, 2184—2188 (1967).

— — — — Venet, W.: Breast cancer found on repetitive examination in mass screening. Amer. J. Roentgenol. (in press).

Urban, J. A., Adair, F. E.: Sclerosing adenosis. Cancer (Philad.) **2**, 625—634 (1949).

Venet, L., Strax, P., Venet, W., Shapiro, S.: Adequacies and inadequacies of breast examinations by physicians. Cancer (Philad.) **24**, 1187—1191 (1969).

Vogel, W.: Die Röntgendarstellung von Mammatumoren. Surg. Clin. Leipzig Univ., given as an address before the Society on Dec. 15, 1931.

Wellens, P., Jansen, W.: Une methode tres simple pour l'obtention de cliches mammographiques parfaitement lisible dans les conditions normales. J. Radiol. Électrol. **40**, 340 (1959).

Witt, H., Bürger, H.: Mammadiagnostik im Röntgenbild. Ein Atlas für die Praxis mit histologischen Schnitten. Berlin: Walter de Gruyter & Co. 1968.

Witten, D. M., Thurber, D. L.: Mammography as a routine screening examination in detecting breast cancer. Amer. J. Roentgenol. **92**, 14—20 (1964).

— The Breast, vol. II in 12-vol. Atlas of Tumor Radiology, Philip J. Hodes, Editor-in-Chief. Chicago, Ill.: Year Book Publishers, Inc. 1969.

Wolfe, J. N.: Mammography as a screening examination in breast cancer. Radiology **84**, 703—708 (1965).

— A study of breast parenchyma by mammography in the normal woman and those with benign and malignant disease. Radiology **89**, 201—205 (1967).

— Mammography. Springfield, Ill: C. C Thomas 1967.

Wynder, E. L., Bross, I. J., Hirayama, T.: A study of the epidemiology of cancer of the breast. Cancer (Philad.) **13**, 559—601 (1960).

Young, G. B.: Mammography in carcinoma of the breast. J. roy. Coll. Surg. Edinb. **13**, 12—33 (1968).

Subject Index

Discussion indicated by roman type, illustrations by **bold face.**

GPSR Compliance

The European Union's (EU) General Product Safety Regulation (GPSR) is a set of rules that requires consumer products to be safe and our obligations to ensure this.

If you have any concerns about our products, you can contact us on ProductSafety@springernature.com

In case Publisher is established outside the EU, the EU authorized representative is:

Springer Nature Customer Service Center GmbH
Europaplatz 3
69115 Heidelberg, Germany

Batch number: 10615099

Printed by Printforce, the Netherlands